DATE			

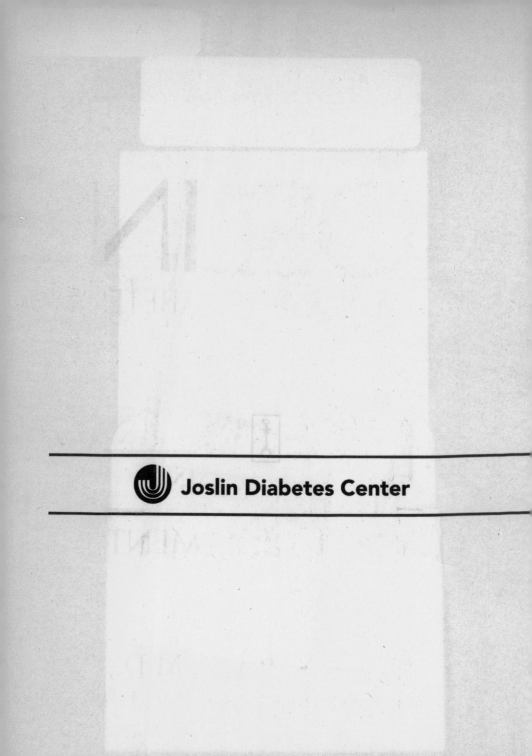

Joslin Diabetes Center

THE JOSLIN

GUIDE TO DIABETES

A PROGRAM

FOR MANAGING

YOUR TREATMENT

Richard S. Beaser, M.D.,
and Amy P. Campbell, R.D., M.S., C.D.E.

A Fireside Book
Published by Simon & Schuster
New York   London   Toronto   Sydney

FIRESIDE
Rockefeller Center
1230 Avenue of the Americas
New York, NY 10020

Revised Fireside Edition 2005

FIRESIDE and colophon are registered trademarks
of Simon & Schuster, Inc.

For information about special discounts for bulk purchases,
please contact Simon & Schuster Special Sales at
1-800-456-6798 or business@simonandschuster.com.

Designed by William Ruoto

Manufactured in the United States of America

10 9 8 7 6 5 4 3 2 1

Library of Congress Cataloging-in-Publication Data
  The Joslin guide to diabetes : a program for managing your treatment / Richard S. Beaser
and Amy P. Campbell.—Rev. Fireside ed.
    p. cm.
  "A Fireside book."
  Includes index.
  1. Diabetes—Popular works.   I. Campbell, Amy, R.D., M.S., C.D.E.   II. Title.
RC660.4.B43   2005
616.4'62—dc22   2005051021

ISBN-13: 978-0-7432-5784-8
ISBN-10:   0-7432-5784-7

ACKNOWLEDGMENTS

Amy and I would like to thank our Joslin colleagues who graciously contributed their time and expertise to this revision of *The Joslin Guide*. They are listed below, along with the particular chapter or chapters with which they assisted:

Elizabeth C. Bashoff, M.D.; Kenneth J. Snow, M.D.—chapter 24

Elizabeth Blair, M.S.N., C.S.-A.N.P., C.D.E.—chapters 21 and 25

Patricia Bonsignore, M.S., R.N., C.D.E.—chapter 12

Florence Brown, M.D.; Suzanne Ghiloni, R.N., B.S.N., C.D.E.—
chapter 23

Lori Laffel, M.D., M.P.H.—chapter 22

Joyce L. Lekarcyk, R.N., C.D.E.—chapters 17, 18, and 19

Catherine Mullooly, M.S., R.C.E.P., C.D.E.—chapters 9 and 10

Jo-Anne Rizzotto, M.Ed., R.D., C.D.E.—chapters 4 and 5

Robert C. Stanton, M.D.; Jerry D. Cavallerano, O.D., Ph.D.;
Ramachandiran Cooppan, M.D., F.R.C.P.(C)—chapter 20

Howard Wolpert, M.D.—chapter 16

John Zrebiec, L.I.C.S.W.—chapters 11 and 26

In addition, we would like to acknowledge the work done by Marion Franz, M.S., R.D., C.D.E., on this current edition; and by Joan V. C. Hill, R.D., C.D.E., L.D.N., who coauthored the first edition of the *Guide;* and thank them for their ongoing contributions to the diabetes community.

CONTENTS

PREFACE

We have certainly come a long way in the treatment of diabetes. In gathering material to write this preface, I looked to my copy of the third edition of *The Joslin Diabetic Manual for the Mutual Use of Doctor and Patient*, the forerunner of *The Joslin Guide*, written by Elliott P. Joslin, M.D., in 1924 and published three years after the discovery of insulin. The book was given to me by my father, Sam Beaser, a diabetes specialist himself.

In the preface to that 1924 edition, Dr. Joslin wrote: "The education of the diabetic was the experiment attempted in the first edition of the manual, but today it is recognized as a necessity." Chapters in that edition describe diabetes and offer a short discussion of what were then recent advances—particularly how people with diabetes could be treated at home rather than in the hospital. The chapter on the treatment of diabetes with medications discusses insulin—period. Subsequent chapters discuss diet, hygiene, and self-care of the teeth and feet. There is even a chapter entitled "Dogs, Diabetics, and Their Friends," which illustrates the good example of self-care that dogs can provide their owners who have diabetes, and also salutes the role dogs played in the early experiments leading to the discovery of insulin.

We have certainly come a long way since 1924, and the benefits to those with diabetes have been tremendous! Urine testing is now replaced with self-monitoring of blood glucose. We now have the AIC test, which is a powerful tool in measuring glucose control and thus evaluating one's risk for complications. With these and other techniques and technologies, such as the insulin pump, along with new, precise, and safer insulins, we can replace insulin action in the body in a manner that comes close to natural patterns. The result is glucose control that is smoother, safer, and more comfortable than could ever have been accomplished in years past. Oral medications to treat type 2 diabetes are also now available and in common and effective use. New methods to prevent or treat the complications of diabetes, now initiated earlier in the course of the disease, have made the quality of life for people with diabetes significantly better than it was back in those early days of the insulin era. Women with diabetes are routinely giving birth to healthy babies.

We know that our concern today about the increasing numbers of people who are overweight or obese, particularly young people, is key to preventing diabetes and some of its major complications, such as heart disease and other vascular problems. Thanks to our evolving understanding of nutrition and the way foods affect our blood glucose, we now know that it's not necessary for those with diabetes to eat a "diabetic diet" of bland food and no sugar. We know that it's important that everyone, whether they have diabetes or not, eat a varied, healthy diet.

And there is an even brighter outlook for the future. New insulins are being developed that may be even more precise, and perhaps, at some point in the future, will be delivered without injections. Meters to measure blood glucose levels may soon not require a pinprick. Newer medications are being developed to replicate more completely and accurately natural insulin action and glucose metabolism. New means to block the development of complications are on the near horizon. Treatments for complications that do develop are becoming ever more effective and easier to use.

Some things, however, do stay the same: Education is just as important in 2005 as it was in 1924—if not more important, because there is so much more to learn! Read through this book, perhaps starting with chapters or sections most relevant to you now. Come back to it, and reread some sections, and delve into others. Look beyond this book, using the information it provides as a basis of understanding new information about current and future research and treatment as it becomes available. Both education about diabetes and the care of one's diabetes should be seen as a continuum—an ongoing process that evolves as one gains experience and new perspectives.

Dr. Joslin would have been pleased with the progress we have made. Read on, with hope and optimism!

Richard S. Beaser, M.D.
Boston, 2005

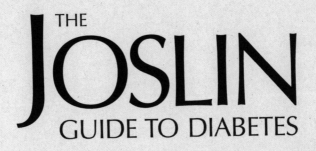

THE

JOSLIN

GUIDE TO DIABETES

CHAPTER 1

Join the Team!

When you have diabetes, you become a member of a very important team. Teams need players and coaches, and, in many ways, having diabetes is similar. It's hard to manage diabetes alone. You need a coach or coaches to help you learn the skills necessary to do the very best you can and to help guide your skill development. Others, such as family members, significant others, and friends, cheer your successes and provide support when things are not going well. But coaches and others can't do it for you. *You* have to learn about diabetes and be the one who controls your health and your diabetes care.

The first step in joining the team is to acquire the skills you need. Any time you want to learn about a medical problem or condition, it helps to approach it in two steps. First, learn how the body functions normally. Then learn what happens when something goes wrong. This is the best way to learn about diabetes too. *The Joslin Guide to Diabetes* will help you learn how your body works—what happens to it when you have diabetes—and how to keep your body working as normally as possible.

If you have been diagnosed with diabetes, you may wonder: "Why do *I* need to know about diabetes? After all, isn't my doctor the one responsible for my treatment?" The answer to this isn't as simple as it seems. The care provided by your doctor and your healthcare team is a very important part of managing diabetes. But to properly control your diabetes, you are the one who must be primarily responsible.

You will also need to know your treatment goals and how to achieve them. For many individuals this may mean acquiring some new skills so you can put into action the information you have learned. This action plan is called your *diabetes treatment program*. However, you also need coaches. That's where your healthcare team becomes important. It can help you take the information, goals, and skills you gain from reading and practicing and put them into an individual "game plan."

And once you understand the importance of a treatment program and your role in carrying it out, you're on the way to being a successful team player. The other players are only there to assist you to do the best you can. They are important because they have a lot to share with you.

Diabetes—an Old Disease, but Many New Remedies

Medical descriptions of diabetes date back to at least 1500 B.C., more than 3,500 years ago. Writings from ancient cultures in China and the Middle East describe the classic signs of diabetes, such as passing large quantities of urine through the body. The ancient Greeks gave us the name *diabetes*, which means "to flow through." Later the Latin word *mellitus* (meaning "sweet urine") was added to form the present medical name *diabetes mellitus*. Physicians actually diagnosed diabetes in ancient times by tasting the urine, but modern physicians have developed newer methods to accomplish this!

Until recent times, people with diabetes could use only diet, exercise, or weight control for treatment. But in 1921, a major breakthrough occurred that changed the outlook and saved the lives of millions of individuals with diabetes—insulin was discovered. Later in this book you will learn a lot about how insulin is used today. Research in diabetes has continued to make major strides. In the late 1970s it became possible for someone to check his or her blood glucose without the help of a doctor or nurse—one of the most important advances in the care of diabetes since the discovery of insulin. Once self-monitoring of blood glucose became available, research studies of people with type 1 and type 2 diabetes were undertaken, and these studies proved that controlling one's blood glucose makes a difference. By maintaining near-normal blood glucose levels, you can prevent or slow the progression of the long-term complications of diabetes. These include problems with the eyes, nerves, kidneys, feet, skin, heart, and blood vessels. The list of advances in diabetes management goes on and on, and all of them help you to gain increased control of your diabetes and thus reduce the risk of developing complications.

Discovering Your Diabetes

If you think back to the time just before you learned you had diabetes, you may have noticed some physical symptoms and some changes in your health. For example, you may have felt very tired and sluggish because your body was unable to properly use food for energy. For some of you, the symptoms were severe enough to cause you to see your doctor to find out what the cause was. For others of you, the symptoms were mild and you had little reason to suspect anything was wrong. But what is important is that at some point you discovered you have diabetes and now you want to learn more about it.

No doubt, you felt some type of stress even before the diagnosis of diabetes. And once you realized that you had diabetes, the stresses associated with its symptoms probably didn't go away. Questions occurred to you, such as How did this happen? What causes diabetes? Can it be cured? How will it affect my daily life? Can I keep my job? What will it cost? What lies ahead? Will I still be healthy enough to do the things in life that I enjoy? Such questions are steps in the right direction. They mean you are concerned about your health. To help you with your feelings about diabetes, it's often a good idea to find someone in whom you can confide—perhaps your physician, a healthcare professional, a family member, or a good friend.

It is extremely important that you gain a complete understanding of diabetes and methods of treatment. Diabetes is a uniquely personal condition. At first you may ask yourself, "Can I really handle this?" But your skills and confidence will grow as the weeks pass and as you learn about and have more experiences living with diabetes. Understanding diabetes will happen over time—you don't have to learn it all at once. However, by becoming more actively involved in your diabetes management, you will feel more confident about your own ability to solve problems, less angry and fearful about diabetes, and more motivated to keep up the effort. *The Joslin Guide to Diabetes* will help you develop that confidence.

This book is designed to be used as a reference tool for people with diabetes who are under the care of a physician and other healthcare professionals. It was written and reviewed by a team of experts in the field of diabetes care and education here at Joslin Diabetes Center in Boston, Massachusetts. Founded in 1898 by Elliott P. Joslin, M.D., a pioneer in diabetes research and care, Joslin Diabetes Center is affiliated with Harvard Medical School and has treated over a quarter of a million people with diabetes. Healthcare providers and educators at Joslin are dedicated to making sure that people with diabetes have the very latest information and know how to use this information to improve their diabetes care. We want you to live healthfully and well with diabetes, and we think this book will help.

PART ONE

Understanding Diabetes

CHAPTER 2

Deciphering Diabetes:
What Type of Diabetes Do You Have?

Do you know someone besides yourself who has diabetes? These days the answer is likely to be yes. That's because diabetes has become one of the most common health problems in the United States and in the world. About 18 million Americans—8.4 percent of the population—have diabetes. That seems like a large number, but it is often hard for us to visualize what these large numbers mean. To do this, think of the last time you were in a sports stadium, concert hall, or theater. Estimate about how many groups of 100 were with you, and then realize that out of every 100 people, approximately 10 have diabetes. If 200 people attended a concert with you yesterday evening, that would mean that besides you, there were 19 persons with diabetes. Even more of a concern is that about a third of those, or 6 people in that group of 20 who have diabetes, are not even aware that they have it. They have not been diagnosed yet, but they have the condition.

The risk of developing diabetes increases with age—nearly 19 percent of adults 65 or older are reported to have diabetes. But of great concern is the fact that today more—and younger—adults, and even children and adolescents, are developing diabetes. It's reported that the number of people in their thirties with diabetes increased by 76 percent during the 1990s. And among children with newly diagnosed diabetes, the number with type 2 diabetes has increased from less than 4 percent before 1990 to as high as 45 percent among certain racial and ethnic groups who are at increased risk of developing diabetes. So if you or someone close to you has diabetes, you are not alone—there are a lot of people with diabetes!

It is very important to discover diabetes as early as possible. If left untreated or uncontrolled, it can lead to serious health problems—heart disease, stroke, blindness, amputations, kidney failure, and even death. If you have diabetes, a lifestyle that includes healthy food choices and healthy eating habits along with physical activity can help you keep it under control and reduce your risk of developing serious complications. For many individuals, this means that medications such as diabetes pills will need to be combined with lifestyle changes. For other individuals it may mean combining insulin with diabetes pills and lifestyle changes, or insulin alone and lifestyle changes. The good news is that advances in treatment options, medications (new diabetes pills and different types of insulin), and medical devices are making it easier than ever before for you to live a healthy life with diabetes.

To understand diabetes, you first need to know how the human body works without diabetes. Understanding how the body normally uses blood glucose (blood sugar), the body's main source of energy, and the role that insulin plays, makes it easier to understand how a breakdown in this process leads to diabetes. Diabetes—high blood glucose levels—develops when your body either can't make any or enough insulin or can't properly use the insulin that it does make.

How the Body Normally Metabolizes Food

Your body needs food to survive. Food is both fuel and building material. *Metabolism* is the process by which the cells of the body change food so that it can be used for energy or to build or maintain cells. To do this, the body breaks food down into basic nutrients. Three basic nutrients—carbohydrate, protein, and fat—will be discussed first because they all require insulin for the body to use them normally.

Carbohydrate is the main source of fuel for the body. Carbohydrate includes starches and sugars and is found in bread, pasta, fruits, vegetables, milk, and sweets. It is broken down into a sugar called *glucose*. During digestion, glucose passes through the wall of the intestine into the bloodstream to the liver and eventually into the general circulation, where it can enter individual cells or tissues throughout the body to be used for fuel to provide energy. Insulin is the key that lets glucose into cells to be used for energy.

Protein is found in meats, poultry, fish, eggs and dairy products such as milk and cheese, and some vegetable foods, such as peas, beans, legumes, and soy foods. Protein breaks down into amino acids, which are used to build and repair body tissues; some protein can also be stored for use as a secondary source of energy. Protein also requires insulin in order to be used properly.

Fats are found in foods such as oils, salad dressings, meats, some dairy products, and nuts. They break down into triglycerides, which are a combination of three fatty acids, and travel to the liver and eventually to fat cells to be used or stored for energy. Fat is burned differently than glucose and can produce a by-product called *ketones*. Fats also require insulin to be used properly. They can also contribute to *insulin resistance*, which is a condition that makes it harder for the cells to use insulin correctly.

After eating, all three of these nutrients are digested, or broken down, in the stomach and intestines, and glucose from carbohydrate enters the bloodstream. If one has diabetes, because there is insufficient insulin, possibly combined with insulin resistance, the body is not able to use this glucose the way it should. Since protein and fat also require insulin, if one has diabetes, they are not used properly either.

The Role of Insulin

You can see that insulin is essential in order to use the foods we eat correctly, but insulin is important for other body processes as well. Insulin is a *hormone*. Hormones are chemical messengers made in one part of the body to transfer "information" through the bloodstream to cells in another part of the body. Your body makes many types of hormones, and insulin is a specific kind. It is made in the organ called the *pancreas*.

The pancreas is a small gland located below and just behind the stomach. It is shaped like a cone lying on its side, with the end tapering off into a "tail." Within this tail are tiny cells known as *islets of Langerhans*. A normal pancreas has about 10,000 islets of Langerhans. These islets are clusters of various types of cells. The most important are the *beta cells*—the tiny "factories" that make insulin. The beta cells also serve as "warehouses," storing insulin until it's needed.

The pancreas has other important functions as well. Cells called alpha cells produce *glucagon*. Glucagon, also a hormone, has the opposite action of insulin—it raises blood glucose levels. It does this by causing glucose stored in the liver or muscles (called *glycogen*) to be released into the bloodstream. The balance between insulin and glucagon keeps blood glucose levels in the normal fasting range (first thing in the morning and before eating), which is approximately 70–100 milligrams (mg) of glucose per deciliter (dl) of blood.

When the beta cells sense that the level of glucose in the blood is rising, they respond by releasing just the right amount of insulin into the bloodstream. Insulin binds to receptors on the body's cells and signals substances in the cells to produce a chemical passageway that allows glucose to enter the cells. After one eats, the beta cells are triggered to make more insulin. When functioning normally, the beta cells release just enough insulin to maintain the level of glucose in the blood within the normal range after eating, which is less than 140 mg/dl. However, even when you are not eating, such as at night when you are asleep, the beta cells release a constant, low level of insulin.

Generally when you eat, you don't need to use all the glucose from your food immediately. The body, with the help of insulin, removes excess glucose from your bloodstream and stores it as glycogen in your liver and muscles. Glycogen is used when your body needs extra glucose—for instance, when blood glucose levels are low or during exercise. In addition, glycogen will release glucose overnight to take care of your energy needs when you're not eating. Insulin helps convert some of the extra glucose into fat, which is stored in the body's fat cells.

Insulin is also needed for amino acids from protein to repair and build new body tissues and for the storage of triglycerides from food fats in the fat cells.

You can see how important insulin is for the normal use and storage of food fuels and why there would be serious problems if insulin is missing or does not work properly.

The beta cells of the pancreas release another hormone, called *amylin*. Amylin is secreted with insulin, and its main function is to slow stomach emptying. It also suppresses the release of glucagon, and both of these actions help keep blood glucose levels normal after eating. Amylin is a hormone you will hear more about later.

Other cells in the pancreas produce substances called *enzymes*. Enzymes help in digestion by splitting foods into simpler substances that can be absorbed through the intestinal walls into the bloodstream.

What Causes Diabetes?

Diabetes is caused by a breakdown in the normal processes described above. This breakdown can occur because the body produces little or no insulin, or because cells are resistant to the action of insulin ("insulin resistance"), or because both of these problems develop. Instead of glucose entering cells throughout the body, excess glucose builds up in the bloodstream.

The most common forms of diabetes are type 1 and type 2 diabetes. Type 1 diabetes results when no insulin or very little insulin is produced, whereas type 2 diabetes is a problem of both *insulin resistance* and *insulin deficiency*. There are similarities between type 1 and type 2 diabetes, and some people have characteristics of both.

Symptoms of Diabetes

Below are the symptoms of diabetes:

- **FREQUENT URINATION AND EXCESSIVE THIRST.** This is caused by *hyperglycemia*, or high blood glucose levels. Blood circulates through the kidneys, which remove waste materials from the blood and expel them into the urine. The kidneys also act like a "dam" to keep and recycle important nutrients such as glucose, sending them back into the blood. But in diabetes, blood glucose rises to excessively high levels and the kidneys can't send all the glucose back into circulation. The kidneys try to "wash out" excessive amounts of glucose from the blood, and glucose spills over the "dam" into the urine. But it takes water to get rid of the glucose, and this results in large amounts of urine. As you lose fluids, you get very thirsty, your body's signal to take in more fluids.

- **LACK OF ENERGY.** If your body can't use the food you have eaten to create energy, you feel tired.

- **WEIGHT LOSS.** When you lose glucose in the urine, you are also losing a lot of calories that your body would normally use for energy. Your body next turns to its stored fat for energy. As you lose glucose (calories) in urine and as fat is used up, you lose weight.

- **CONSTANT HUNGER.** When you can't get energy from the glucose in your blood, your body sends out hunger signals for more food. Of course, a lack of glucose isn't the real problem. The problem is that your body can't use the glucose that is already there.

- **BLURRED VISION.** Glucose can also build up in the fluids of your eyes. The excess glucose draws water with it, causing the eye's outer lens to swell, which distorts your vision. Once you begin your diabetes treatment and your blood glucose gets back to normal levels, your vision will clear.

- **OTHER SYMPTOMS.** Perhaps you had other symptoms of diabetes before your problem was identified. You may have experienced *nausea, vomiting, abdominal pain, weakness,* or *rapid, shallow breathing.* Or you may have experienced what is called *diabetic ketoacidosis* or a *diabetic coma.* Any of these symptoms can occur when the body uses stored fat instead of glucose as an alternative source of energy.

Some people with type 2 diabetes may not have any of the symptoms of diabetes, or the symptoms may be so mild that unless they are regularly tested for diabetes, they can have it for many years before it is detected. It may not be detected until it has caused damage to the heart, blood vessels, eyes, or kidneys.

To help you understand your treatment options, it is important to know what type of diabetes you have. This may seem simple. But as you will discover, for many it isn't so easy. The following sections will describe and explain type 1 and type 2 diabetes.

Type 1 Diabetes

Type 1 diabetes, which accounts for only 5 to 10 percent of all diabetes, was once called "juvenile onset" diabetes because it was thought to develop most often in children and young adults. It is now known, however, that this type of diabetes can occur in people of any age, including adults in their seventies and eighties.

Type 1 diabetes develops when the pancreas makes little, if any, insulin. Individuals with this type of diabetes must take daily doses of insulin to survive, which is why this type has also been called *insulin dependent*. Insulin can be injected with a standard syringe or an insulin "pen" containing a supply of insulin ("an injection") or by means of an insulin pump that is attached outside the body and is programmed by the user to give some insulin around the clock, and more with meals and snacks. In the future, inhaled insulin may also be available. Insulin can't be taken by mouth, because stomach acids render it ineffective.

Type 1 diabetes is known as an autoimmune disease because, for many people with this type of diabetes, the body's own immune system—which normally fights off infections—attacks the pancreas and destroys the insulin-producing beta cells. It's not clear why this happens, but researchers believe genetics and exposure to certain viruses or other chemical toxins may be involved in triggering the disease. It is known that there is a tendency for type 1 diabetes to occur more frequently in certain families. Studies show that if the father has type 1 diabetes, there is a 6 percent chance of the child developing it. If the mother has type 1 diabetes, the chance is between 1 and 4 percent. The risk is about two times higher if either parent was diagnosed with type 1 diabetes before age 11. To put this into perspective, if there is no diabetes in the family, there is only a 1 percent chance of an individual developing type 1 diabetes by age 50.

Although the symptoms seem to appear suddenly—for example, rapid weight loss often occurs in just a couple of days—in most cases beta cells are gradually destroyed over several years before symptoms appear and diabetes is diagnosed.

When type 1 is diagnosed, individuals usually have one or more circulating *autoantibodies* to pancreas islet cells, insulin, or other cell parts. Antibodies are proteins that the body makes to protect itself from foreign substances such as bacteria and viruses. (*Auto* simply means that they are self-produced.) In diabetes, something goes wrong, and instead of these antibodies protecting the cells against destruction, they actually act themselves to destroy the body's cells. For example, there are islet cell autoantibodies, which destroy the beta cells, and autoantibodies to insulin itself, which destroy the insulin being produced. Over time, after the diagnosis of type 1 diabetes, these antibodies decrease and may not be detectable. However, detecting them in people who, perhaps because of genetics, are at risk of developing type 1 diabetes may in the future help predict who will develop type 1 diabetes.

You can see that the cause of type 1 diabetes is a complex and complicated process. But the result is that the body's lack of insulin causes the various symptoms of diabetes described in the section above—the outward signs that let you know that something is wrong.

Type 2 Diabetes

Type 2 diabetes is the more common form of diabetes. About 90 to 95 percent of people diagnosed with diabetes have type 2. It's caused by a combination of problems, but it usually begins with *insulin resistance*. Recall that insulin acts as a sort of key to let blood glucose into the cells, where it is converted to energy. When things are working well, the pancreas produces enough insulin to handle the blood glucose produced by the food you eat. When someone has insulin resistance, however, the cells don't respond to the insulin and blood glucose can't enter the cells to make energy. In the early stages of the disease, the pancreas responds by making more insulin than normal in an attempt to overcome the insulin resistance, and as long as it can do so, the blood glucose levels remain normal. In fact, early on in the course of type 2 diabetes, the insulin-producing beta cells in the pancreases of people with type 2 diabetes are often able to secrete large amounts of insulin into the bloodstream. Eventually, however, the beta cells become sluggish in their response. They lose the ability to secrete insulin immediately after the glucose begins to rise from incoming food. This results in a delay in the release of insulin after food is eaten, while at the same time the glucose level is rising significantly. By the time the beta cells respond, the blood glucose level can be quite high, and then the insulin that is secreted has to play "catch-up" to bring the glucose level back to normal. This pattern of glucose rise after a meal, and then rapid fall, is an important first sign of diabetes. The resulting increase in insulin secretion is called *hyperinsulinemia*, or increased insulin production. Nevertheless, even though the body makes more than a normal amount of insulin, it is still not enough to keep the glucose levels normal. This condition is referred to as *relative insulin insufficiency*.

Eventually, the body can't produce enough insulin to overcome this resistance and the problem becomes an absolute *deficiency in insulin*. The longer you have diabetes, the more likely the reason blood glucose levels are elevated is because of insufficient insulin. One of the signs of insulin deficiency is a high blood glucose level in the morning. Normally your liver releases stored glucose in the early-morning hours to provide energy to your body, and at this time your body also makes more insulin so the glucose can be used correctly. If it can't release enough insulin, your blood glucose level will be elevated.

Effect of High Blood Glucose

High blood glucose levels can make all of the problems worse. How? Excess glucose in the blood may further damage the beta cells, making them less able to produce insulin. Or maybe because they have to work harder and produce more insulin to keep blood glucose levels normal, the beta cells simply become exhausted sooner. It is a vicious cycle—the higher your blood glucose goes, the more difficult it is for the body to bring it back to normal. This condition is referred to as *glucose toxicity*. This is why, whatever the cause, the secret to keeping your beta cells producing insulin normally and longer is to keep your blood glucose levels as close to the "normal" range as you possibly can.

Progression of Treatment

When type 2 diabetes is first diagnosed, many individuals can control their glucose by making and maintaining some changes in food and eating habits and in physical activity (together these are called *lifestyle changes*). But over time the disease progresses and these lifestyle changes may need to be combined with diabetes pills and, for many, eventually, insulin. Many people think that if this happens to them, they must have done something wrong. But it's not their fault. The problem is simply that when one has type 2 diabetes, the beta cells of the pancreas will, over time, "fail." The best thing you can do to keep your beta cells working longer is to keep your blood glucose under control. We will discuss more about managing type 2 diabetes later, but for now, remember that the goal is to help you control your blood glucose levels.

Role of Genetics

Genetics plays an important part in determining who develops type 2 diabetes. This type of diabetes "runs" in families. Studies show that if one parent has type 2 diabetes, his or her children have a 7 to 14 percent chance of developing the disease. If both parents have type 2 diabetes, this increases to a 45 percent chance. If an identical twin has type 2 diabetes, there's a 58 to 75 percent chance that the other will too. Again, to put this into perspective, if there is no diabetes in the family, there is an 11 percent chance that a person will develop type 2 diabetes by age 70.

Risk Factors for Type 2 Diabetes

Following are the risk factors for developing type 2 diabetes:

- Family history of diabetes
- Age 45 years or older

- Overweight
- Habitually inactive
- Belong to a high-risk ethnic group, including African Americans, Hispanic Americans, Asian Americans, Native Americans, and Pacific Islanders
- Have been told that you have impaired glucose tolerance (IGT) or impaired fasting glucose (IFG)
- History of gestational diabetes or delivery of a baby weighing more than 9 pounds
- Hypertension greater than or equal to 140/90 mmHg in adults
- HDL cholesterol less than or equal to 35 mg/dl (0.90 mmol/l) and/or a triglyceride level greater than or equal to 250 mg/dl (2.82 mmol/l)
- Polycystic ovary syndrome
- History of vascular disease (narrowing of blood vessels)
- Type 2 (and probably some type 1) diabetes is more common in people with schizophrenia or bipolar disorders, likely due to genetics, lifestyle, and possible side effects of some of the antipsychotic medications.

Epidemic of Type 2 Diabetes

As you can see above, obesity is one of the risk factors for developing type 2 diabetes. In the United States, there are widespread and growing epidemics of both obesity and diabetes in adults and children. Before 1990, it was rare for a child to be diagnosed with type 2 diabetes. The last decade, however, has seen an epidemic rise in the occurrence of childhood obesity and the emergence of type 2 diabetes in children. With this current trend of increasing childhood obesity, the Centers for Disease Control and Prevention estimates that one out of every three Americans born in the year 2000 will develop diabetes during his or her lifetime. Type 2 diabetes is also more common among many ethnic groups, such as African Americans, Native Americans, Latinos, and Asian Americans. For example, 15 percent of American Indians and Alaska native adults have diabetes, as do 11 percent of African American adults and 8 percent of Hispanic adults. Although it's not known why, type 2 diabetes is slightly more common in women than men.

Other Types of Diabetes

Gestational diabetes is defined as any degree of elevated blood glucose that occurs or is first recognized during pregnancy. It develops in about 7 percent of all pregnant women. Although it typically disappears after delivery, studies have shown that close to 40 percent of women with a history of gestational diabetes eventually develop type 2 diabetes. In rare cases, type 1 diabetes can develop during pregnancy. It's important to manage gestational diabetes to avoid complications for the mother and the baby.

Other, less common types of diabetes can be caused by certain pancreatic problems, the surgical removal of the pancreas, use of certain medications (including corticosteroid drugs such as prednisone), and an iron overload in the body (hemochromatosis). These types of diabetes are rare and account for less than 2 percent of all diagnosed cases.

Pre-Diabetes

Pre-diabetes is a condition in which either your fasting or two-hour post-meal blood glucose levels are higher than normal, but not high enough for a diagnosis of type 2 diabetes. Studies show that most people with pre-diabetes will develop type 2 diabetes within ten years if they don't change their lifestyle. They also have a higher risk of developing cardiovascular (heart and vessel) disease.

People with pre-diabetes usually do not have the classic symptoms of diabetes and as a result may not be screened. This is unfortunate because having pre-diabetes doesn't mean you will necessarily develop type 2 diabetes. In several studies, researchers have found that a moderate weight loss of 10 to 20 pounds and regular physical activity for 30 minutes a day can *prevent* or *delay* the onset of diabetes in those with pre-diabetes.

Diagnosing Diabetes and Pre-Diabetes

Methods for diagnosing diabetes and pre-diabetes include testing a blood sample for glucose, and, less commonly, a glucose tolerance test. We all have glucose in our blood at all times. The question is, how much?

The normal range for blood glucose first thing in the morning (called a fasting plasma glucose), or if you have not eaten for several hours, is 70 to 100 mg/dl. After eating, the normal glucose value is less than 140 mg/dl.

There are three ways to diagnose diabetes, and each must be confirmed on another day—unless the symptoms of diabetes are present and so obvious that another test does not need to be done. One way to diagnose diabetes is to do a blood test any time during the day regardless of when you have eaten (this is referred to as a *casual* or *random* blood test). If you have any of the symptoms of diabetes listed above and your blood test is 200 mg/dl or higher, and if it is confirmed with another test on another day, then you have diabetes.

In two other tests, a sample of your blood is drawn after an overnight fast to measure whether your blood glucose is above the normal range of 100 mg/dl. This is called a fasting glucose test. In the glucose tolerance test, additional blood tests are done every hour or at the two-hour point after drinking a sugar-filled liquid. If you have diabetes, after two hours your blood glucose rises to over 200 mg/dl. Generally one of the first two tests described—a casual or fasting test—is used to diagnose diabetes; a glucose tolerance test (GTT) is not done very often. However, it may pick up diabetes earlier in its development than the fasting or casual glucose test, so your healthcare provider may want to do a GTT if the other tests are not conclusive and you are at high risk for developing diabetes based on the criteria listed below in the section on screening.

Pre-diabetes is diagnosed if your fasting glucose level is between 100 and 125 mg/dl. Fasting blood test results between these levels mean that you have impaired fasting glucose (IFG). If after a two-hour glucose tolerance test your blood glucose level is between 140 and 199 mg/dl, you have impaired glucose tolerance (IGT). Both IFG and IGT are medical terms for pre-diabetes.

Screening for Diabetes and Pre-Diabetes

Generally, before people who have type 1 diabetes are diagnosed, they have symptoms and relatively high blood glucose levels. But many people who have type 2 diabetes do not have symptoms and frequently are not diagnosed until complications of diabetes appear. Therefore, it is recommended that all adults have a fasting blood glucose test at age 45. If your blood glucose levels are normal after taking the test, you should be retested again in three years. If you have pre-diabetes, you should be tested every one to two years. You should be tested sooner and more frequently, however, if you are overweight and have one or more of the following diabetes risk factors:

- a sedentary lifestyle
- a first-degree relative with diabetes
- are a member of a high-risk ethnic population (African American, Latino, Native American, Asian American, Pacific Islander)
- have delivered a baby weighing more than 9 pounds or have been diagnosed with gestational diabetes
- high blood pressure (greater than 140/90)
- HDL cholesterol less than 35 mg/dl and/or a triglyceride level greater than 250 mg/dl
- polycystic ovary disease
- any signs of insulin resistance, such as acanthosis nigricans (velvety brownish gray skin patches that are often on the neck or in skin folds)

Children who are overweight and have two of the following risk factors should also be screened:

- a family history of type 2 diabetes
- are a member of a high-risk ethnic population
- show signs of insulin resistance, such as acanthosis nigricans (thickening and darkening of the skin, typically found on the back of the neck)

The American Diabetes Association recommends that such high-risk children be screened beginning at age 10 or at the onset of puberty. If the test is normal, they should be screened again in two years.

What Type of Diabetes Do You Have?

If you know you have diabetes, what type of diabetes is it? If you are not sure, check with your healthcare provider at your next visit. While a diagnosis of diabetes is never good news, it is not cause for panic. But it is cause for concern and immediate action.

If you have any of the risk factors for type 2 diabetes, be sure to be tested at your next visit with your healthcare provider to see if you have pre-diabetes or diabetes so that you can begin treatment or start making lifestyle changes.

If you have pre-diabetes, work with your healthcare team to make lifestyle changes that can prevent or delay the development of diabetes. If you have diabetes, once you have gained a better understanding of what diabetes is and how it affects your body, you must then learn what you can do to keep your body working as normally as possible. But remember, you can have diabetes and still be healthy! Read on—the rest of this book will help you learn how to live a healthy life with diabetes.

CHAPTER 3

Goals and Tools for Treatment

Diabetes is a chronic condition that requires treatment for a lifetime. We are fortunate today to have better methods and medications to help you manage your diabetes. It is important to treat diabetes for two reasons. First, you want to feel better—to gain relief from the immediate and uncomfortable symptoms caused by high blood glucose. Second, you want to prevent or minimize the long-term complications that can result if your blood glucose remains high for months and years.

An important goal of treatment is to help you gain the necessary knowledge and skills so that you can achieve the best possible control of your glucose, lipids (blood fats), blood pressure, and other risk factors for developing the complications of diabetes.

Blood Glucose Goals

Two landmark studies demonstrated without a doubt the clear link between good control of blood glucose and the development of complications in type 1 and type 2 diabetes. The first study, the Diabetes Control and Complications Trial (DCCT) was designed to test the question, Will normalization or near normalization of blood glucose levels in people with diabetes help to delay or prevent diabetes complications? The answer was yes. The study involved approximately 1,400 persons with type 1 diabetes who were treated with either intensive (multiple injections of insulin, or use of an insulin pump guided by blood glucose monitoring) or conventional (one or two injections a day) insulin regimens. The lesson learned: individuals who achieve tight control similar to that of the intensively treated patients and achieve an A1C of 7 percent or less can reduce the risk of eye, kidney, or nerve complications by 50 to 75 percent. The second study, the United Kingdom Prospective Diabetes Study (UKPDS), followed for an average of 10 to 11 years approximately 5,000 patients newly diagnosed with type 2 diabetes, who were treated either conventionally or intensively. With intensive therapy that lowered A1C to 7 percent, eye and kidney complications decreased by 25 percent and the risk of heart and blood vessel disease by 16 percent compared with conventionally treated patients. The UKPDS study also documented the importance of lowering blood pressure for reducing the risk of stroke, eye and kidney complications, and other diabetes-related deaths.

Although the optimum level of glucose control for each individual isn't always known, it is known that achieving the best control possible is crucial. Both Joslin Diabetes Center and the American Diabetes Association make the following recommendations for adults with diabetes:

- A1C: less than 7 percent
- Pre-meal plasma glucose: 90–130 mg/dl
- Post-meal plasma glucose (1–2 hours after the beginning of the meal): less than 180 mg/dl (Joslin recommends less than 160 mg/dl)

Other organizations may have other targets, such as an A1C of 6.5 percent. However, healthcare professionals should determine a specific target for each individual. For some individuals, an A1C of less than 6 percent may be appropriate. However, a lower A1C goal is not recommended if it can't be achieved without increasing the risk of frequent hypoglycemia (low blood glucose levels). Control of the post-meal glucose level is also important, but the best value for this number is also unclear. It is important that you discuss your individual glucose goals with your healthcare team.

Lipid and Blood Pressure Goals

You should also be aware of lipid and blood pressure goals. *Lipid* refers to blood fat, and lipid goals are those for cholesterol, and its different components, and triglycerides. Treatment to lower lipid levels and blood pressure will be discussed in later chapters. Achieving lipid and blood pressure goals is important for the prevention of heart and blood vessel diseases. Over the years, like blood glucose goals, the goals for low-density lipoprotein (LDL) cholesterol—the "bad" cholesterol—triglycerides, and blood pressure have been lowered, while high-density lipoprotein (HDL) cholesterol—the good cholesterol—goals are higher. The American Diabetes Association makes the following recommendations for adults with diabetes:

- LDL cholesterol: less than 100 mg/dl (although recent studies suggest that aiming for a value of 70 mg/dl in high-risk individuals such as those with diabetes may be preferable)
- Triglycerides: less than 150 mg/dl
- HDL cholesterol: greater than 40 mg/dl for men, and greater than 50 mg/dl for women
- Blood pressure: less than 130/80 mmHg

Protecting Your Blood Vessels

Other means of protecting your blood vessels are also available. Your healthcare provider may recommend the use of aspirin, either a baby aspirin (81 mg) or a full-size dose (325 mg). Research has suggested that the use of other treatments, such as medications called *ACE-inhibitors* and some of the medications used to lower cholesterol levels, may also protect your blood vessels. These treatments will be discussed later. Another good way to protect your blood vessels is to avoid smoking, or stop smoking if you currently do so.

Understanding Your Treatment Program

Just as it is important that goals be individualized for you, the same is true for your treatment program. But whatever treatment program is designed for your diabetes, the overall goal is the same—to keep your blood glucose, lipids, and blood pressure in control. To help you accomplish your treatment goals your program will include four basic approaches:

- **FOOD AND MEAL PLANNING.** You will use a food and meal plan to balance the foods and nutrients you need to maintain good health and manage your blood glucose levels. Your meal plan will also help you meet your lipid and blood pressure goals. It will be important for you to share with your healthcare providers your usual meal and activity schedules, the types of foods you like or dislike, and goals you may have for weight loss or maintenance.

- **REGULAR PHYSICAL ACTIVITY.** Becoming or staying physically active helps everyone, whether they have diabetes or not. Not only does it make you feel better, but it also preserves and increases your muscle tone and strength, gives your heart a workout, increases your lung efficiency, and helps you maintain a healthy weight. If you have diabetes, there are extra benefits from physical activity. It helps you use insulin better by increasing the body's sensitivity to insulin, thereby lowering the amount of glucose in your blood, which often enables you to use smaller doses of insulin and oral diabetes medications. Some recent research also showed that people with diabetes who are fit, which means they engage in regular physical activity, have a lower risk of death from diabetes complications, regardless of their weight.

- **MEDICATIONS.** If you have type 1 diabetes, you will need insulin injections to stay alive. If you have type 2 diabetes, you may initially be able to meet your goals with meal planning and physical activity. Later you may need to combine your lifestyle strategies with diabetes pills that stimulate your body to produce additional insulin or to use insulin better. But for many people with type 2 diabetes, the body in time becomes less able to produce enough insulin, and they will eventually need to combine insulin injections with lifestyle changes and perhaps some diabetes pills or other injected medicines to keep their blood glucose in a healthy range. We are fortunate today to have newer medications and insulin available to better help you manage your diabetes well.

- **SELF-MONITORING.** Monitoring your diabetes involves checking your blood for glucose and thinking about what the level is in relation to your medication, eating, and activity. Doing this tells you how well you are managing your diabetes. Monitoring is essential because it helps you and your healthcare providers decide what changes need to be made in your treatment program in order to meet your treatment goals.

To one degree or another, diabetes will affect nearly all aspects of your life. That's why it is so important that a treatment program be "customized" to meet your individual needs and lifestyle. Education is also a vital part of diabetes management: attend educational programs offered at your local hospital, clinic, or diabetes center. Your treatment program should also include professional support to deal with the impact of diabetes on your emotional and social well-being. Talk with mental health professionals about your concerns. Many persons find support groups helpful as well. By gaining appropriate knowledge, skills, and attitudes, you will be able to manage your diabetes with competence and confidence.

Your Role in the Treatment Program

We started the book by suggesting that you, your healthcare providers, and your family members were like members of a team. Unlike some other serious conditions, diabetes necessitates that you take an active part in the treatment. But because you have a team, you are not alone. You will play an important role in designing your treatment program, but your "coaches" will be there to help you. However, once the program is in place, you are responsible for actually carrying it out. It is your responsibility to maintain and monitor the program. And when you have questions or problems, you will need to alert your healthcare team so that adjustments can be made in your meal plan, your physical activity program, or your medications.

Actively participating in your treatment will also enable you to achieve a far greater level of freedom and control in your everyday life. With the best equipment—and with the help of your team members—you will do well.

The Role of the Healthcare Team

Once you are diagnosed with diabetes, it is very important to look for a physician who is knowledgeable about the disease and its complications. As with other complex medical problems, even the best family practitioner or primary-care physician may not be aware of all the concerns that need to be addressed in diabetes. Though the primary-care provider is an important person to help you sort out day-to-day medical issues and should be a key part of your healthcare team, it is also important to have access to other specially trained team professionals who will play a significant role in your care. These generally consist of the following:

■ DIABETOLOGIST—a physician who is an expert in treating diabetes. This physician may also be a board-certified endocrinologist (hormone specialist).

■ NURSE EDUCATOR OR DIABETES NURSE SPECIALIST—a nurse who is trained in the management of diabetes and is also skilled in teaching diabetes care. Look for the initials C.D.E. (certified diabetes educator) or B.C.-A.D.M. (board-certified advanced diabetes manager) after her or his name.

■ REGISTERED DIETITIAN OR DIABETES NUTRITION SPECIALIST—a professional who is trained to provide medical nutrition therapy for diabetes and who is also skilled in teaching food and meal planning for people with diabetes. Look for the initials C.D.E. or B.C.-A.D.M. after her or his name (a dietitian will probably also have R.D. after her or his name).

- **EXERCISE PHYSIOLOGIST**— a person trained to help people with diabetes develop and implement an effective physical activity program.

- **MENTAL HEALTH SPECIALIST**— someone who can help you and your family deal with the emotional and social impact of a chronic condition such as diabetes. This person could be a social worker, a psychiatrist, a psychologist, or a licensed therapist.

- **OTHER PROFESSIONALS** — these include *ophthalmologists* (eye doctors) and *podiatrists* (foot doctors).

Additional resources you may need at times include other medical specialists—for example, a nephrologist (kidney specialist), a neurologist (nerve specialist), or a cardiologist (heart specialist). Your healthcare team may refer you to these or other specialists either to prevent or to treat such complications.

Many people continue to see their primary-care physician for their other medical needs, and the diabetes treatment team to help manage their diabetes. The diabetes team works with you and your primary-care physician to develop and monitor your individualized treatment plan. It's comforting to know that a team of experts is ready to assist you.

To help you identify qualified physicians, the American Diabetes Association and the National Committee for Quality Assurance (an independent organization that assists the public in distinguishing among health plans and physicians based on quality of care) cosponsor a Diabetes Physician Recognition Program (DPRP). Physicians may voluntarily apply, and if they achieve "recognition," it means that their medical care of adults with diabetes meets certain high standards. Below are the indications of quality care that the DPRP recognizes. Even if your physician has not applied for recognition, he or she should still be doing the following:

- Regularly measuring your A1C level and helping you achieve a level less than 7 percent. It is recommended that you have an A1C test at least two times a year if you are meeting your treatment goals, and quarterly if your diabetes treatment program is changed or if you are not meeting glycemic goals.

■   Measuring your blood pressure level at every visit and helping you achieve a level less than 130/80 mmHg.

■   If you have type 2 diabetes, screening for eye problems *(retinopathy)*. This should be done by an ophthalmologist shortly after your diagnosis or, if you have type 1 diabetes, within three to five years after the onset, and repeated annually. Less frequent exams (every two to three years) may be considered if your eye care professional determines you had a normal eye exam.

■   Asking you if you smoke and, if you do, giving you advice or treatment to help you stop.

■   Completing a lipid profile at least once a year, and more often if needed to achieve your lipid goals. If your LDL cholesterol is at your goal—less than 100 mg/dl and perhaps even closer to 70 mg/dl if you are considered to be at high risk—your HDL is greater than 50 mg/dl, and your triglycerides are less than 150 mg/dl, the tests can be repeated every two years.

■   Performing a test for the presence of microalbuminuria (protein in your urine) every year. This test is done to see if there are any problems with your kidneys *(nephropathy)*. If you have type 2 diabetes, you should have the test for the first time at diagnosis, and if you have type 1 diabetes, you should be tested after you have had diabetes for five or more years.

■   Performing a comprehensive foot exam every year (your physician and/or a podiatrist) and a visual inspection of your feet at each routine visit.

(Note: The clinical measures above are slightly different for pediatric patients. If you have a child with diabetes, check with your pediatrician to see what the differences are.)

   Although the following are not clinical measures, it is important that your healthcare provider:

- Provide you with self-management education or refer you to a diabetes educator (a C.D.E.) so that you will be better able to manage your diabetes day to day.

- Refer you to a dietitian who can help you design a meal plan.

- Explain self-monitoring of blood glucose, regardless of whether you are treated with insulin or not.

- Making sure you are satisfied with your overall diabetes care, that you are receiving answers to your diabetes questions, that you know what to do or who to call in case of an emergency, that your laboratory results are explained to you, and that you are being treated in a courteous and respectful manner.

If you can answer the following questions, you are off to a good start:

- Do you know what your blood glucose goals are?
- Have you seen or been referred to a diabetes team for education?
- Has your doctor taken or talked to you about all of the measures listed above?

Even if your doctor is doing everything right and even if you are surrounded by a caring, supportive team, remember: *you* are still the most important member of the team. You are the person who ultimately will be responsible for achieving success.

PART TWO

Treating Diabetes with Nutrition Therapy and Physical Activity

CHAPTER 4

Nutrition and
Meal Planning Basics

Good nutrition is important for everyone. We need to eat foods for energy, to build and repair body parts, and to regulate hundreds of body processes. It is especially important for those with diabetes because what, when, and how much you eat play an essential role in controlling blood glucose. It is helpful for you to know about the nutritional values of food because you can use this information to develop a meal plan that will provide you with the energy and nutrition you need and at the same time keep your blood glucose in control. An additional benefit is that the more you know about foods, the more you will be able to eat the foods you enjoy while managing your diabetes well.

All of us benefit and improve our health by choosing and eating healthful foods and by participating in regular physical activities. Studies involving healthy people and people at risk for developing chronic diseases, such as diabetes and heart disease, support the benefit of eating fruits, vegetables, whole grains, low-fat dairy foods, lean meats and meat substitutes, and healthy fats. Studies also support taking care in using saturated fats and sodium.

If you have diabetes, however, there are other important considerations. The first is to have a meal plan to help you decide when and how much to eat. When you go on a vacation, you use a map to help guide you to your destination. You also plan special activities to make your trip a success. In a similar manner, if you have diabetes, following a meal plan will help you keep your blood glucose in your target range while at the same time allowing you to enjoy your favorite foods. In addition, if you need to lose weight or would like to maintain your current weight, a meal plan can help you meet your goal. It is recommended that you see a dietitian who will work with you and provide what is called *medical nutrition therapy*. This involves an individual assessment of your food and nutrition needs and working with you to develop a meal plan that will be right for you. It is also important to meet regularly with a dietitian as part of your overall diabetes care. You will no doubt have questions that need answers, and your nutrition needs will change over time. There's a lot to learn about food and meal planning, and it takes time to process and use the information. If your medical goals are not being met, your dietitian may have suggestions for some changes you can make to help achieve these goals, or it may be time to change medications or combine them with your meal plan. Your dietitian will also help you evaluate how nutrition therapy contributes to your overall diabetes treatment program.

Why Do Food and Meal Planning Matter?

Your body changes much of the food you eat into glucose, or blood sugar, so the amount of food you eat is very important. The basic strategy behind your meal plan is to coordinate your food intake with the action of insulin in your body. It doesn't help your cells to have blood glucose "knocking on the door" if there is no insulin "key" to let it in. Insulin interacts with glucose circulating in your bloodstream, which comes from the food you eat or from glucose stored in your body. The body can store glucose as *glycogen* in the liver and muscles so that when your blood glucose levels decrease, the body has a source of glucose it can use to keep them within a normal range. The balance between glucose, insulin, and other body hormones, such as glucagon, is what keeps blood glucose levels within your target range. So when insulin is missing or isn't working properly, blood glucose levels increase. The idea is to match as closely as possible each side of this equation:

Glucose in your bloodstream = insulin in your bloodstream

For example, if you have type 1 diabetes, you must take insulin either by injection or by means of an insulin pump to replace the insulin no longer produced by your pancreas. However, the good news today is that because there are many types of insulin, if your healthcare providers know your schedule of meals and activities, an insulin regimen can almost always be designed to cover your choice of foods and lifestyle. For this to work, you have to let your dietitian know what you like to eat and when. Together, the two of you will design a meal plan that will work for you; it will then be shared with the healthcare provider who is designing your insulin regimen.

Your meal plan will start with the number of carbohydrate servings you choose to eat at meals. This is because the amount of insulin you take at mealtimes, which is usually a *rapid-acting insulin* such as lispro or aspart, is determined by the amount of carbohydrate you eat at the meals. The mealtime dose is called your *bolus* or *mealtime insulin*. You also need some background insulin to meet the needs of all the other body processes that insulin regulates—this is called *basal insulin*. (Chapters 14 and 15 cover insulin regimens in more detail.)

If you have type 2 diabetes, you might manage it by lifestyle alone; lifestyle and diabetes pills; lifestyle, diabetes pills, and insulin and/or other injected medications; or lifestyle and insulin. You can see there are many options, but with all of them, what and how much you eat is still important. Following a meal plan can help reduce the *insulin resistance* often associated with type 2 diabetes. Insulin resistance occurs when the body's cells "resist" the action of available insulin. Insulin resistance is linked to heredity and excess weight, so if you shed a few pounds, your cells will be better able to use insulin. But just being careful of how much food and the types of food you eat, and eating at the right time, also helps your body combat insulin resistance. This can happen before you lose a single pound, or even if you are not able to lose weight.

Type 2 diabetes also involves a decline in insulin production, which usually occurs with or without insulin resistance. This is often referred to early on in the process as *relative insulin deficiency,* and later on, when a more significant loss of insulin production occurs, as *absolute insulin deficiency.* You may need diabetes pills or injected medication to boost insulin production or to improve your body's ability to use insulin, or you may need to take insulin to supplement the small amount still being produced by your pancreas. Meal planning can help manage two factors associated with insulin deficiency—*defective beta cells* and/or a *reduced number of beta cells* in the pancreas. (Remember that beta cells are special cells within the pancreas that produce and secrete insulin.) When you follow a meal plan, your beta cells will be able to respond more quickly to your body's needs for insulin—immediately after a meal, for example. This is because your meal plan calls for you to select the appropriate foods in the appropriate amounts—amounts that your pancreas can still produce enough insulin to handle. While you may need injected insulin (or diabetes pills) to boost your body's natural insulin production, the dose(s) may be smaller.

By following a meal plan, you gain short- and long-term benefits that come with maintaining your blood glucose at the proper levels. You will feel better and have more energy. People who have had diabetes for many years are susceptible to serious complications, some that can even be life-threatening. In years past, one's chances of developing such complications were high. Following a meal plan can help reduce that risk for people with both type 1 and type 2 diabetes by helping to keep blood glucose levels in as normal a range as possible. Even if you have developed some complications from your diabetes, following a meal plan can help to slow their progression.

Food Groups

Before carpenters can build a house, they must first learn some basic facts about building materials. Then they learn how all the pieces fit together into the framework of a building. In similar fashion, before your meal plan can be developed, you must learn the basics of food and meal planning. You can then use this knowledge to develop a healthy eating style through your meal plan—a style that will help keep your blood glucose in your target range.

The first basic is to learn the food groups. Generally, foods fall into one of the following groups or in a combination of these groups:

- *Carbohydrate*
- *Protein*
- *Fat*

Carbohydrate

Carbohydrate provides energy to the cells in the body. There is now a Recommended Dietary Allowance for carbohydrate of 130 grams a day for adults and children. This amount is based on the average minimum amount of glucose that is used by the brain. The two basic types of carbohydrate are sugars and starches. Historically, people with diabetes were advised to avoid sugars because it was believed that sugars would be rapidly digested and absorbed into the bloodstream and thereby cause blood glucose to soar. It was such a widely held belief that for many years no research was done to see if it was true. Needless to say, the medical community and people with diabetes were surprised to find that if you substituted an equal amount of sucrose for starch, the blood glucose response was very nearly the same. For example, 50 grams of carbohydrate from a sugar such as maple syrup has the same effect on blood glucose as 50 grams from a starch such as bread. However, note the portion sizes—¼ cup of maple syrup contains about 50 grams of carbohydrate whereas three slices of bread contain about the same amount. There are now more than 20 research studies showing that when individuals choose a variety of foods containing either starches or sugars in meals, if the total amount of carbohydrate eaten is similar, glucose response will also be similar. Because foods containing either sugars or starches are broken down or digested into glucose at about the same rate, it is important to control *all* of the carbohydrate you eat, not just the sugars. This is the basis of *carbohydrate counting*—a meal-planning method commonly used by people with diabetes.

The balance between the amount of carbohydrate foods you eat and the available insulin determines how much your blood glucose level goes up after meals or snacks. To help control your blood glucose, you need to know what foods contain carbohydrate, what average serving sizes are, and how many carbohydrate servings to eat. There's no magical number of carbohydrate servings that is right for everyone. Instead, it is important that you work with a dietitian to determine what will be a good number for you. One of the main determinants is the number of carbohydrate servings you think is reasonable for you to eat throughout the day. By checking your blood glucose, you can monitor the response and see whether changes are needed. If your blood glucose levels are too high, you may need to do one of the following:

- eat fewer carbohydrate servings
- be more physically active
- work with your diabetes team to add or make adjustments in your diabetes medications

The following foods contain carbohydrate:

- grains, pasta, rice
- breads, crackers, cereals
- starchy vegetables such as potatoes, corn, peas, winter squash
- legumes such as beans, peas, and lentils
- fruits and fruit juices
- milk, yogurt
- sweets and desserts such as cookies and ice cream; sugars; jams, jellies, and syrups

Nonstarchy vegetables such as broccoli, salad greens, and green beans are so low in carbohydrate and calories that they are usually considered "free."

Carbohydrate in foods is measured in grams (g). One carbohydrate serving is the amount of a food that contains 15 grams of carbohydrate. You may also hear one portion of food that contains 15 grams of carbohydrate called one "carb choice." The Nutrition Facts panel on food labels also lists the total grams of carbohydrate in one serving size of the food. The following are some examples of one carb choice, or serving:

Starches

⅓ cup cooked pasta or rice
½ cup starchy vegetables (corn, peas, potatoes)
½ English muffin or 1 oz. bagel
1 slice bread or small roll
6 saltines or 4–5 snack crackers

½ cup cooked beans or lentils
¾ cup dry cereal
½ cup cooked cereal
3 cups popcorn, plain

Fruit

1 small fruit
½ cup juice
½ cup canned fruit
1 cup berries

Milk

1 cup skim or low-fat milk
⅔ cup (6 oz.) fat-free yogurt, flavored, sweetened with nonnutritive
  sweetener

Sweets

½ cup ice cream, frozen yogurt
1 tbsp. jam, sugar, honey
2 small cookies

Additional food choices are provided in the Appendix.

Protein

Meats, poultry, and fish are good sources of protein. Because they are usually the primary source of protein in most people's diets, they are often called proteins. However, there are really very few foods that contain only protein. For example, most meats and meat substitutes, such as cheese and eggs, contain both protein and fat. Many of these foods have more calories from fat than from protein. Other good sources of protein, such as milk, yogurt, and beans, contain both protein and carbohydrate, which is why you often find them on carbohydrate lists. Grains, legumes, and nuts also contain varying smaller amounts of protein. Tofu and other soy products, such as soy burgers, are vegetarian protein sources.

The word *protein* is derived from a Greek word meaning "of first importance," which is indicative of protein's role as the basic building material of life. The body uses protein to build and repair its tissues. Muscles, organs, bones, skin, and many of the hormones in the body are made from protein. As a secondary role, protein can also provide energy if carbohydrate is not available.

In general, most adults should limit the total amount of protein (weight after cooking) in a day to about six ounces, or two servings of three to four ounces. A serving is a portion of meat about the size of a deck of cards or the palm of your hand. You should choose meats and cheeses that are low in fat. Lean beef, fish, pork, and poultry without skin are good choices. Examples of protein servings are listed later in this chapter.

Fat

The third group of foods your body needs is fat. That's right—your body needs fat! Contrary to what you may have been led to believe, fat is not all bad. It's only when we eat too much fat or the wrong kind that it becomes a problem. The different types of fat—saturated and unsaturated—are discussed in Chapter 6.

Fats can be in either a solid or a liquid form and are found in meats; dairy products such as whole milk, butter, and cheese; margarine; and vegetable oils such as corn, sunflower, canola, and olive oil. Fat is used to maintain healthy skin and hair and serves as a "vehicle" to carry fat-soluble vitamins throughout your body. In addition, fats are changed into fatty acids—an important source of energy. However, any extra calories that your body does not use immediately are stored as body fat *(adipose tissue)*.

When it comes to fat, eat less animal fat and control all portions of added fats to keep your heart healthy and your weight in a healthy range. Heart-healthy choices of added fats include olive, peanut, and canola oils, and nuts such as walnuts, almonds, and peanuts.

"Free Foods"

You may have heard the term "free food." A free food is one that has fewer than 20 calories and 5 grams of carbohydrate in a serving. The following are examples of "free foods."

- Diet (sugar-free) sodas and beverages
- 1 cup raw vegetables
- 1 tbsp. fat-free cream cheese
- ¼ cup salsa
- 2 tsp. "lite" or low-sugar jam
- 1 tbsp. nondairy creamer
- Sugar-free gelatin
- 1 tbsp. catsup
- Herbs, spices, seasonings

How Foods Affect Blood Glucose

Carbohydrate, protein, and fat affect your blood glucose in different ways. Most of the carbohydrate you eat turns into blood glucose, and the effect it will have depends on the amount of available insulin. Without enough insulin, you will have high blood glucose levels. Protein and fat also require insulin to be metabolized but have minimal effect on your blood glucose levels. Protein is used to build and repair body tissues, and some protein and fat is stored for future energy needs. However, eating too much fat can cause insulin resistance, which may lead to prolonged high blood glucose levels.

Developing a Meal Plan

Your dietitian will develop your meal plan with you, based on the following factors:

- the type of diabetes you have
- whether you are taking diabetes pills or insulin
- your usual day's activities
- your usual eating schedule
- the types of food you like
- your physical activity patterns
- other medical conditions, such as high blood pressure or high cholesterol
- your weight goals

Figure 4-1

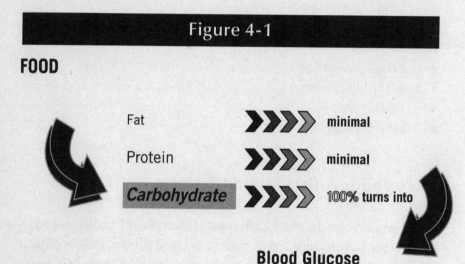

FOOD

Fat   ⟫⟫ minimal

Protein   ⟫⟫ minimal

Carbohydrate ⟫⟫ 100% turns into

Blood Glucose

Your meal plan will be tailored so that you feel confident in your ability to implement it. That's why it's important that you share your concerns with your healthcare providers. The goal is for you to have a realistic meal plan that you can follow day to day to help guide your food choices and food portions.

In creating a meal plan, don't think of it as a "diet." That term usually implies a drastic and temporary eating strategy often used to lose weight. Instead, the goal is to develop a healthy and lifelong "eating style" that will help you control your diabetes as well as contribute to optimum health.

In designing a meal plan, you should consult with a registered dietitian who is an expert in food and diabetes nutrition therapy. You and your dietitian will consider all of the factors listed above in creating a plan. Your meal plan will look something like the one in Figure 4-2, Sample Meal Plan. The Meal Plan includes a place for your name as well as the name and telephone number of your dietitian.

In the top section is a space labeled Total Calories. A calorie is a way of measuring the amount of energy supplied by food. Your dietitian will write in the approximate number of calories your body needs each day to balance the calories you burn. The amount is determined by your height, weight, age, gender, and level of physical activity. If you need to lose weight, the number of calories will be reduced so that you burn more calories than you eat. However, you don't need to count calories, because by following your meal plan you will be eating the right amount.

Be sure to let your dietitian know if you are having difficulty following your meal plan. Remember that this is a guide for you to use to help control your diabetes. Your meal plan should be created especially for you with your preferences in mind; it should be realistic and easy to follow.

Carbohydrate Counting

Carbohydrate counting not only can help you improve your diabetes control, it offers more flexibility than more "traditional" methods of meal planning. For example, if you take rapid-acting insulin before your meals, carb counting allows you to vary the amount of carb you consume on a day-to-day and meal-to-meal basis. You're not "locked in" to eating a set amount of carb at your meals every day. You might eat 45 grams of carb one night for supper, but the next night 80 grams. This is an added bonus if you eat out or travel frequently. In addition, you can decide if you want to eat a snack or not. However, if your goal is to lose weight, you may still want to aim for a certain amount of carb at your meals and snacks. And, if you take diabetes pills, you will need to eat a *consistent* amount of carb at your meals and snacks. Remember that calories count, and portion control is the key to successful weight loss.

Most people find carb counting easy to do. Look at the left-hand column of the sample meal plan. The three meals that you eat each day—

Figure 4-2   Sample Meal Plan

 Joslin Diabetes Center

Name: *Wilomena Burke*

Date: *5/20/05*

— MEAL PLAN —

Daily Guidelines: Total Calories: *1803*   Carbohydrate: *221g*   Protein: *106g*   Fat: *55g*

Meal	Sample #1	Sample #2

Breakfast Time: _7 a.m._
 4 Carb choices or
     Carb grams *60*
     2 Starch
     1 Fruit
     1 Milk
 1 Meat / Protein choices
 0–1 Fat choices		

Snack Time:		

Lunch Time: _12 noon_
 4 Carb choices or
     Carb grams *60*
     2 Starch
     1 Fruit
     1 Milk
 1–2 Vegetables
 3 Meat / Protein choices
 0–1 Fat choices		

Snack Time: _3 p.m._ *15* grams of carb		

Dinner Time: _6:30 p.m._
 4 Carb choices or
     Carb grams *60*
     2 Starch
     1 Fruit
     1 Milk
     2 Vegetables
 3–4 Meat / Protein choices
 1 Fat choices		

Snack Time: _9 p.m._ *15* grams of carb		

Christina Martin

Registered Dietitian

Registered Dietitian's Phone Number

breakfast, lunch, and dinner—are listed there. The time of day you usually eat each meal is also listed. Look next at the line in the left-hand column under breakfast, lunch, or dinner. That number will tell you how many carbohydrate servings or choices to select for that meal. It will also list the total carbohydrate grams in that meal and give you some suggestions as to what types of carbohydrate to choose. For example, 4 carbohydrate choices could be 2 servings of starch, 1 serving of fruit, and 1 serving of milk. After the carbohydrate choices, the number of meat/protein and fat servings are listed.

Turn now to the Food Choice Lists (Appendix) or look at the food lists your dietitian has given you. Find the Carbohydrate Foods and look under Starch: Grains/Breads/Starchy Vegetables. The meal plan you have been looking at lists two starch servings for breakfast. If this was your meal plan, you could choose any two foods from this list in the amount listed beside each food. You could choose half an English muffin and half a cup of cooked cereal. Or you could use both of your breakfast starch servings to have twice as much of one of the foods. You could have a whole English muffin or a whole cup of cooked cereal. If you don't want these foods, you can choose from the other foods on the carbohydrate list, such as fruit and milk. You can choose breakfast items from the other food groups in the same way. There are spaces on your meal plan for snacks between meals and at bedtime. Your dietitian may advise you to eat a snack at these times or you may simply prefer to have snacks at one or more of these times. It's also possible that you won't have any snacks on your meal plan—in part, because of your own preferences, and also because of your blood glucose levels.

This type of food and meal planning is called *carbohydrate counting*, or carb counting. You can decide to carb count either by counting actual grams of carbohydrate or by using carb choices, as in the breakfast example above. Either way is acceptable. However, if you take rapid-acting insulin and eventually plan to "match" your insulin to your carbohydrate intake (see Chapter 15), counting grams of carbohydrate is a more precise method. (Chapter 5 will discuss more advanced carb counting, including how to calculate your insulin-to-carbohydrate ratio and your insulin sensitivity factor.) Other individuals may use *exchange lists* or *fat-gram counting*. The important thing is that you have a method for planning what to eat and when.

Until You See a Dietitian . . .

Perhaps you are wondering what you should eat while you are waiting for your appointment with a dietitian. The "plate method" shown below in Figure 4-3 will give you an idea of how much of each food group you should eat at each meal.

Figure 4-3   Plate

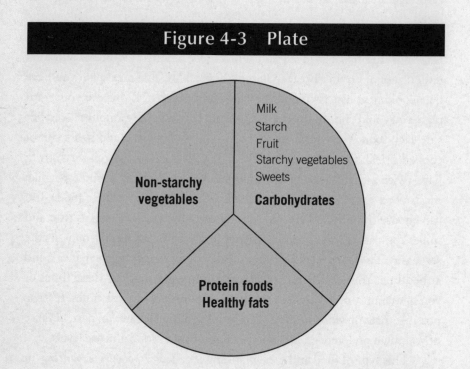

Another method is to follow a temporary "starter" meal plan. The following sample meal plan can be used until you meet with a dietitian.

"Starter" Meal Plan

Breakfast

Eat 3 to 4 carbohydrate servings, or choices (45–60 grams). Include a low-fat protein source like milk or yogurt as 1 carbohydrate serving.

Sample Breakfast Menus

30 grams carb or 2 carb choices

½ cup oatmeal
4 oz. skim milk
1 tbsp. raisins
	½ small bagel
	½ grapefruit
	1 tbsp. low-fat
	  cream cheese
		1 cup light-style
		  yogurt
		½ cup Fiber One
			1 slice toast
			4 oz. juice
			¼ cup low-fat
			  cottage cheese

½ English muffin
½ banana
1 tbsp. peanut
  butter
	¾ cup Cheerios
	4 oz. skim milk
	½ banana
		1 low-fat waffle
		sugar-free syrup
		1 cup berries
		1 tsp. low-fat
		  margarine
			2 slices light
			  toast
			6 oz. light yogurt
			1 tbsp. low-fat
			  margarine

45 grams carb or 3 carb choices

1 cup oatmeal
4 oz. skim milk
1 tbsp. raisins
	1 small bagel
	½ grapefruit
	1 tbsp. low-fat
	  cream cheese
		1 pkt. instant
		  breakfast drink
		8 oz. skim milk
			2 slices toast
			4 oz. juice
			1 egg
			1 tbsp. low-fat
			  margarine

1 English muffin
½ banana
1 tbsp. peanut
  butter
	1½ cups Cheerios
	4 oz. milk
	½ banana
		2 low-fat waffles
		sugar-free syrup
		1 cup berries
		1 tbsp. low-fat
		  margarine
			2 slices light
			  toast
			6 oz. light yogurt
			¼ cantaloupe
			1 tbsp. low-fat
			  margarine

60 grams carb or 4 carb choices

1 cup oatmeal
4 oz. skim milk
½ small bagel
1 tbsp. raisins
1 tsp. margarine
	1 (4-oz.) bagel
	1 tbsp. low-fat
	  cream cheese
	¼ cup egg
	  substitute
		1 pkt. instant
		  breakfast drink
		8 oz. milk
		1 banana
			3 slices toast
			4 oz. juice
			1 egg
			1 tbsp. low-fat
			  margarine

3 pancakes
  (4-inch diameter)
sugar-free syrup
1 med. orange
1 tbsp. low-fat
  margarine
	1½ cups
	  Cheerios
	8 oz. skim milk
	½ banana
		blender breakfast:
		8 oz. skim/soy
		  milk
		½ cup plain yogurt
		½ banana
		¼ cup wheat germ
		1 tbsp. peanut
		  butter
			2 slices whole-
			  grain toast
			6 oz. light yogurt
			2 small tangerines
			1 tbsp. low-fat
			  margarine

Lunch and Dinner

Eat 3 to 4 carbohydrate servings, or choices (45–60 grams). Be sure to include some fruit and a nonstarchy vegetable. Choose small portions (3 ounces) of low-fat meat, poultry, or fish. Include 1 or 2 servings of fat.

Sample Lunch Menus

45 grams carb or 3 carb choices

2 slices whole-grain bread	2 slices light bread	1 cup vegetable soup	1 med. potato
lettuce, tomato	lettuce, tomato	6 saltines	½ cup broccoli
1 small apple	10 baked chips	15 grapes	6 oz. light yogurt
2–3 slices lean luncheon meat	½ large pear	1 oz. low-fat cheese	2 oz. shredded cheese
1 tbsp. reduced-fat mayo	2–3 slices lean ham		2 tbsp. light sour cream
	1 tbsp. reduced-fat mayo		

2 cups salad	⅔ cup pasta	1 plain fast-food hamburger	2 cups Caesar salad
¼ cup chickpeas	½ cup tomato sauce	1 garden salad	½ cup croutons
½ cup tuna, plain	salad	1 pkg. fat-free herb vinaigrette	2–3 oz. grilled chicken
½ med. pita	2–3 oz. ground turkey		1 tbsp. Caesar dressing
1 cup fruit salad	2 tbsp. light dressing		½ cup froz. yogurt
2 tbsp. light dressing			

60 grams carb or 4 carb choices

2 slices whole-grain bread	2 slices light bread	2 cups vegetables	1 "wrap" sandwich with lean filling
lettuce, tomato	lettuce, tomato	6 saltines	salad
1 small apple	½ large pear	17 grapes	2 tbsp. light dressing
3 small gingersnaps	10 baked chips	1–2 oz. low-fat cheese	6 oz. light yogurt
2–3 slices lean luncheon meat	2 reduced-fat Oreos		
2 tsp. light mayo	2–3 slices lean ham		
	2 tsp. light mayo		

2 cups salad	1 cup pasta	1 fast-food broiled chicken sandwich (no sauce)	1 low-fat frozen entrée
½ cup chickpeas	½ cup tomato sauce		salad
½ cup tuna, plain	salad	½ cup frozen yogurt	2 tbsp. light dressing
½ med. pita	2–3 oz. ground turkey		½ cup sugar-free pudding
1 cup fruit salad	2 tbsp. light dressing		
2 tbsp. light dressing			

Sample Dinner Menus

45 grams carb or 3 carb choices

⅔ cup pasta	1 cup cooked rice	1 cup mashed	1 (4-oz.) sweet
½ cup spaghetti	1 cup broccoli	potato	potato
sauce	3–4 oz. baked	½ cup corn	1 cup green beans
2 tbsp. Parmesan	chicken breast	½ cup carrots	3–4 oz. broiled fish
cheese	1 tbsp. low-fat	3–4 oz. turkey	½ cup applesauce
salad	margarine	2 tbsp. gravy	1 tbsp. low-fat
2 tbsp. light	sugar-free Jell-O		margarine
dressing			

1 cup vegetable	2 tortillas	⅔ cup brown rice	1 hamburger bun
soup	½ cup refried beans	1 cup stir-fry	3–4 oz. lean
2 slices bread	½ cup salsa	vegetables	hamburger patty
3 oz. tuna	lettuce, tomato	3–4 oz. light tofu	lettuce, tomato
lettuce, tomato	2 tbsp. light sour	½ cup light ice	10 baked french
1 tbsp. reduced-fat	cream	cream	fries
mayo			

60 grams carb or 4 carb choices

1 cup pasta	1 cup cooked rice	1 cup mashed	1 (4-oz.) sweet
½ cup spaghetti	1 cup broccoli	potato	potato
sauce	3–4 oz. baked	½ cup corn	1 cup green beans
2 tbsp. Parmesan	chicken	½ cup carrots	3–4 oz. broiled fish
cheese	1 small apple	1 small roll	½ cup applesauce
salad	1 tbsp. low-fat	3–4 oz. turkey	8 oz. skim milk
2 tbsp. light	margarine	2 tbsp. gravy	1 tbsp. low-fat
dressing			margarine

2 cups vegetable	2 small tortillas	1 cup brown rice	1 hamburger bun
soup	½ cup refried beans	1 cup stir-fry	3–4 oz. lean
2 slices whole-grain	⅓ cup rice	vegetables	hamburger patty
bread	½ cup salsa	3–4 oz. light tofu	lettuce, tomato
3–4 oz. tuna	lettuce, tomato	½ cup light ice	10 baked french
lettuce, tomato	2 tbsp. light sour	cream	fries
1 tbsp. reduced-fat	cream		½ cup pineapple
mayo			chunks

75 grams carb or 5 carb choices

1 cup pasta	1⅓ cups cooked	1 cup mashed	1 (4-oz.) sweet
1 cup spaghetti	rice	potato	potato
sauce	1 cup broccoli	1 cup corn	1 cup green beans
2 tbsp. Parmesan	3–4 oz. baked	1 cup carrots	3–4 oz. broiled fish
cheese	chicken	1 small roll	½ cup applesauce
salad	1 small apple	3–4 oz. turkey	4 small gingersnaps
2 tbsp. light	1 tbsp. low-fat	2 tbsp. gravy	8 oz. skim milk
dressing	margarine		1 tbsp. low-fat
			margarine

continued on next page

75 grams carb or 5 carb choices (*continued*)

2 cups vegetable soup	2 small tortillas	1⅓ cups brown rice	1 hamburger bun
2 slices bread	½ cup refried beans	1 cup stir-fry vegetables	3–4 oz. lean hamburger patty
3–4 oz. tuna	⅔ cup rice	3–4 oz. light tofu	lettuce, tomato
lettuce, tomato	½ cup salsa	½ cup light ice cream	15 baked french fries
½ cup sugar-free pudding	lettuce, tomato		½ cup pineapple chunks
1 tbsp. reduced-fat mayo	2 tbsp. light sour cream		

Snack

If you need a snack, eat 1 to 2 carbohydrate servings, or choices (15–30 grams).

Snack Ideas

15 grams carbohydrate or 1 carb choice:

1 small fruit

6 oz. light yogurt

2 popcorn cakes

3 cups low-fat microwave popcorn

3 small gingersnaps

5 vanilla wafers

¾ ounce pretzels

15–20 baked potato or tortilla chips

6 saltines

3 graham cracker squares

1 granola bar

2 sugar-free fudgesicles

30 grams carbohydrate or 2 carb choices:

6 oz. light yogurt and ¼ cup low-fat granola

1 cup sugar-free pudding

16 animal crackers

8 melba toast

12 saltines

6 graham cracker squares

1 Nutrigrain bar

1 large piece fruit

1 cup cereal and 8 ounces milk

30 baked potato or tortilla chips

1 English muffin

1 small (2 ounces) bagel

Keeping Food Records

Paying attention to what you eat is important. Many people report that keeping food records helps them do this. If you haven't met with a dietitian, it's a great idea to write down what and when you eat and drink for three days. Take the record with you when you see the dietitian. That way you can plan as much as possible around your usual eating habits and lifestyle.

Once you start following your new meal plan, your dietitian will likely ask you to continue keeping a food record or to keep track of the servings of carbohydrate you eat. To do this, write down the time and everything you eat and drink. Try to estimate the amount or serving size of each food or drink. If you are just keeping track of carbohydrate servings, use the Food Choice Lists in the Appendix. Many individuals find it helpful to note the results of their blood glucose checks in their food or carbohydrate record. Figure 4-4, Sample Food Record, shows how a food record might be kept.

Estimating Portion Sizes

In your own kitchen it is easier and more convenient to measure and, if necessary, weigh foods. This will make your food records more accurate. Using measuring cups and a scale is the best way to keep close tabs on your portion sizes. Use the scale for weighing foods such as meat, poultry, fish, and cheese, and measuring cups for dry foods, such as cereal, pasta, and rice. Be sure to weigh and measure foods *after* you have cooked them. Measuring

Figure 4-4   Sample Food Record

	BREAKFAST		SNACK	LUNCH		SNACK	DINNER		SNACK	COMMENTS
	Before	After		Before	After		Before	After	Bedtime	
Time										
BG										
Food and Amount **DAY 1**										
	Carb _____ gm			Carb _____ gm			Carb _____ gm			
Time										
BG										
Food and Amount **DAY 2**										
	Carb _____ gm			Carb _____ gm			Carb _____ gm			
Time										
BG										
Food and Amount **DAY 3**										
	Carb _____ gm			Carb _____ gm			Carb _____ gm			

spoons should be used for foods eaten in smaller portions, such as peanut butter and salad dressing. With practice, you will be able to estimate accurately and will not need to use the scale all the time. However, it's always a good idea to weigh and measure your foods on an occasional basis, perhaps once or twice a month, since portions have a tendency to grow over time!

Many of your meals are probably eaten away from home. In this case, your hand can be a "handy" tool to help you determine portion sizes. Men may need to estimate down a little bit, since the measures below are based on a woman's hand of average size. The following tips for using your hand will make it easier to estimate portions:

- Your *fist* is about the size of one cup.
- Your *palm* is about the size of three ounces of cooked meat; this is also the size of a deck of cards.

- Your *thumb* is about one ounce of cheese, or one tablespoon of salad dressing or peanut butter.
- Your *thumb tip* (the top joint of your thumb) is about one teaspoon. One teaspoon equals one serving of fat, such as butter, margarine, mayonnaise, and oil.
- Your *whole hand* is a handful of about one to two ounces of a snack food (not a heaping handful). About three handfuls of popcorn equal one ounce (1 carbohydrate serving). For pretzels, two handfuls equal ¾ ounce (1 carbohydrate serving).

Some people find it easier to visualize portion sizes. Try to picture the following:

- 1 ounce of meat looks like a matchbox
- 1 ounce of cheese is about the size of a Ping-Pong ball
- 1 tablespoon of peanut butter is about the size of a walnut
- 1 cup of fruit is about the size of a baseball
- A medium apple or orange is about the size of a tennis ball
- A bunch of grapes equal to a ½ cup serving is about the size of a lightbulb
- A medium potato is about the size of a computer mouse

If you eat out a lot, your idea of a serving tends to grow without your noticing. So when you're at home, it's always a good idea to check your portions periodically and keep your portion-estimation skills strong.

Label Reading

Food labels are another important tool to help you figure out what you are eating. The packaging of almost all foods in your grocery store contains detailed information about nutrition in the Nutrition Facts panel. However, there may seem to be too much information, and you may not be sure what kind will be the most useful for managing your diabetes. Figure 4-5, Nutrition Facts Food Label, is typical of these labels. The following steps will help you decide how to "count" this food.

Figure 4-5   Nutrition Facts Food Label

Whole Grain Cereal

Nutrition Facts

Serving Size: 1 cup (53g/1.9 oz.)
Servings Per Container: About 8

Amount Per Serving

Calories 190	**Calories from Fat** 25

	% Daily Value**
Total Fat 3g*	5%
Saturated Fat 0g	0%
Trans Fat 0g	
Cholesterol 0mg	0%
Sodium 95mg	4%
Potassium 300mg	9%
Total Carbohydrate 36g	12%
Dietary Fiber 8g	32%
Soluble Fiber 3g	
Insoluble Fiber 5g	
Sugars 13g	
Protein 9g	14%

Vitamin A 0%	•	Vitamin C 0%
Calcium 4%	•	Iron 10%
Phosphorus 10%	•	Magnesium 10%
Copper 8%		

* Amount in Cereal. One half cup of fat free milk contributes an additional 40 calories, 65mg sodium, 6g total carbohydrates (6g sugars), and 4g protein.
** Percent Daily Values are based on a 2,000 calorie diet. Your daily values may be higher or lower depending on your calorie needs:

		Calories.	2,000	2,500
Total Fat	Less Than		65g	80g
Sat. Fat	Less Than		20g	25g
Cholesterol	Less Than		300mg	300mg
Sodium	Less Than		2,400mg	2,400mg
Potassium			3,500mg	3,500mg
Total Carbohydrate			300g	375g
Dietary Fiber			25g	30g
Protein			50g	65g

Calories per gram:
Fat 9   •   Carbohydrate 4   •   Protein 4

INGREDIENTS: Soy Grits, Hard Red Winter Wheat, Long Grain Brown Rice, Whole Grain Oats, Barley, Rye, Buckwheat, Sesame Seeds, Evaporated Cane Juice Syrup, Corn Meal, Corn Flour, Soy Protein, Wheat Bran, Oat Flour, Corn Bran, Honey, Natural Flavors, Calcium Carbonate, Salt

CONTAINS SOYBEAN AND WHEAT INGREDIENTS

Serving Size

Begin by looking at the Serving Size. Is this the amount you plan to eat? This is important because the nutrition information on the label corresponds to one serving size. If you are accustomed to eating more than one serving, you will need to account for the extra amount.

Total Carbohydrate

Next, focus on the Total Carbohydrate. This number is used to determine the number of carbohydrate servings in the serving size. The important number to remember is:

15 grams of carbohydrate = 1 carbohydrate serving (choice)

According to the information on the Nutrition Facts food label in Figure 4-5, a ½ cup serving of this food contains 13 grams of total carbohydrate and would be counted as 1 carbohydrate serving (13 divided by 15 = 1 serving; the leftover 2 grams, being less than 5, are not counted as a serving). Ignore the Sugars amount as it is already counted within the total carbohydrate. Note that Sugars and Dietary Fiber are indented and in lighter print than Total Carbohydrate. Often people assume the sugars are simply added sugars. But in fact the sugars comprise both added and naturally occurring sugars, such as lactose in milk, and fructose in fruit.

When counting carbohydrate, most people can also ignore the Dietary Fiber amount as well. However, when people are trying to be very precise with the carbohydrate amount—for example, when determining an insulin-to-carbohydrate ratio for more "advanced" carbohydrate counting (see Chapter 5 for more information on this)—if the dietary fiber amount is greater than 5 grams, it can be subtracted from the total carbohydrate grams. Dietary fiber is not absorbed, but it is unlikely that 5 to 10 grams will have much effect on your blood glucose level unless you eat more than one serving.

Some labels may also list *sugar alcohols*, which are used in some foods as a sweetener. In general, about half the grams of sugar alcohols are digested. Just as for fiber, you can generally ignore the sugar alcohol amount when counting carbohydrate. However, when determining an insulin-to-carbohydrate ratio, if the sugar alcohol is more than 10 grams, you can subtract half of the amount from the total carbohydrate grams. *Net carb, low carb,* and *impact carb* are relatively new phrases on labels. So far, they have not been defined by the Food and Drug Administration, although the agency is currently working to define them. These terms were created by companies to give their products more shelf appeal. The best advice is that consumers should not be fooled by promises on wrappers. Calories still count, and these special "low carb" food products are not calorie free and can affect your blood glucose levels.

Total Fat

The Total Fat is the total number of grams of fat in a serving of this food—*saturated, monounsaturated, polyunsaturated,* and *trans fats.* It's best to choose foods made from monounsaturated and polyunsaturated fats. Avoid products that contain large amounts of saturated fats, and keep trans fats to as small an amount as possible. The different types of fat are discussed in more detail in the next chapter.

Total fat grams per day should be about 40 to 70 grams for women and 60 to 90 grams for men. A food can be labeled low fat if it has 3 grams or less in one serving. A low-saturated-fat food has no more than 1 gram of saturated fat per serving. Look at the total grams of fat in one serving size and select foods with:

- 3 or less grams of fat for every 15 grams of carbohydrate
- 3 grams of fat for every 7 to 8 grams of protein (or one ounce of a protein food)
- ⅓ or less of the total fat as saturated fat

Sodium

Sodium is listed in mg (milligrams) per serving. Look for foods that have less than 400 milligrams in a single serving, or less than 800 milligrams for convenience food and meal entrées. Sodium is also discussed in the next chapter.

Label "Lingo"

Labels that you see on food packaging now have standard definitions, set by the Food and Drug Administration (FDA). Here are some of the most common terms you will see:

- *Fat Free:* less than 0.5 gram of fat per serving
- *Low Fat:* 3 grams of fat or less per serving
- *Low Saturated Fat:* 1 gram of saturated fat or less per serving
- *Low Sodium:* 140 milligrams of sodium or less per serving
- *Low Calorie:* 40 calories or less per serving
- *Lean:* less than 10 grams of fat, 4 grams of saturated fat, and 95 mg of cholesterol per serving
- *Light:* ⅓ fewer calories or ½ less fat of the regular version; or no more than ½ the sodium of the higher-sodium version
- *"Reduced":* 25 percent less of a specific nutrient, or 25 percent fewer calories than the regular version

Vitamins, Minerals, and Dietary Supplements

Carbohydrate, protein, and fat are often called macronutrients, or "major nutrients," because they supply energy, in the form of calories, to your body. Vitamins and minerals (often called micronutrients), such as calcium, iron, potassium, and zinc, are essential nutrients that are present—but only in small amounts—in the foods we eat. Vitamins and minerals do not provide energy, but they are very important because they help the body process foods and are involved in many other body functions, including the metabolism of carbohydrate.

People with diabetes often ask if they should take vitamin or mineral supplements (capsules or tablets) available from drugstores or health food stores. If you are eating a balanced diet, you may not need to take these supplements. But, since many people find it challenging to eat a balanced diet on a daily basis, it may be wise to consider taking a multivitamin and mineral supplement. Other people who may benefit from taking a supplement include the elderly, pregnant or lactating women, strict vegetarians, and individuals on calorie-restricted diets. And newer research has shown that people with type 2 diabetes who take a multivitamin/mineral supplement are less prone to developing infections. If you choose to take a multivitamin, look for one that does not have more than 100–150 percent of the Recommended Dietary Allowance (RDA) for any of the vitamins and minerals in it. Your dietitian can assist you in choosing a supplement that best fits your needs.

Certain groups may benefit from a specific supplement. All women of childbearing age need an adequate amount of folate for the prevention of birth defects. People who don't drink milk are likely to have an inadequate calcium intake—important for the prevention of bone disease—unless they take a calcium supplement. This may be especially important for women with type 1 diabetes, who are at greater risk for developing osteoporosis. Premenopausal women may need extra iron. However, you should discuss the use of iron supplements with your healthcare provider before you start to take them. Older adults are at risk for deficiencies of specific nutrients, such as vitamin B_{12} and vitamin D. If you are an older adult, speak with your healthcare provider or dietitian to learn whether you should take specific supplements.

Currently, there are no vitamin, mineral, or other supplements that have a proven benefit in controlling blood glucose levels. You may have heard or wondered about chromium. There are no accurate ways to test for chromium deficiency in people with diabetes, but because chromium is widely distributed in foods, it is unlikely that individuals are deficient in it. Supplements are most likely to be of benefit when there is a deficiency in a specific vitamin or mineral.

Several small studies had previously suggested that antioxidants—vitamin E, beta-carotene, vitamin C, and selenium—might protect against heart and vessel disease. However, large randomized trials, involving over 81,000 persons, that compared antioxidants with placebos (fake antioxidants) found no benefit from the antioxidants in preventing heart and vessel disease in the general public or in people with diabetes. Of concern are recent studies reporting that antioxidants hampered the beneficial effects of a statin (a medication for lowering cholesterol) and niacin on blood cholesterol values—they appeared to prevent the increase in HDL (the "good") cholesterol usually achieved with these medications. The American Diabetes Association has concluded that routine supplementation with antioxidants is not advised, because of the uncertainties relating to long-term benefit and safety. What is important for the prevention of heart and vessel disease is lifestyle factors (nutrition and physical activity), aspirin, medications for lowering cholesterol and blood pressure, and smoking cessation. However, research does indicate that certain antioxidants may play an important role in the prevention of certain other diseases and conditions. Be sure to talk with your dietitian or other healthcare providers if you are wondering about taking a supplement. They can help you decide what type and amount would be most likely to be beneficial for you.

Herbal and Other Nutritional Supplements

There are a variety of herbal and botanical supplements that in animal studies or in small or poorly conducted studies in humans have been shown to improve glucose levels. However, there is little evidence to suggest a benefit from any of the herbal supplements in persons with diabetes. What minimal evidence there is looks at substances such as cinnamon, which may improve blood glucose and lipid levels in people with type 2 diabetes; some research shows that the antioxidant alpha lipoic acid may help reduce the frequency and severity of symptoms of diabetic neuropathy. You should, however, be cautious about using herbs, botanicals, and nutritional supplements, some of which have the potential to interfere with medications you may be taking. These supplements may also affect your blood glucose levels. It is therefore important that you discuss with your dietitian and physician any supplements you are taking or plan to take. And never substitute a supplement for a prescription drug without first checking with your healthcare providers.

Making the Change to Healthy Eating

For many persons with diabetes, healthy eating means a new way of eating—for a lifetime. If you slip from your meal plan for a few days, don't let it keep you from achieving your target goals. Get back on the road to health. Here's how:

- **ASK YOURSELF WHY YOU GOT OFF TRACK.** Were you feeling stress at home or work? Have you been traveling or on vacation? Do you feel as if you are doing it alone? Find out what triggered your sidetrack—and start again.

- **DON'T WORRY ABOUT A SLIP.** Everyone slips—especially when learning something new. Remember that changing your lifestyle is a long-term process.

- **SEE WHETHER YOU TRIED TO DO TOO MUCH AT ONCE.** Often, those starting a new lifestyle try to change too much at once. This is especially true if you have just been diagnosed with diabetes. Instead, change one or two things at a time. Slowly but surely is the best way to succeed.

- **BREAK THE PROCESS DOWN INTO SMALL STEPS.** This not only keeps you from trying to do too much at once but also keeps the changes simpler. Break complex goals into smaller, simpler steps, each of which is attainable. For example, if you're trying to master carbohydrate counting, focus on one meal at a time, starting with breakfast.

- **WRITE IT DOWN.** This is the key to success in examining your current lifestyle and making appropriate changes. Begin by keeping track of what you eat for at least one week. Besides recording *what* you eat, also record *when* you ate, *where* you were while eating, and *why*—how you felt—while eating. "What" is fairly straightforward. Be sure to record everything. "When" and "where" are also important, especially if your notes reveal a pattern of times and places when you tend to overeat. Do you eat more if you are watching TV? While standing in front of the refrigerator? Driving to work? "Why" is also significant. Are you really hungry when you eat, or do you eat because you are bored or depressed? If you have these feelings, try to find other activities to substitute for eating.

- **ASK YOUR FAMILY AND FRIENDS FOR SUPPORT.** Expect your eating habits to change slowly—they developed over a long time. Support for change from family and friends is essential. Encourage them to develop the same healthy lifestyle. Make it easy to eat what you should. For example, place a bowl of fruit on the kitchen table. Ask your healthcare providers for help as well. Your dietitian can provide new ways to prepare food, new recipes, and encouragement. Using blood glucose monitoring results, you can learn how to incorporate into your meals foods you previously thought you couldn't eat.

- **SEEK SUPPORT FROM YOUR HEALTHCARE TEAM.** If you find that you're not getting support at home, ask your provider or dietitian for help. Consider joining a support group for people with diabetes who are dealing with similar issues.

- **CELEBRATE SUCCESS.** Treat yourself to a nonfood reward, such as a new best-selling novel or a pair of sneakers, for your accomplishments. Remember, you are not trying to follow a short-term diet—you are developing a lifelong eating style that will help you manage your diabetes and benefit your overall health. So reward yourself along the path to success.

Studying the "Food Map"

This chapter began by comparing a meal plan to a nutritional "road map" that will help get you to your "destination" of blood glucose control. It focused on the importance of having a meal plan and on food groups and basic carbohydrate counting. This information is essential if you have any type of diabetes—type 1, type 2, gestational—or prediabetes. Learning portion sizes and reading food labels are important skills for making accurate food choices. But to more fully understand the direction in which you are headed, it's important to learn a few more facts about food. The next chapters will provide those details.

CHAPTER 5

More About Carbohydrate

Nature's building blocks are the *nutrients* in the foods we eat. They provide the body with the substances it needs for maintenance and growth, to stay warm, and to perform a wide range of other functions—in short, what we need to live! The three major nutrients, introduced in Chapter 4, are *carbohydrate, protein,* and *fat.* This chapter moves from the basics of carbohydrate counting to advanced carbohydrate counting, which involves the use of insulin-to-carbohydrate ratios and the calculation of your sensitivity factor. Fiber and whole grains, the glycemic index and glycemic load, and caloric and noncaloric sweeteners are also discussed in this chapter. Chapter 6 covers the basics of food's effect on blood fats and blood pressure. Other food-related topics important in the care of diabetes—alcohol, vitamins and minerals, and eating out—are covered in Chapter 7.

Advanced Carbohydrate Counting: Insulin-to-Carbohydrate Ratios

Everyone with diabetes should understand how carbohydrate affects his or her blood glucose levels and know the basics of carbohydrate counting. However, some individuals with diabetes also benefit from learning about *insulin-to-carbohydrate ratios,* a more advanced level of carbohydrate counting. This is especially important for anyone using *physiologic insulin therapy,* which is discussed in Chapter 15. An insulin-to-carbohydrate ratio tells you how much rapid-acting insulin, such as lispro, aspart, or glulisine you need to cover the carbohydrate you eat at a meal or snack. Knowing how to match your insulin dose to what you eat helps increase your flexibility in food choices and the timing of meals. There are several ways for you to determine your insulin-to-carbohydrate ratio. The simplest entails the following steps:

1. With the help of your dietitian, look at your food records and determine the total amount of carbohydrate at each meal and snack for at least three days. Determine either your average intake over the three days or your range of carbohydrate intake (e.g., 30–45g) for each meal and snack.

2. Decide on a carbohydrate goal for each meal and snack, and then eat consistent amounts of carbohydrate for three days or more.

3. Study your glucose records. Identify some meals when both the before-meal and after-meal (two hours after the start of eating) measurements were within your target range.

4. Use those meals to figure your insulin-to-carbohydrate ratio: divide the number of grams of carbohydrate by the units of mealtime insulin. For example, you took 3 units of rapid-acting insulin, ate 45 grams (3 servings) of carbohydrate, and your post-meal glucose was within your target range. Divide 45 by 3, which gives 1 unit of insulin per 15 grams of carbohydrate, or a 1:15 insulin-to-carbohydrate ratio (or 1 unit of insulin per 1 carbohydrate serving).

For the best results, figure your ratio for several meals on other days to be sure it is correct. Your ratio may vary by meal, on workdays versus weekend days, or on active days versus sedentary days. Fine-tuning your ratio(s) may take some time and may require the assistance of your diabetes educator.

Another method for calculating your insulin-to-carb ratio involves using what is called the 450 Rule. Here's how this works:

1. Determine your total daily dose of insulin. This includes both your rapid-acting and long-acting, or basal, insulin. If you're not sure how

to figure this out, ask your diabetes educator or healthcare provider to help you.

2. Divide 450 by your total daily insulin dose. For example, let's assume your total daily dose is 50 units. If we divide 450 by 50, we get 9. This means that your starting insulin-to-carbohydrate ratio is 1:9. One unit of your fast-acting insulin "covers" every 9 grams of carbohydrate you eat.

3. To use your ratio, first calculate how many grams of carbohydrate you plan to eat at a meal. For example, assume you will eat 45 grams of carbohydrate for breakfast. Using your ratio of 1:9, divide the 45 grams by 9, which equals 5. This means you need to take 5 units of insulin to cover your 45 grams of carb.

Your ratio may be slightly different at different times of the day. You may find that you need more insulin for the amount of carbohydrate you eat at breakfast compared with that same amount at lunch or dinner—your ratio at breakfast might be 1:9, but for lunch and dinner the ratio might be 1:12.

Sensitivity or Correction Factor

Before you calculate and start using your own insulin-to-carb ratio, you need to learn one other key component of carbohydrate counting: the *sensitivity factor*, also known as the *correction factor*. Your insulin-to-carb ratio, if it's correct, will cover the amount of carb you eat at your meal. But what if your blood glucose is above target before you even start eating? You need insulin to help bring that high blood glucose back to target in addition to the amount you'll take to cover the carbs in the food you're eating. That's where the sensitivity factor comes in.

The *insulin sensitivity factor* is also called the *correction factor* or *supplemental factor*. It is defined as the amount of blood glucose in mg/dl that is lowered by 1 unit of rapid-acting or regular insulin. The insulin sensitivity factor is used to calculate the amount of insulin you need to return blood glucose to within your target blood glucose range. Your healthcare team may provide you with an insulin sensitivity factor, or you may work with them to calculate it. In general, most adults use an insulin sensitivity factor of 50 mg/dl. This means that 1 unit of insulin should lower your blood glucose by about 50 mg/dl or "50 points."

Commonly accepted formulas called the 1800 Rule and the 1500 Rule are used as starting points in determining insulin sensitivity factors. The 1800 Rule is sometimes used for rapid-acting insulin, and the 1500 Rule for regular insulin or for people who may be insulin resistant. At Joslin Diabetes Center, the 1500 Rule is typically used to calculate an initial sensitivity factor that will later likely need to be adjusted.

To calculate insulin sensitivity factors, use the following steps:

- Start with your total daily insulin dose. In the example above, it was 50 units.
- Divide 1,500 by the total daily insulin dose for your insulin sensitivity factor (1500 ÷ 50 = 30).
- Your insulin sensitivity factor is 30 mg/dl. This means 1 unit of rapid-acting insulin decreases your blood glucose by about 30 points.

Here's an example of when you might use your insulin sensitivity factor:

- Your target blood glucose before meals is 90 to 130 mg/dl.
- Your glucose check before lunch is 205 mg/dl, which is 75 mg/dl above your target (205 − 130 = 75).
- Divide 75 by your insulin sensitivity factor (75 ÷ 30 = 2.5, round to 3). (If you're very sensitive to insulin, you can take 2.5 units.) You would need to add a correction dose of 3 units of rapid-acting insulin to your usual mealtime dose to bring your glucose level within target range.

Again, it's very important that you work closely with your healthcare team as you start to use your insulin-to-carb ratio and your sensitivity factor. Don't be surprised if they both change as you start to count carbs. You will also need to reevaluate your ratio and sensitivity factor to determine whether they are correct. Finally, your healthcare team will provide further guidance on more advanced topics, such as how to make a "reverse correction," or how to adjust your sensitivity factor for sick days.

EXAMPLE   Let's look at an example to help explain how you would use both your insulin-to-carb ratio and your sensitivity factor. Remember: you must use your sensitivity factor if your pre-meal blood glucose level is above your target range. Also, don't forget that you adjust only your rapid-acting insulin when using your insulin-to-carb ratio and sensitivity factor, never your long-acting or basal insulin.

Here is an example of the information you will need to have:

Your insulin-to-carb ratio: Let's say you calculated it using the formula provided above and found that your ratio is 1:15, which means 1 unit of insulin covers 15 grams of carbohydrate.

Your sensitivity factor: Let's say you calculated it using the formula provided above and found that your sensitivity factor is 40, which means that 1 unit of insulin lowers your blood glucose by 40 points

Your pre-meal blood glucose: 200

Your target blood glucose: 120

It's time for you to eat dinner.

1.   When you check your blood glucose, it is 200, although your pre-meal target blood glucose is 120. To figure out how much insulin you'll need to lower your blood glucose to the target, subtract your target from your actual blood glucose.

$$\begin{array}{r} 200 \text{ (actual blood glucose)} \\ - 120 \text{ (target blood glucose)} \\ \hline 80 \text{ mg/dl} \end{array}$$

This means that you must lower your blood glucose by 80 points. In this example, we are supposing that your sensitivity factor is 40. If you divide 80 by 40, you get 2. This means you must take 2 units of insulin to lower your pre-meal blood glucose to its target level of 120.

2. You determine how many grams of carb you plan to eat. Let's assume you'll be eating 75 grams of carbohydrate. Using your insulin-to-carb ratio of 1:15, determine how much insulin you will need to cover the 75 grams of carb. To do this, divide the 75 grams of carb in your meal by the amount of insulin needed to cover 1 gram of carb: 75 ÷ 15 = 5 units of insulin.

    This means you need 5 units of insulin to cover the 75 grams of carb you'll be eating.

3. Add the 5 units of insulin needed to cover the carbs you will eat and the 2 units needed to lower your blood glucose to its target level for a total of 7 units that you will take before eating dinner.

4. To determine whether your insulin dose was correct, check your blood glucose two hours after your meal, and again four hours after your meal. If your blood glucose is approximately 40 to 80 points higher than your target two hours later but has returned to "normal" four hours later, your calculations were correct! If your blood glucose is higher or lower, you may need to adjust your insulin-to-carb ratio or your sensitivity factor, or both. Work with your healthcare team to determine how to make adjustments.

Now that you know how to calculate your insulin-to-carb ratio and your sensitivity factor (so that you know how much insulin you will need to cover the amount of food you are eating), you can be much more flexible with regard to your food choices and the timing of your meals.

Fiber and Whole Grains

Fiber is the structural portion of fruits, vegetables, grains, nuts, and legumes. Structural fibers cannot be digested or absorbed by your body. Therefore, fiber does not provide calories. Some fibers add "bulk" to your meals, helping you feel full. Other fibers have a laxative effect on the digestive system. Common sources of fiber are wheat, corn, and oat bran; legumes (cooked dried peas and beans); nuts; and vegetables and fruits, especially when raw.

Very large amounts of fiber, approximately 50 grams per day, have been shown to improve glucose, lipid (fat), and insulin levels. Because the average fiber intake in the United States is about 10 to 13 grams per day, it isn't known if most people with diabetes can consume enough fiber on a regular basis to improve their blood glucose control. However, there are other benefits of eating a diet high in fiber and whole grains, including a lower risk for heart disease and some types of cancer, improved digestive health, and even weight control. In addition, foods high in fiber typically contain more of the important vitamins and minerals that may be missing in refined or processed foods.

Fiber and whole grains go hand in hand. Whole grains include all three parts of the grain—bran, germ, and endosperm. The fiber, vitamins, minerals, and hundreds of phytonutrients (health-protective substances in plant foods) found in grains work together to help protect against heart disease and diabetes, and may help with blood glucose control. The best way to identify whole grain foods is to look at the ingredients list on packages. Look for foods with the whole-grain ingredient listed first—for example, whole-wheat flour, whole oats, whole-grain corn, and brown rice.

Tips for Increasing Fiber and Whole Grains

The goal is to increase your intake of fiber to between 20 and 35 grams per day. If you're not used to eating much fiber, you should increase your intake gradually to allow your digestive system time to "adjust." Eating too much fiber at once can lead to gas, cramps, and even diarrhea. Also, be sure to increase your fluid intake as you increase your fiber intake in order to avoid constipation.

Here are ways you can increase the fiber content of your meals:

- Dietary fiber is listed just beneath Total Carbohydrate on the Nutrition Facts label. Foods that are an excellent source of fiber have 5 grams or more per serving; good sources have 2½ to 5 grams.

- Choose foods with a high-fiber content: whole-grain cereals, breads, and crackers; grains such as oats, barley, bulgur, and buckwheat; acorn and butternut squash; cooked peas, beans, and lentils; berries; and dried fruit and nuts.

- Look for whole-grain bread that contains 3 grams of fiber per serving and whole-grain crackers that contain at least 2 grams of fiber per serving.

- Baked products, such as muffins or cookies, can be prepared with whole-wheat flour. If a recipe calls for all-purpose flour, use ½ whole-wheat flour and ½ all-purpose flour. To use only whole-wheat flour, substitute 1 cup of whole-wheat flour minus 1 tablespoon for every 1 cup of all-purpose flour.

Glycemic Index and Glycemic Load

Have you ever noticed that even though you carefully measure your carbohydrate servings, you still can't always explain your blood glucose after a meal? The glycemic index (GI) of foods may shed some light on this. While different foods may have the same number of carbs, they may not have the same effect on blood glucose. The glycemic index is a system of ranking foods containing equal amounts of carbohydrate according to how much they raise blood glucose levels. For instance, the carbohydrate in a slice of 100 percent stone-ground whole-wheat bread (a low glycemic index food) may have less impact on your blood glucose than that in a slice of processed white bread (a high glycemic index food). The GI is an additional meal-planning tool that may help you understand how carbohydrate foods can differ in their effects on your blood glucose.

Researchers measure the GI of carbohydrate foods and assign them a GI number that typically ranges from 0 to 100. Foods with lower values have less of an effect on blood glucose than do foods with higher values. Researchers determine the effect on blood glucose of a reference food— either 50 grams of glucose or 50 grams of bread—and then compare that effect with the effect of 50 grams of various other carbohydrate foods. The result of this comparison is expressed as a percentage. When using glucose—which has a GI of 100—as a reference, a food is considered to be "low GI" if it is ranked from 0 to 55, "intermediate GI" if it is ranked from 56 to 69, and "high GI" if it is ranked 70 or greater. The methods by which GI is calculated are not always standard, so knowing the exact GI number is not as important as knowing in general if a food has a ranking that is low, moderate, or high (that is, if the food has a low, moderate, or high effect on blood glucose). Table 5-1 lists examples of low, moderate, and high GI foods.

TABLE 5-1   Examples of Low, Moderate, and High Glycemic Index (GI) Foods

Low GI Foods	Moderate GI Foods	High GI Foods
Whole-grain breads	Rye bread	White bread
Bran cereals	Frosted Flakes	Corn Chex
Green grapes	Fruit cocktail	Watermelon
Cooked barley	Canned sweet corn	Instant mashed potatoes
Milk	Soft drinks	Sports drinks

Many factors affect how the carbohydrate in foods ranks on the GI scale. For example, highly processed foods, such as white bread, generally have higher GI values than foods that are not as processed. Fiber, fat, and acidity all slow digestion and lower a food's GI value. Interestingly, sugars, fruit, and fruit juice usually have lower GI values as well. Because sugars, either natural or added, are half glucose and half fructose, and fructose is primarily stored in the liver, 50 grams of a sugar will raise blood glucose levels only about half as much as a similar portion of glucose. *If a food has a low GI, it does not mean that people with diabetes can eat unlimited amounts without it affecting their blood glucose levels.* Nor does it mean you have to eliminate all high GI foods—rather, try to combine them with low or moderate GI foods. Generally, when a high GI food is combined with a low GI food, the meal will be within the moderate GI range; for example, milk (low GI) and a cereal made primarily from corn (high GI) will together have a moderate GI.

The glycemic index can be difficult to apply to everyday eating situations because foods are compared with one another not in usual portions, but in equivalent amounts of carbohydrate. For example, a pound and a half of carrots and one cup of spaghetti have 50 grams each of carbohydrate, and this amount is used to determine their GI even though it is very unlikely that anyone would consume that many carrots at one time.

Because of the difficulty of relating GI with portion sizes, some researchers are suggesting the use of another approach, the *glycemic load*. The glycemic load (GL) combines the GI value and the carbohydrate content of an average serving of a food, of a meal, or of a day's worth of food. Table 5-2 lists some foods and their GI and GL.

TABLE 5-2	Glycemic Index (GI) and Glycemic Load (GL) of Some Common Foods			
Food	Serving Size	Grams of Carbohydrate	GI	GL
Pizza	1 slice	78 g	86	68
White rice	1 cup	45 g	102	46
Potatoes	1	37 g	102	38
Orange juice	6 oz.	20 g	75	15
White bread	1 slice	13 g	100	13
Carrots	½ cup	8 g	131	10
Milk	8 oz.	11 g	46	5

The glycemic load is calculated by multiplying the GI number of a food by the actual number of grams of carbohydrate in a single serving and then dividing that number by 100: GL = (GI x the number of carb grams per serving) divided by 100.

A GL of 10 or less is low; 11–19 is medium; and 20 or more is high. In the preceding chart, carrots have a high GI (remember, the GI for carrots is arrived at by comparing 50 grams of carbs in carrots with 50 grams of carbs in the reference food—and it would take one and a half pounds of carrots to get 50 grams); you might therefore think you need to avoid them. However, the GL (based on both the GI and the amount of carb in *one serving* of carrots) is only 10, which puts them in the low category.

The American Diabetes Association concludes in its evidence-based nutrition recommendations that research does not support the glycemic index as a primary method of meal planning for people with diabetes. Placing the initial focus on the total amount of carbohydrate eaten is deemed more beneficial. However, you can see why carbohydrate counting alone is not always perfect either. Some individuals find the GI or the GL can be used to help fine-tune glucose control. For example, some people may benefit from choosing low GI foods, especially at breakfast; others may not. Only by checking your blood glucose levels before and after meals can you determine whether some foods raise your blood glucose levels more than others. For accuracy, blood glucose levels must be in the target range before the meal, and the total amount of carbohydrate in the meals tested must be the same. You can't compare a meal that contains 45 grams of carbohydrate, for example, with a meal that has 75 grams of carbohydrate. Information gained from testing foods can help you decide whether you need to choose smaller portions of the foods that raised your blood glucose levels more than others. Or you may have to cover foods with the right amount of diabetes medication. Something everyone can do is to replace highly processed carbohydrates with more whole grains, fruits, low-fat milk, legumes, and nonstarchy vegetables. These foods all have lower GI values and contribute valuable nutrients important for a healthy diet. If you're interested in learning more about either the GI or the GL, ask your dietitian for information.

Sweeteners

Sweeteners can be divided into those that contribute calories (called *nutritive* or *caloric sweeteners*) and those that contribute few, if any, calories and are therefore called *noncaloric* or *nonnutritive sweeteners*. If you have diabetes, a wide range of sweeteners will fit into your eating program. Not all sweeteners are alike—they can have different effects on your blood glucose. Table 5-3, Sugars, Sweeteners, and Sweets, lists most of the sweeteners available today and the common or brand names by which they are known.

TABLE 5-3 Sugars, Sweeteners, and Sweets

Caloric Sugars, Sweeteners, and Sweets	Common Names	Comments/Applications
Carob	Carob flour Carob powder Carob chips	75% sucrose, glucose, and/or fructose; tastes like chocolate
Chocolate	Bittersweet Bitter Milk chocolate	40% to 43% sucrose
Fructose	Fruit sugar Levulose	100% fruit sugar
Glucose	Corn sugar Dextrose Grape sugar	Not as sweet as sucrose
Honey	Creamed honey Honeycomb	About 35% glucose, 40% fructose plus water
Lactose	Milk sugar	50% glucose, 50% lactose; not as sweet as sucrose
Maltose	White crystalline sugar formed from starches	100% glucose; not as sweet as sucrose
Molasses	Blackstrap Golden syrup Refiners' sugar	50% to 75% sucrose and invert sugar
Sucrose	Beet sugar Brown sugar Cane sugar Confectioners' sugar Dehydrated cane juice (Sucanat) Invert sugar Powdered sugar Raw sugar	50% glucose, 50% fructose

continued on next page

TABLE 5-3 Sugars, Sweeteners, and Sweets
(continued)

Caloric Sugars, Sweeteners, and Sweets	Common Names	Comments/Applications
Sucrose *(continued)*	Table sugar Turbinado	

Sugar alcohols (polyols)	Ducitol
	Isomalt
	Maltitol
	Mannitol
	Sorbitol
	Xylitol
	Hydrogenated
	  starch
	  hydrolysate
		Add sweetness and bulk to foods; not as sweet as sucrose, with about half the calories of other sugars because they are not completely absorbed; may cause abdominal pain, cramping, gas, bloating, and diarrhea, especially in children

Syrups	Corn syrup Corn syrup solids and/or fructose High-fructose syrups Honey maple syrup Molasses Sugar cane syrup Sorghum syrup	Primarily glucose
Acesulfame-K	Sweet One Sunette	200 times sweeter than sucrose; can be used in baking and cooking
Aspartame	Equal NutraSweet Sweet Mate	180 times sweeter than sucrose; loses sweetening effect when heated; prolonged cooking at high heat may result in loss of some sweetness

continued on next page

Caloric Sugars, Sweeteners, and Sweets	Common Names	Comments/Applications
Neotame		8,000 times sweeter than sucrose; only very small amounts are needed to sweeten foods and beverages; can be used alone or in combination with other noncaloric or caloric sweeteners
Saccharin	Sweet'n Low Sugar Twin Sweet Magic Sucaryl	375 times sweeter than sucrose; can be used in baking and cooking
Sucralose	Splenda	600 times sweeter than sucrose; can be used in cooking and baking; pours, measures, and bakes like sugar

Caloric Sweeteners

These sweeteners are carbohydrates and affect your blood glucose levels. Most of them contain 4 calories per gram, just like other carbohydrates. This means you need to count caloric sweeteners the same as you count other carbohydrate servings. The main problem with nutritive sweeteners is that they contribute calories without any other nutritional value, so, like everyone else, people with diabetes should be careful about how much they eat or drink of sweetened foods.

One simple way to keep "sweetness" in your meals without adding extra amounts of carbohydrate is to cut back on the amount of sugar used. With most recipes, you can reduce the sugar by at least one third without changing taste and texture. For example, if a recipe calls for 1 cup of sugar, use ⅔ cup instead, and the next time try ½ cup.

Be aware! "Sugarless," "sugar free" and "no sugar added" usually mean that sucrose (table sugar), dextrose, corn syrup, honey, and other sugars have been replaced with sweeteners known as *sugar alcohols* or *polyols*, which cause a slightly lower rise in blood glucose. This does not mean that these foods are better for people with diabetes, as they are usually not reduced very much in calories. And many people don't realize that "sugar free" foods still contain carbohydrate—often, just as much carbohydrate as the "regular" versions! These foods often contain higher amounts of fat, which can increase their calories per serving. Bloating, gas, diarrhea, and stomach upset are also common side effects of the sugar alcohols.

There are some general guidelines for carbohydrate counting with sugar alcohols:

- Sugar alcohols are usually combined with other carbohydrates, therefore subtract half of the sugar alcohol's grams from the total carbohydrate grams and count the remaining carbohydrate grams.

- If ALL the food's carbohydrate and calories are from sugar alcohols, and there are less than 10 carbohydrate grams per serving, it is considered a free food.

- If ALL the carbohydrate is from sugar alcohols, and there are 10 or more grams of carbohydrate per serving, divide the number of grams in half and count as carbohydrate.

Noncaloric Sweeteners

Five noncaloric sweeteners are currently approved by the FDA. Four are listed in Table 5-4. Neotame was the latest to be approved. Other than saccharin, which was on the market before the FDA food additive approval process was established, these sweeteners were all approved through FDA's rigorous safety process. Saccharin, which in very large quantities was linked to cancer, was dropped from the FDA's cancer-causing chemical list in 2000, and labels of saccharin-containing products no longer require a health warning. Articles questioning the safety of aspartame are often circulated on the Internet. Aspartame has been the subject of more than 200 studies since 1965. These studies have concluded that eating products sweetened with aspartame is not associated with any adverse health effects.

After extensive testing, all approved noncaloric sweeteners were determined to be safe for the general public, including people with diabetes, and pregnant and lactating women. The following recommendations have been set by the FDA for acceptable daily intake (ADI) and include a 100-fold safety factor. The World Health Organization's Joint Expert Committee on Food Additives has set the ADI for saccharin.

TABLE 5-4 Noncaloric Sweeteners, Acceptable Daily Intake (ADI), and Amounts in Soda and Packets

	ADI (mg/kg body weight)	Average amount (mg) in 12-oz. can of soda*	Number of cans of soda to reach ADI for a 100-pound person	Amount (mg) in a packet of sweetener	Number of packets to reach ADI for a 100-pound person
Acesulfame-K	15	40†	17	50	13
Aspartame	50	200	11	35	63
Saccharin	5	140	1.6	40	6
Sucralose	5	70	3.2	5	45

* This number represents an average; different brand names and fountain drinks may have different amounts of sweeteners.

† Based on the most common blend, with 90 mg aspartame.

Table adapted from *American Diabetes Association Guide to Medical Nutrition Therapy for Diabetes,* 1999.

The benefit of noncaloric sweeteners is that they can be used in foods and beverages without adding carbohydrate or calories, particularly advantageous in the case of sodas and soft drinks. Consider that 12 ounces of regularly sweetened soda contains about 155 calories and 40 grams of carbohydrate (the equivalent of 10 teaspoons of sugar). A soda with a noncaloric sweetener contains 0 calories and 0 grams of carbohydrate. Often the first step in improving glucose levels is to substitute diet drinks for regular sodas and soft drinks.

In baking, you can't substitute noncaloric sweeteners for sugar completely. Why? Because sugar provides bulk as well as sweetness in these recipes. In some recipes, you can add nutmeg, cinnamon, vanilla, or almond extract in place of some of the sugar. These flavorings give foods a sweet taste without adding sugar or calories.

CHAPTER 6

Heart-Healthy Eating

A strong link between diabetes and heart disease is now well established. People with diabetes are more likely to develop cardiovascular complications (problems with the heart and blood vessels) than people without the disease. These are the most common long-term problems that develop among those with diabetes. Further, women with diabetes have an even greater risk of heart disease compared with those of similar age who do not have diabetes. There are two reasons for the connection. First, high blood glucose levels damage blood vessels, making the walls thicker and less elastic so blood has a harder time passing through. Second, people with diabetes tend to have higher fat levels in their blood. Higher blood glucose can cause this. These fats, or lipids, clog and narrow the blood vessels, sometimes clogging them completely. These problems are referred to as *atherosclerosis*. Any blood vessel in your body can become narrow and clogged, and this can lead to a heart attack, angina (heart pain), stroke, or painful legs.

There's no certain way to avoid heart disease and circulation problems. But there are a number of things to do to cut your risk.

- Lose weight if you are overweight
- Get regular physical activity

- If you smoke, stop
- Keep your blood glucose under control
- Keep your blood pressure in the proper range
- Keep your blood fats and cholesterol levels in a healthy range

In this chapter we'll discuss the food-related ways you can minimize the risk of heart disease.

The types and amounts of fat you eat and your sodium (salt) consumption play a major role in the development of heart disease, stroke, and atherosclerosis. To reduce the risk of developing these problems, you and your healthcare providers should pay close attention to your lipid (blood fat) and blood pressure numbers.

Fat is high in calories, so eating less fat can help you control your weight. Fat packs a double punch of calories into every gram: a gram of fat contains nearly 9 calories, compared with only 4 calories for every gram of carbohydrate or protein. Extra pounds put a strain on your heart and also make your body's cells more resistant to insulin. Eating less fat, especially saturated fat, can help lower blood cholesterol and triglyceride levels. Changing the type of fat you eat can also help keep your heart and blood vessels healthy—which applies not just to people with diabetes, but everyone.

Lipids (Blood Fats)

Fat and cholesterol are often mentioned together, but they are not the same. Cholesterol is not a fat, but it does act together with fats in the body. Cholesterol is a waxy, fatlike substance made in your liver. Your body uses it to make bile and a number of hormones. If your body has too much cholesterol, it can be deposited on the walls of your arteries, a process probably related to inflammation in the artery wall, or "endothelium." This process results in the buildup of plaque, leading to blood vessel narrowing. Cholesterol and other substances are contained in the plaque. Plaques can rupture, exposing the cholesterol and other materials to the flowing blood, which then clots on the site of the rupture. This clot formation can cause a heart attack or stroke because blood can no longer travel freely forward through that vessel. To help reduce the buildup of these plaques, your total blood cholesterol should be *less than 200 mg/dl*.

More important than your total cholesterol, however, is the *type* of cholesterol made by your body—good and bad. LDL (which stands for *low-density lipoprotein*) cholesterol is considered "bad" because it can be deposited in the arteries. Your LDL cholesterol should be *less than 100 mg/dl*. If you already have heart disease or are otherwise deemed to be at high risk for it (if you have diabetes, for example), your healthcare provider may recommend that your LDL cholesterol be closer to 70 mg/dl. If your LDL level is above target, work with your dietitian on ways to reduce your saturated fat, trans fat, and cholesterol intake. In addition, your doctor may prescribe one or more medications to help lower your LDL level. If you do start on medication, remember that you must continue to limit your intake of harmful fats and cholesterol.

HDL *(high-density lipoprotein)* cholesterol, on the other hand, is considered "good" because it actually sweeps cholesterol from the arteries and carries it back to the liver, where it is reprocessed or eliminated. Ideally, men's HDL cholesterol should be above *40 mg/dl*, and women's above *50 mg/dl*. If your HDL level is below target, try the following suggestions to help increase it:

- If you smoke, stop.
- Aim to be physically active most days of the week, as exercise can raise HDL levels.
- Use monounsaturated fats, such as olive or canola oil, for cooking and for adding to foods.
- Lose weight if you need to.

While alcohol may actually help raise HDL levels, it's not a generally recommended treatment. However, if you do drink alcohol, be sure to limit your servings to two drinks per day (for men) or one per day (for women). Always discuss the use of alcohol with your healthcare provider.

People with diabetes also need to be concerned with blood levels of *triglycerides*, stored in fat cells as body fat and burned for energy. High levels of triglycerides are linked with an increased risk of heart and blood vessel disease. Your triglyceride level should be *150 mg/dl or lower*. Since high blood glucose levels due to insufficient insulin availability, as well as insulin resistance itself, can increase triglyceride levels, keeping your blood glucose levels as near normal as possible also improves your triglyceride levels. Further, shedding a few extra pounds and doing regular physical activity to help reduce insulin resistance can also be beneficial. Of course, limiting saturated fat intake also helps improve triglycerides.

Developing an eating pattern that reduces your risk of heart and blood vessel disease involves reducing your intake of some types of food fats and food cholesterol, and substituting and using healthy food fats. Reducing your intake of sodium, shedding a few pounds, and doing regular physical activity will also lower your blood pressure.

Food Fats

There are three types of food fat: *saturated fat, unsaturated fat* (both *polyunsaturated* and *monounsaturated*), and *trans fat*. Saturated fat is solid at room temperature. Foods that contain saturated fat include butter, shortening, fatty meats, whole milk, cheese, hydrogenated fats, and tropical oils. Saturated fats raise blood cholesterol levels by interfering with the entry of cholesterol into cells. This causes cholesterol to remain in the bloodstream longer and to become a part of the plaque that builds up in the blood vessels. *Trans fat* is a type of fat formed from *hydrogenation,* a chemical process that changes a liquid oil into a solid fat. The process involves adding hydrogen to the unsaturated liquid oil and changing it into a saturated solid fat. *Trans fats* are found in processed foods, such as snack foods, cookies, fast foods, and some stick or solid margarines. Both saturated fats and *trans fats* can raise cholesterol levels and should be eaten in as small amounts as possible.

Unsaturated fats come primarily from vegetables and are liquid at room temperature. Polyunsaturated fats, contained in safflower, corn, sunflower, and soybean oils and fish, can help lower cholesterol levels. Another important type of polyunsaturated fat is omega-3 fatty acids, found in fish, flaxseed, and walnuts. This kind of fat can help lower triglyceride levels and lower the risk of heart disease. Monounsaturated fats include olive, canola, and peanut oils, peanuts, olives, avocados, and nuts. Monounsaturated fats

also help lower blood cholesterol levels and may help raise HDL cholesterol levels.

Cholesterol, which acts like saturated fat in the body, can be manufactured in the liver or intestines but is also found exclusively in animal foods,
such as eggs, milk, cheese, liver, meat, and poultry. Because eating too much
may increase your blood cholesterol levels, the goal is to limit your intake to
no more than 300 mg per day. If your LDL cholesterol is higher than 100
mg/dl, you may benefit from lowering your cholesterol intake to less than
200 mg per day. However, saturated fat and trans fat actually raise your
blood cholesterol more than does cholesterol found in food. Therefore,
your first step in lowering your cholesterol level is to limit foods high in saturated fat and trans fat. And the good news is that when you lower your intake of saturated fat (which is typically found in animal foods), you usually
lower your intake of food cholesterol as well.

You may have noticed margarinelike spreads in the supermarket that
contain *plant stanol esters* or *plant sterol esters* and wondered whether they
were beneficial. Plant stanol and sterol esters block the absorption of cholesterol in the intestine. Plant stanols are made from substances in plants
that are combined with canola oil to form stanol esters, while plant sterols
are made from soy. The FDA studied their safety and their ability to lower
cholesterol extensively before they were allowed to be marketed, and they
were found to be equally effective in lowering cholesterol. Research shows
that eating about 2 grams (2 teaspoons) per day decreases total and LDL
cholesterol by about 10 percent. They are not a drug and can be used safely
in combination with cholesterol-lowering drugs such as statins. One orange juice producer adds plant sterols to its juice. However, keep in mind
that 8 ounces of orange juice contains approximately 30 grams of carbohydrate!

Remember that eating foods containing soluble fiber, though it's not
a fat, can also lower blood cholesterol levels, because it can bind cholesterol
in your intestines. Foods high in soluble fiber include oatmeal, oat bran,
dried beans and peas, some fruits and vegetables, barley, and psyllium. For
tips on increasing fiber in your diet, see Chapter 5.

Tips to Reduce Your Intake of Saturated Fat and Cholesterol

Eating less saturated fat and cholesterol may help treat and prevent high blood cholesterol and triglyceride levels. An eating plan low in saturated fat can even help you treat and prevent high blood pressure. Below are some tips that will help:

- Read Nutrition Facts labels and choose foods with no more than 1 gram of saturated fat per serving.

- Use nonfat or low-fat dairy products, such as skim or 1 percent low-fat milk, nonfat or low-fat yogurt, and lower-fat cheeses.

- Limit your protein portions at meals to 3 to 4 ounces. Most adults should limit total protein intake to about 6 oz. after cooking per day. Some women need only 4 to 5 oz. per day. People on meal plans of 2,000 calories or more may be able to have up to 8 oz. of protein per day.

- Choose leaner cuts of meats, such as beef and pork tenderloin. Look for luncheon meats with 3 grams or less of fat per ounce.

- Limit high-fat meat choices, including regular luncheon meats, other processed meats, frankfurters, sausage, bacon, and prime cuts of meat.

- Eat poultry without skin.

- Eat seafood, including fish and shellfish, often—at least two to three servings a week.

- Use olive, canola, and peanut oil for cooking instead of butter, lard, bacon fat, and solid shortenings.

- Limit fatty snack foods, such as cookies, chips, and some crackers.

- Use low-fat cooking methods such as baking, broiling, and roasting. When frying or sautéing foods, use a small amount of vegetable oil or a vegetable oil spray.

- Remove the fats from gravy and soup, using a fat separator (a small pitcher with a specially designed spout). Or refrigerate the food until the fat hardens. Remove the fat layer, reheat, and serve.

- Use plain nonfat yogurt (2 tbsp. contain fewer than 20 calories) instead of sour cream (2 tbsp. contain 50 calories) or mayonnaise (2 tbsp. contain 200 calories) as a condiment or in recipes for dips and salad dressings.

- Use a soft tub margarine or one made with a plant stanol or sterol ester instead of butter, but be careful with amounts. The number of calories in margarine and butter are the same, but because butter is primarily a saturated fat, margarine is recommended. Look for margarine that lists a liquid oil such as corn, safflower, canola, or soybean as the first ingredient. A soft or tub margarine is a better choice than solid or stick margarine. Better yet, look for a light (lower-fat and lower-calorie) tub margarine that is also free of *trans fat*.

- Check food labels for the terms *hydrogenated* or *partially hydrogenated fats*. If present in a food, these types of fat should be listed near the bottom of the ingredients, not near the top.

- Choose low-fat or fat-free salad dressings: 1 tablespoon of a low-fat or fat-free dressing generally has fewer than 20 calories and is considered a "free food"; 2 or 3 tablespoons make up one fat serving. One tablespoon of a regular dressing is one fat serving, which is 5 grams of fat and 45 calories.

- Many fat-free products, such as salad dressings and sour cream, contain carbohydrate. Check the nutrition label to determine whether your serving size should be counted as a carbohydrate serving.

Sodium

A lower-sodium eating plan is important for preventing and treating high blood pressure *(hypertension)*. Most of the sodium we eat comes from *sodium chloride* (table salt) added to processed foods or sprinkled on foods during preparation or eating. It also occurs naturally in a wide variety of foods—meats, dairy foods, and some vegetables.

Sodium is a mineral that is necessary for the proper functioning of several body processes, including regulating the fluid balance in your body and helping maintain blood pressure. Most Americans however eat far more sodium than they need. Research shows that sodium may contribute to some types of high blood pressure, a problem that many people with diabetes either have or are at greater risk of developing. In persons with either normal blood pressure or high blood pressure, reducing sodium intake lowers blood pressure. Because it is so important for people with diabetes to control blood pressure, daily intake of sodium should be limited to less than 2,400 milligrams (mg) per day—that's equal to about a teaspoon of salt. By doing this, you may reduce your chances of aggravating high blood pressure and the risk of heart and blood vessel disease.

Tips for Reducing Sodium

Obvious ways to reduce sodium intake are to eliminate the use of table salt at meals and use minimal amounts of salt in cooking. There are salt substitutes that taste like salt but have little or no sodium—some people find the taste bitter, so try using a smaller amount than usual and experiment with different brands to find one you like. Although salt substitutes may be fine to use, you will probably do better limiting them as well as salt. After a while, you will probably find you don't miss the taste. Some salt substitutes contain potassium chloride, and people with kidney disease need to be careful about using products containing this mineral. If you have kidney disease, check with your healthcare provider before using a salt substitute.

The Nutrition Facts panel on food labels lists the amount of sodium in one serving size in milligrams. By definition, a low-sodium food is one that contains no more than 140 mg of sodium per serving. However, a good rule of thumb is to look for foods with 400 mg or less of sodium per serving, and 800 mg or less of sodium per convenience dinner or entrée.

- Always taste your food before adding salt. Remove the saltshaker from the table.

- Eat fewer high-sodium smoked or cured meats, such as bacon, hot dogs, and cold cuts. Instead, choose chicken, sliced turkey, and lean roast beef.

- Rely less on canned, packaged, and convenience foods. Rinsing canned foods with fresh water for about 30 seconds reduces their sodium content by one half to three fourths.

- Cook with less salt. Try herbs, spices, lemon juice, garlic, onion, and vinegar to flavor food. Substitute onion and garlic powders for onion and garlic salts.

- Limit high-sodium foods such as dill pickles, sauerkraut, chips, canned soups, and sauces such as ketchup, soy sauce, and steak sauce.

- Switch to low-sodium snacks. Instead of salted potato chips, salted nuts, and crackers, eat raw vegetables, fruits, and lower-salt crackers and nuts.

- Limit fast foods, which tend to be higher in sodium than foods at sit-down restaurants.

Mediterranean-Type Diet

Perhaps you have been reading or hearing about the benefits of a *Mediterranean-type diet,* a moderate-fat diet low in saturated fat and cholesterol that also emphasizes controlling portion sizes to help in reducing overall calories. This eating plan encourages the use of olive oil (or other unsaturated fats) for salad dressings and for sautéing or stir-frying vegetables.

Nuts such as almonds, peanuts, and walnuts in moderate portions are included, along with generous servings of vegetables. More servings of fruits, grains, legumes, and low-fat and fat-free dairy products are recommended than animal-based foods. Fish and lean meats provide variety and enhance taste. A meal plan based on a Mediterranean-style diet may help you lower your risk of developing heart disease and high blood pressure.

So how do you put all this together with the information on carbohydrate counting discussed in Chapter 4 so as to design a meal plan that's right for you? As you work with your dietitian, the two of you can decide on the number of servings from the different food groups that will work for you. It will also be important for you to spread the carbohydrate servings throughout the day to better balance them with diabetes medications you may be taking and to help control your blood glucose levels.

Arriving at Your Destination

We have compared your meal plan to a map that can help guide you to your destination—control of your diabetes. When you use a map, there are often different routes you can take to help make your trip a success. The same is true with food and meal planning: there are different "routes" you can take to help you reach your goal. Carbohydrate counting is usually the starting point, but combining the principles of a Mediterranean-style diet with carbohydrate counting can also be a route. The bottom line is to decide with a dietitian or diabetes educator what is the best "route" for you.

CHAPTER 7

Dining Out

The old adage "You are what you eat" applies to everyone. But it takes on special meaning for people with diabetes. That's because what you eat and when you eat can have a dramatic effect on your blood glucose, lipid (blood fat) levels, and blood pressure—topics covered in the previous three chapters. As a result, food can also be an important factor in the prevention of long-term complications from diabetes.

Eating Out

One of the most enjoyable aspects of eating out has absolutely nothing to do with food. It's the pleasure of spending time with people important to you. By focusing on the social part of the dining-out experience, you will develop a healthier mind-set. Part of this mind-set is to adapt to the unexpected—food that isn't prepared right, slow service, or the temptation to eat foods you know you probably shouldn't. If the unexpected happens, your meal will still be enjoyable because you have already decided that the most important part of eating out is to enjoy the company of your friends and family. And people with diabetes can and should enjoy dining out just as much as people who don't have diabetes.

Eating out doesn't just mean going to a restaurant. It can mean a drive-up window at a fast-food restaurant, eating at a ball park, food courts, or during an after-work meeting. Or it can be food you purchase at a deli or restaurant and take home to eat, such as a chicken dinner, pizza, or Chinese food. Unfortunately, the foods that are available away from home are usually higher in total and saturated fat, cholesterol, sodium, and sugars. And whole grains, fruits, and vegetables are often not available.

Of course, eating good foods should still remain high on your list. Even though you are away from your own kitchen, you can still follow your eating plan. By adapting guidelines you've learned for managing your diabetes at home, you can develop a strategy for eating out. Here are a few tips that may help you enjoy both your food choices and your friends and family.

- **KNOW YOUR MEAL PLAN AND THE NUMBER OF CARBOHYDRATE SERVINGS OR GRAMS YOU HAVE AT MEALS.** When eating out, try to adhere to your meal plan as much as possible, especially your number of carbohydrate servings or grams.

- **CHOOSE A RESTAURANT CAREFULLY.** Look for restaurants that offer a wide selection of broiled and baked foods, especially fish and poultry. Avoid restaurants that offer only large portions of fatty meats and fried foods, like large prime steaks and fried chicken and fish. Call the restaurant ahead of time to ask about the menu, or search the Internet—many restaurants now post their menus online.

- **PLAN WHAT YOU WILL ORDER.** It's helpful if you are familiar with the menu offerings and can plan what you might order ahead of time. Try to be the first to order so you're not tempted to change your mind when you hear what your friends are ordering. Choose dishes that are grilled, baked, broiled, poached, steamed, roasted, or lightly sautéed. See Table 7-1, Healthy Choices for Dining Out, for other menu suggestions.

- **BE AWARE OF THE DANGERS OF "ALL YOU CAN EAT" RESTAURANTS.** You may think an all-you-can-eat buffet is a good option.

After all, you will be able to see the food, determine how it is prepared, and serve your own portions. If you have fantastic self-control, this strategy may work. But remember, these places are billed as "all you *can* eat," not "all you *should* eat." Too often, people are tempted to pile far too much food on their plates, especially if the food all looks so good that it's hard to resist. Salad bars pose a similar temptation. If you stick to fresh vegetables and low-calorie dressings, you'll do fine. But watch out for all the prepared salads, cheese, eggs, gelatins, and high-fat salad dressings.

- **ASK FOR SAUCES AND DRESSINGS ON THE SIDE.** By controlling how much salad dressing and gravy you use, you'll end up using less and reducing your fat and calorie intake.

- **EYEBALL THE PORTIONS.** Large portions are a fact of restaurant dining. Consider sharing an entrée with a companion. Practicing portion control at home (weighing and measuring your foods periodically) will help you control portions when you're away from home. And don't forget the system restaurants have long used to help you with portion control—the doggie bag! Ask your server to package half your meal in the kitchen before it's served to you.

- **SHARE AN ENTRÉE WITH YOUR DINING COMPANION OR ORDER OFF THE APPETIZER MENU (AS LONG AS THE CHOICES ARE HEALTHY).** Some restaurants offer half portions of entrées as well.

- **MAKE REQUESTS.** Restaurants are in the business to serve people and usually try to comply with reasonable requests made in a pleasant and nonthreatening manner.

- **LOOK UP NUTRITION INFORMATION FOR CHAIN AND FAST-FOOD RESTAURANTS BEFORE LEAVING HOME.** Many of these restaurants post their information on the Internet. In addition, many books are available that compile the information for you—ask your dietitian for a good reference at your next visit.

- **BE REALISTIC.** Accept the fact that nobody is perfect all the time. Whether you are eating at home or away, do the best you can. And if you have a momentary lapse, keep it a momentary lapse. Just pick up where you left off and continue your diabetes management with a positive outlook. If you've overeaten, don't feel guilty; instead, go for a walk or do some other physical activity after the meal that will help lower your blood glucose and burn off calories.

- **CONSIDER EATING A SMALL SNACK IF YOUR MEAL WILL BE LATER THAN USUAL.** If you prefer to take your diabetes pills before you leave for the restaurant, and you expect your meal to be later than usual, you may need to eat a small snack to "hold you over" and prevent the possibility of low blood glucose. Your healthcare team can give you guidance on the timing of your medications and your meals.

- **AND FINALLY, IF YOU ARE TAKING RAPID-ACTING INSULIN AT MEALS, LEARN HOW TO ADJUST YOUR DOSE TO APPROPRIATELY COVER THE CARBOHYDRATE YOU EAT.** You can use your insulin-to-carbohydrate ratio to make adjustments based on the number of carbohydrate servings you plan to eat. You can take your insulin (and diabetes pills) after you get to the restaurant or even, for the rapid insulins, when the food is being brought to the table, in case your meal is served late. Check your blood glucose more often whenever you eat meals at different times than you usually do.

Alcohol

Alcoholic beverages are a common part of many individuals' social lives. Each adult must decide, in conjunction with his or her healthcare team, whether or not to drink alcohol. When you make this decision, you should understand the potential effects of alcohol on your diabetes control. Perhaps you are someone who has routinely enjoyed having an occasional drink on social occasions or a glass of wine with dinner. Now that you have diabetes, you may wonder whether you should continue doing this.

Alcohol recommendations for adults with diabetes are similar to

TABLE 7-1 Healthy Choices for Dining Out

BREAKFAST: cereal with skim or 1% low-fat milk; whole-grain toast, bagels, or English muffins; omelets made with egg substitutes; pancakes or waffles with fruit; Canadian bacon

APPETIZERS: shrimp or crab cocktail; chicken teriyaki; raw vegetables; fresh fruit cup; bouillon or consommé; broth-based soups

FAST FOODS: regular-size burgers without cheese or sauces; grilled chicken sandwiches; small servings of fries; salads with low-calorie dressings

PIZZA: thin-crust pizza with vegetable toppings; cheeseless pizzas

DELIS: sandwiches made with turkey or chicken breast, lean roast beef, lean ham; vegetables, hummus; mustard instead of mayonnaise

MEXICAN: fajitas, burritos, or soft tacos with chicken or bean fillings; Mexican rice, black beans on the side; salsa, chopped vegetables

ITALIAN: minestrone, pasta fagioli soup; plain Italian bread; pasta with chicken or seafood in a vegetable marinara (tomato), or light wine sauce

CHINESE: wonton, hot-and-sour soup; stir-fried vegetables with meat, seafood, or poultry (not deep-fried); mu-shu dishes; vegetarian dishes; steamed vegetables and brown rice

AMERICAN: broiled, grilled, or stir-fried poultry, seafood, and lean meat dishes; baked potatoes, or brown or wild rice; steamed or lightly sautéed vegetables (without added butter)

those for the general public: men should limit alcoholic drinks to two or less per day, and women one or less per day. One drink contains about 15 grams of alcohol and is defined as

- 12 oz. of beer (preferably light)
- 5 oz. of wine
- 1½ oz. of distilled spirits ("hard liquor," such as scotch, whiskey, and vodka)

If you drink alcohol in moderation and with food, it will have minimal, if any, effect on your blood glucose or insulin levels. However, if you take insulin or certain diabetes pills, and if alcohol is consumed without food, it can cause low blood glucose reactions. Alcohol is absorbed directly from the stomach into the bloodstream and carried to the liver, where it is broken down (metabolized). While the liver is processing alcohol, its ability to release glucose is blocked. In essence, the liver is "distracted" from doing its regular job. This can cause blood glucose to drop, especially if no food is eaten, with the resultant risk, for up to 10 to 12 hours after drinking, of a low blood glucose reaction.

That's why you should follow your usual meal plan when drinking an alcoholic beverage, and no food should be omitted. Food in the stomach also slows down the absorption of alcohol into the bloodstream and lowers the amount of alcohol that reaches the liver at one time. The liver can perform better while processing smaller amounts of alcohol. In addition, if you drink alcohol in the evening, be sure to check your blood glucose before you go to sleep. You may need to eat a snack to prevent your blood glucose from dropping during the night. Also, be aware that if you exercise *and* drink alcohol (for example, having a few beers after playing a game of basketball), your risk of having a low blood glucose reaction later on increases. For this reason, it's important to monitor your blood glucose levels more often whenever you drink alcohol.

As a general guideline, two alcoholic beverages may be an occasional addition to your regular meal plan. No food should be omitted in exchange for an alcoholic drink. Because 12 ounces of regular beer contains about 15 grams of carbohydrate, a light beer may be a better choice. Some alcoholic beverages contain higher amounts of sugar, such as wine coolers and liqueurs. Use these sparingly as they may increase your blood glucose levels. Twelve ounces of nonalcoholic beer also contains about 15 grams of carbohydrate and should be counted as one carbohydrate choice in your meal. If you're trying to lose weight, remember that alcohol contributes calories even if it doesn't affect blood glucose. For example, a 12-ounce light beer, a 5-ounce glass of wine, and a 1½-ounce "shot" of hard liquor each contain about 100 calories. In fact, alcohol contains 7 calories per gram, almost as much as fat, at 9 calories per gram. Table 7-2, Alcoholic Beverages, lists the calories and grams of carbohydrate in common alcoholic drinks.

Some people with diabetes should not drink, including pregnant and lactating women, and people with medical problems such as pancreatitis, advanced neuropathy, and alcohol abuse. Incidentally, recent research has also shown that while moderate amounts of alcohol do not raise triglyceride levels, alcohol should be avoided if triglyceride levels are extremely high. Excessive amounts of alcohol may increase blood pressure and may also worsen retinopathy (diabetic eye disease). Finally, if you take metformin to help control your diabetes, do not drink large amounts of alcohol. This may increase your risk of developing lactic acidosis, a rare but serious metabolic complication.

While there may be beneficial effects from drinking small to moderate amounts of alcohol—for example, in adults with type 2 diabetes, one to two drinks per day is associated with decreased risk of heart disease and increased insulin sensitivity—the research is not strong enough to recommend that adults who don't drink now should start. Alcohol also appears to increase HDL (or "good") cholesterol, which has a protective effect against heart disease, but regular exercise can have the same potential benefit and, for many adults, will be more appropriate.

Guidelines for Alcohol

The message is always the same. Avoid large amounts of alcoholic beverages. But if you choose to have a drink now and then, the following guidelines can help you safely enjoy the occasion:

- Consume alcoholic beverages along with food. This is especially important if you use insulin or take diabetes pills. Signs and symptoms of low blood glucose and intoxication are similar, and your companions may just think you are a little "tipsy" rather than hypoglycemic. Make sure your friends know you have diabetes and know how to treat low blood glucose.

- For men, limit alcohol to 2 drinks or less per day, and for women, 1 drink or less per day. A drink is defined as a 12-ounce beer (preferably light beer), a 5-ounce glass of wine, or 1½ ounces of a distilled beverage, such as whiskey, rum, vodka, and gin.

- Limit alcohol if you are trying to lose weight. Even if it doesn't affect your blood glucose, alcohol can still contribute significant calories.

- Mix hard liquor such as gin, rum, whiskey, bourbon, scotch, and vodka with water or sugar-free beverages rather than juices, regular sodas, or regular tonic water.

- Check with your healthcare providers to see if you are taking medications that might interact with alcohol or if there are other reasons you should avoid alcoholic beverages.

- Drink safely and smartly. Carry or wear identification that states you have diabetes.

- Follow all precautions that are encouraged for all adults—drink in moderation, and don't drink and drive.

Holidays and Special Occasions

Holidays are special occasions for all of us, and on such occasions it is permissible to allow some flexibility with meal planning. Certainly for those counting carbohydrate, the adjustment of insulin doses to compensate for variations in carbohydrate intake will occur as part of the built-in dose selection process. However, even for those who do not make such adjustments, reasonable deviations from your meal plan on a few important days will certainly not drastically compromise your long-term health, provided that the next day you get back on track.

Vacations can also be difficult times, with variations in eating not focused on one day but over a week or more. While the excess seen on Thanksgiving or one's birthday is not recommended throughout a week's vacation, it is recognized that less-than-optimal consumption may occur. Try to limit the "excursions" from the meal plan to foods that are "worth it,"

TABLE 7-2 **Alcoholic Beverages**

Beverage	Amount (ounces)	Calories	Carbohydrate (grams)
Beer			
Regular beer	12	150	14
Light beer	12	100	5
Nonalcoholic beer	12	70	15
Distilled spirits			
Gin, rum, vodka, whiskey, scotch, bourbon	1.5	105	Trace
Wine			
Red or rosé	5	105	3
White	5	100	1
Sweet wine	2	90	7
Wine coolers	12	190	22
Champagne	4	100	4
Vermouth	3	105	4
Cocktails			
Gin and tonic	7.5	225	16
Martini	2.5	160	0
Daiquiri	4	220	2
Bloody Mary	5	115	5
Liqueurs/cordials	1.5	160	18

such as a special dinner, but keep on target then for breakfast and lunch. Certainly, when back home, making a concerted effort to get back on track immediately is crucial to restoring your ongoing nutritional control. Here are some other tips to help get you through the holidays and special occasions:

■   Plan ahead. Think about the types of foods that may be served at Thanksgiving dinner or a holiday party, and decide what you'll have before you start eating. If you want a piece of pumpkin pie, for example, determine how many grams of carb it has and substitute it for another carb food at your meal (or adjust your insulin dose accordingly). Offer to bring a dish to a party that you feel comfortable eating.

- Try to eat at your regular mealtimes as much as possible. If your meal is delayed, eat a small snack at your regular mealtime.

- If you're baking for the holidays, reduce the amount of sugar and fat the recipes call for.

- Check your blood glucose levels more often than usual to help you stay in better control.

- Avoid lingering at the buffet table at parties.

- Limit your intake of alcohol; if you do drink, be sure to eat some food with your cocktail.

- Be as active as possible! Rather than taking a nap after a huge holiday meal, go out for a walk. Regular activity is important any time of the year, but it's especially important on holidays and vacations.

- Create new traditions. Instead of baking twelve dozen cookies to give as holiday gifts, try your hand at making ornaments. Set a good example for your family and plan an annual skating party, or plan something active after a summer holiday cookout.

- Ask your dietitian for help—he or she can help you figure out how to fit favorite foods into your meal plan, how to determine how many carbs are in certain foods, and how to alter recipes to make them more healthful.

- Keep a record. Many people find it helpful to keep a food and activity record, especially during busy holidays. It's one way to help you evaluate your blood glucose levels in response to the different food and activity patterns that crop up at these times.

Now you're prepared to go out and have a wonderful time. Bon appétit!

CHAPTER 8

Losing Weight—
Gaining Control

Being overweight affects every system in your body—and not for the better. Carrying around extra pounds makes the heart work harder and less efficiently; you tire quickly and become short of breath. But most important for people who are at risk for or have type 2 diabetes, being overweight affects your body's ability to use insulin. That's why your healthcare providers may advise you to lose weight—to get your body as close to a good weight for you as possible.

The combination of a proper meal plan and a physical activity plan is the most effective way to lose weight. You may also need to change some of the behaviors that may be preventing you from shedding some unwanted pounds. Your healthcare team can help you develop a game plan based on sound medical principles for weight loss.

Why Lose Weight?

Many people who are at risk of developing or have type 2 diabetes are advised to lose weight. If this is you, your body produces insulin, but being overweight makes you resistant to its actions. However, research has shown that if your body is resistant to insulin, losing even a small amount of weight will help. The insulin your body produces will be more effective in allowing blood glucose to enter your cells, which results in lower blood glucose and more energy.

People who are at risk of developing diabetes benefit the most from losing modest amounts of weight. A large study called the Diabetes Prevention Program reported that individuals who on average reduced their weight by about 15 pounds delayed or prevented diabetes from developing by 58 percent compared with individuals in a control group who were told to lose weight but weren't successful. To be successful required an intensive lifestyle program emphasizing a low-fat, low-calorie eating plan and 150 minutes a week of physical activity with regular contact with "coaches" throughout the three years of the program.

Weight loss can also affect your use of insulin and diabetes pills. If you take medication to control your blood glucose, even small amounts of weight loss may decrease your need for diabetes medication significantly. If you take insulin, your insulin needs will probably change as you lose weight. Plan to check your blood glucose daily, then discuss the results with your healthcare providers. They will adjust your insulin dose or show you how to adjust it. Not doing so, and having low blood glucose reactions, would make it necessary to eat more, which would sabotage your efforts to lose weight! If you are losing weight and having low blood glucose reactions and are not sure what to do, ask your healthcare provider about an adjustment to your treatment.

There are other reasons to lose weight. Everyone can reduce the risk of heart and blood vessel disease by following a heart-healthy meal plan and getting plenty of physical activity. Losing weight also lowers blood pressure and may reduce the amount of blood pressure medication you need to take. If you have diabetes, you run a higher risk of developing heart and blood vessel problems and high blood pressure. That's why it's important to get on board with a healthy eating plan and regular physical activity. Additional health benefits are associated with weight loss: decreased back and knee pain, lower risk of some types of cancer, and decreased risk of gout and gallbladder disease. Weight loss can also improve your quality of life. You may not be as short of breath when climbing stairs, may be more able to keep up with your children or grandchildren, and may be able to enjoy travel again.

A Two-Part Equation

To lose weight you need to burn more calories than you eat. There are two basic ways to do this:

- Increase your activity—the reason for regular physical activity
- Cut back on your food intake—the reason for your eating plan

What's the best way to go about losing weight? You've probably seen ads and books for many fad diets, and while they may claim dramatic results, the reality is that the majority of them do not work in the long term. You may indeed be able to shed pounds quickly—but you'll probably gain them back just as quickly. Most weight-loss gimmicks are too extreme for people to follow long enough to achieve true fat loss. Often you very quickly lose a lot of body fluids, not body fat. Although the numbers on the scale look great, the body resists being dehydrated and quickly replaces the lost fluids.

A pound of body fat stores approximately 3,500 calories. This means that to lose a pound of body fat, you either have to eat 3,500 calories fewer than your body needs for energy; burn up, through physical activity, an extra 3,500 calories; or follow a combination of eating fewer calories and increasing physical activity. On average, most adults need about 2,000 calories a day for energy and to maintain their weight. Walking or running a mile burns about 100 calories, so to lose a pound of body fat you have to walk or run 35 miles. You can see that to truly lose body fat takes time and effort.

People have varying degrees of success in losing weight, but often the greater challenge lies in maintaining the weight loss. Research has shown that people lose weight on almost all plans or programs that reduce calories. Weight loss generally peaks at about six months, after which it tends to level off. At this point compensatory, internal mechanisms that protect against "starvation" take over, and if the weight-loss program stops, the lost weight is regained. What we eat, how many calories we expend, and body weight are all centrally regulated in our brain in an area known as the *hypothalamus*. When we cut back on food, a series of messages are sent to the brain telling it that the fat cells are becoming empty. Another series of messages leave the brain, signaling that it is time to eat. Thus, when you restrict food intake and increase physical activity, you also have to override a powerful biological system set up to protect you against weight loss. Part of this complex biological system of weight control involves hormones, including *leptin*, which is produced by your adipose, or fat, tissue. Leptin stimulates other chemicals in the body that control appetite and metabolism. *Ghrelin*, also a hormone, relays messages between your digestive system and your brain. It works to stimulate appetite, slow metabolism, and decrease your body's ability to burn fat. Some studies show that dieters who lose weight and try to maintain that weight loss actually make more ghrelin than they did before they dieted, which can partially explain why maintaining weight loss can be challenging. Researchers are currently exploring ways to target the effects of these hormones and other related substances with medication. This doesn't mean that you can't lose weight, but it does help explain why it takes so much effort to maintain the weight loss. Reducing calories also slows your body's metabolism—the rate at which you burn calories. That makes it even harder to lose and maintain weight loss. Women tend to have a slower metabolism than men—in part because women have less lean body mass than men. However, metabolism for both men and women decreases every decade that we age. One of the reasons you should plan to make physical activity an important part of your program is that it helps slow this decrease in metabolism. Research studies have provided support for the following important points:

- Individuals must have realistic expectations about weight-loss efforts. Intensive weight-loss programs have shown that within six months, individuals can lose on average about 7 percent to 10 percent of their starting weight. Some people lose more, and some less, but for most the loss will be about 15 to 20 pounds.

- At this point, if you go back to your usual eating habits and stop physical activity, lost weight is rapidly regained. However, by continuing to follow your eating plan and engaging in regular physical activity, you can maintain your new weight.

■   The good news is that even a weight loss that is small to moderate (5 percent to 7 percent of your starting weight) has major health benefits. Small amounts of weight loss lower blood pressure, improve blood fats, and help prevent or delay type 2 diabetes. If you have diabetes, a small amount of weight loss can also make your blood glucose easier to control.

Keep these three points in mind if you are beginning a weight-loss program. A healthy eating plan, combined with physical activity, can help you achieve and maintain a healthy weight.

Since one of the greatest challenges with any weight-loss plan is maintaining the loss, below are a few tips from the National Weight Control Registry, a national database containing information on a large number of people who have lost approximately 60 pounds and have sustained that weight loss for two years.

■   Eat breakfast every day.
■   Weigh yourself regularly.
■   Be active every day, ideally for 60 minutes.
■   Follow a low-fat eating plan, and eat healthy carbs.
■   Get support. People who joined a support group maintained their weight loss, those who didn't regained almost half the weight.

How to Determine a Healthy Weight: The Body Mass Index

A commonly used method to determine a healthy weight is to calculate your body mass index (BMI), which evaluates weight in relation to height. The actual calculation is obtained by dividing your weight in kilograms (kilograms = pounds divided by 2.2) by your height in meters (meters = inches multiplied by 0.0254) and then squaring that figure. Table 8-1 has already done the calculation for you to give you an approximate BMI. Find

TABLE 8-1 **Body Mass Index (BMI)**

Height	120	130	140	150	160	170	180	190	200	210	220	230	240	250
4'10"	25	27	29	31	34	36	38	40	42	44	46	48	50	52
5'	23	25	27	29	31	33	35	37	39	41	43	45	47	49
5'2"	22	24	26	27	29	31	33	35	37	38	40	42	44	46
5'4"	21	22	24	26	28	29	31	33	34	36	38	40	41	43
5'6"	19	21	23	24	25	27	29	31	32	34	36	37	39	40
5'8"	18	20	21	23	24	26	27	29	30	32	34	35	37	38
5'10"	17	19	20	22	23	24	26	27	29	30	32	33	35	36
6'	16	18	19	20	22	23	24	26	27	28	30	31	33	34
6'2"	15	17	18	19	21	22	23	24	26	27	28	30	31	32

(Weight)

☐ Underweight   ▨ Healthy weight   ▨ Overweight   ☐ Obese

Note: This chart is for adults 20 years of age or older.

TABLE 8-2 **Interpreting the BMI**

	BMI
Underweight	Less than 18.5
Normal weight	18.5 to 24.9
Overweight	25 to 29.9
Obesity	30 or greater

your height in feet and inches on the side, and your weight in pounds at the top. The number at which they intersect is your BMI.

Waist Circumference Method

Another method to determine a healthy weight is the *waist circumference method.* Too much body fat in the abdomen, when this is not in proportion to your total body fat, is considered a predictor of risk factors and conditions associated with obesity, such as heart disease. Men who would be considered at risk have a waist measurement greater than 40 inches. Women at risk have a waist measurement greater than 35 inches.

Talk to your healthcare provider to determine what your healthy weight should be based on weight goals that are realistic and achievable.

Food and Meal Planning— Half the Equation

If you have diabetes, your healthcare providers have probably advised you to follow a meal plan. A well-designed meal plan can be an ideal way to achieve and maintain both your target blood glucose goals and a healthy weight.

As you learn to modify your eating habits by checking your blood glucose levels and boosting your activity, you can gradually lose weight and achieve good blood glucose control. When you have diabetes, it is especially important to consult with a dietitian. In general, if you are trying to lose weight and maintain weight loss, your dietitian will devise a meal plan based on a simple concept: your total intake of calories should be less than what you now eat, assuming that what you now eat is maintaining your current weight. Your weight loss should be slow and steady. The goal is to lose about a half to one pound a week.

Mind over Matter

A big part of the weight battle is changing how you think about maintaining your weight. One way is to change the words you use:

- Rather than "losing weight," think of gaining the overall benefits that come from being physically active every day and eating fewer high-fat foods.
- Instead of feeling "deprived" of foods, think of enjoying more lower-calorie and low-fat foods.
- Rather than the word *diet*, use *healthy eating pattern* or *meal plan*.

You may also have to change some behaviors that are standing in your way to success. No one can lose weight for you, and it's important that you personally accept the responsibility for managing your weight program. It will be harder to follow a program if you shift the responsibility to other people or allow them to take it upon themselves. You should be directly involved in your food and meal planning decisions and in planning and preparing your meals and snacks. That doesn't mean your family has to stay completely out of the picture. In fact, it is essential that they provide support and help you with your new eating habits. So be sure to invite them to meetings with your healthcare providers when weight and eating plans are discussed.

Fat-Gram Counting

The three main nutrient groups—carbohydrate, protein, and fat—are all important sources of calories, but every gram of fat contains twice as many calories as carbohydrate and protein. If you are trying to lose and maintain weight, it is helpful to eat fewer calories from fat. (For ways to reduce fat, see Chapter 5.) You already know how to count carbohydrate servings (see Chapters 4 and 5), but for controlling calories, it is also important to be aware of fat grams. And there's another good reason to reduce food fat: recent studies have shown that a high-fat diet contributes to insulin resistance—even if you don't eat an excess number of calories.

One way to cut back on food fat is with a meal-planning technique called fat-gram counting. With this method, your dietitian looks at your individual needs and determines the total amount of fat grams that you should eat in a day. Table 8-3 gives an approximation. Try to keep your fat intake to no more than 30 percent of your total calories (the second column in Table 8-3), which is actually what's recommended for everyone. Your dietitian may recommend you follow a low-fat meal plan, which is the third column in Table 8-3. You can keep a daily record of your fat intake and use a fat-gram counter, a chart that lists the number of grams of fat in different foods, to choose foods that are lower in fat. You can also use the Nutrition Facts food label; it lists the total grams of fat in a serving size of the food.

TABLE 8-3	Daily Recommendations for Total Fat Intake	
Calories	Grams of Fat for a Lower-Fat Eating Plan	Grams of Fat for a Low-Fat Eating Plan
1,200	40	30
1,500	50	35
1,800	60	45
2,100	70	50
2,400	80	60

If you are at risk for developing diabetes, it is very important that you pay attention to the amount of fat you eat. If you have either type 2 or type 1 diabetes, combining carbohydrate and fat-gram counting can help you control both your blood glucose and weight. If you're interested in learning more about fat-gram counting, discuss it with your dietitian.

Making Healthier Food Choices

When you are careful about portion sizes and understand fat and calorie content, you can eat just about anything. But the following advice will help you make healthier food choices:

- Eat a total of five servings of fruits and vegetables every day. Include a variety of colors: green, red, orange, and yellow.

- Aim for at least six servings of unrefined or unprocessed starches like bread, cereal, and starchy vegetables daily. Starchy vegetables include peas, dried beans, and lentils, as well as potatoes. Try replacing white rice and white bread with brown rice and whole-grain bread. Read bread labels carefully and look for "whole grain" on the ingredients list—many breads that appear to be whole grain contain mostly refined white flour.

- Eat foods high in fiber, as fiber has bulk that makes you feel full. Fiber also helps lower your cholesterol. Good sources of fiber are whole grains, fruits, vegetables, and dried beans and legumes. For ways to increase the fiber content of your meals, see Chapter 5.

- Eat sugars, sweets, and desserts in moderation. These foods tend to be high in calories and fat and contain few vitamins and minerals. Often just a bite or two will satisfy your need for something sweet.

- Drink more fluids—water is the best choice, but sugar-free beverages are acceptable as well.

Figuring It Out

How many calories a day should you eat to lose weight? Your dietitian can help you determine that number. The answer will depend on your present weight, how active you are, and the medications you take.

Table 8-4, 1,200-Calorie Daily Menus, and Table 8-5, 1,500-Calorie Daily Menus, are two sample eating plans. The total calories in each are generally the daily amounts recommended for adults trying to lose weight—1,200 to 1,500 calories for women, and 1,500 to 1,800 calories for men. The first column shows a high-fat, low-fiber menu. The second column shows a menu that has the same calorie count but includes more low-fat, high-fiber foods. Compare the two menus and you'll quickly see the low-fat, high-fiber version is more balanced and filling—a model for healthy eating.

Facts About Snacks

You might be wondering whether you should include snacks in your eating plan. You should work with your dietitian to determine if, when, and how often to snack. For example, if you control your diabetes with lifestyle alone and prefer to eat just three meals a day, don't add snacks. If, however, you take insulin, and your meals are more than four to five hours apart, you may

TABLE 8-4   1,200-Calorie Daily Menus

High Fat, Low Fiber	Lower Fat, Higher Fiber *(Recommended)*
Breakfast	
1 boiled egg	1 boiled egg
1 slice bacon	1 slice Canadian bacon
1 slice white toast with 1 tsp. butter	1 slice whole-wheat toast with 1 tsp. trans-fat-free margarine
4 ounces orange juice	1 cup cantaloupe chunks
Lunch	
1 fast food hamburger	1 oat-bran pita bread
1 order small french fries	2 oz. turkey breast
	lettuce, tomato, mustard
	1 raw carrot, cut into sticks
	1 small apple
Snack	
½ cup fruit cocktail	6 oz. light yogurt
Supper	
2 oz. broiled pork chop	3 oz. broiled salmon
⅓ cup white rice	⅔ cup brown rice
½ cup corn	1 cup steamed broccoli
2 tsp. butter	1 tsp. olive oil

need to include snacks to prevent low blood glucose. Many people find that they become hungry more often when they're trying to lose weight, and prefer to eat snacks throughout the day. If you like to snack, the best are those that are high in fiber and low in fat and contain approximately 15 grams of carbohydrate per serving. Table 8-6 offers a list of snacks that can keep you on the path to a healthy weight.

TABLE 8-5   1,500-Calorie Daily Menus

High Fat, Low Fiber	Lower Fat, Higher Fiber (Recommended)
Breakfast	
8 oz. reduced-fat milk	8 oz. fat-free milk
1 bakery-style blueberry muffin	½ small banana
	½ cup bran flakes
	1 boiled egg
Lunch	
2 slices white bread	2 slices multigrain bread
2 oz. deli-style ham	3 oz. tuna, packed in water
1 oz. Swiss cheese	2 tsp. light mayonnaise
lettuce, tomato, mustard	lettuce, tomato
1 oz. potato chips	1 oz. baked chips
	6 oz. light yogurt
Snack	
1 medium pear	1 small orange
	2 tbsp. almonds
Supper	
3 oz. steak	4 oz. baked chicken breast
1 medium baked potato	1 medium baked potato
½ cup green beans	1 cup green beans
1 tsp. butter	1 tbsp. trans-fat-free margarine
	2 cups salad
	2 tbsp. light Italian dressing

TABLE 8-6   Lower-Calorie Snacks

The following snacks are equal to 15 grams of carbohydrate (1 carb choice) and contain about 60–80 calories per serving:

Starches

4–6 whole-wheat crackers
3 cups air-popped or low-fat
    microwave popcorn
2 rice/popcorn cakes
1 oz. baked potato chips
1 oz. baked tortilla chips
¾ oz. pretzels
½ English muffin
4 melba toast
3 2½-inch-square graham crackers
3 gingersnaps
5 vanilla wafers
2 fig bars
6 saltines
4–5 crispbreads
43 Goldfish crackers
1 granola bar
¾ cup unsweetened ready-to-eat cereal

Fruit

1¼ cup strawberries
1 small banana
12 cherries
1 small apple, orange, peach
1 kiwi
¼ cup dried fruit
17 grapes
½ cup unsweetened apple sauce
½ cup unsweetened canned fruit
1 frozen fruit juice bar
8 oz. tomato/vegetable juice

Milk

8 oz. fat-free or low-fat milk
6 oz. light yogurt
2 no-sugar-added fudgesicles
½ cup sugar-free pudding
1 packet no-sugar-added hot cocoa (mixed with water)

Protein Choices

The following foods contain about 5–8 grams of protein and 55–75 calories per serving. Low-fat items have no more than 3 grams of fat per serving.

1 oz. low-fat cheese
¼ cup 1 percent milk-fat cottage cheese

continued on next page

TABLE 8-6   Lower-Calorie Snacks *(continued)*

¼ cup low-fat ricotta cheese
¼ cup canned tuna, packed in water
1 hard-boiled egg
1 tbsp. peanut butter
1 oz. low-fat luncheon meat

Fat Choices

The following foods contain about 5 grams of fat and 45 calories per serving.

10 peanuts
6 almonds
4 walnut halves
1 tbsp. sunflower seeds
10 green olives
⅛ avocado

Healthy Food Tips

The following strategies can help you stick to a meal plan and lose weight:

- **MONITOR PORTION SIZES.** Since the amount of food you eat is critical to weight loss, it's a good idea to weigh and measure your food. Keep a food scale, a calculator, and measuring cups and spoons in a handy spot in your kitchen. When eating away from home, remember that most restaurant portions are large. Practice "eyeballing" your food at home to so you can gauge restaurant portions and avoid overeating. Estimating a serving size can be challenging—the following tips can help you size up your meal:
  - **A ONE-CUP SERVING OF CARBOHYDRATE,** which includes fruit, vegetables, pasta, and rice, is about the size of your fist.
  - **ONE THREE-OUNCE SERVING OF MEAT, FISH, OR POULTRY** is about the size of a deck of playing cards or the palm of your hand.

- **A ONE-OUNCE SERVING OF CHEESE** is equal to the size of your thumb.

- **EAT AT EVERY MEAL AND PLANNED SNACK TIME.** Never skip a meal. Though this is a common weight-loss ploy, it can have a negative effect on your blood glucose. If you don't eat a meal and your insulin or oral medications are still active, your blood glucose may drop too low and you will have to eat more to bring it back up. Above all, be sure to eat breakfast. Research studies have shown that people who eat breakfast do better in controlling food intake during the rest of the day.

- **USE REMINDERS.** These notes can keep you true to your eating plan. Place them in a conspicuous spot—on the refrigerator door or the bathroom mirror. Always write a positive message. Instead of "Stay out of the refrigerator after work," write "Snack on the carrot sticks in the crisper drawer." Notice that the message is quite specific. It steers you directly to the proper snack without giving you the chance to think about other options.

- **BREAK THE CHAIN OF EVENTS THAT LEADS TO OVEREATING.** Lifestyle patterns that cause you to overeat often have nothing to do with food. For example, heavy traffic may lead to stress, causing you to stop at an ice cream parlor and overeat. This chain could be broken by taking an alternative route home to avoid the heavy traffic *and* the ice cream parlor.

- **BREAK HABITS ASSOCIATED WITH OVEREATING.** You may have developed behaviors that automatically lead to overeating. If watching TV prompts you to snack, confine eating to areas away from the TV. If you tend to eat very quickly—faster than the time your body needs to signal that you are satisfied—put the utensils down between bites. Or pace your meal by serving salad as a first course.

- **FIND ACTIVITIES TO DEAL WITH THE EMOTIONS THAT CAN LEAD TO OVEREATING.** Do you use food as a "comforter" when sad? As an "entertainer" when bored? As a "distracter" when under stress? Try to substitute some activity for eating at these times. Run errands when feeling restless, read a light novel when under stress, or telephone a friend when feeling lonely.

- **ASK FOR THE SUPPORT OF FAMILY AND FRIENDS.** If you tend to eat when preparing foods, perhaps others can help with the cooking. Or ask someone to encourage you with your weight-loss program. In sharing your goals with a friend, your commitment may rise dramatically.

- **PLAN OBSTACLES TO UNHEALTHY EATING.** Make it hard to eat what you shouldn't. Place high-fat foods purchased by other family members in hard-to-reach places—at the back of a lower shelf of the refrigerator, or at the top of the kitchen cabinets, reachable only with a step stool. Or put foods in containers you can't see through. Better yet, keep tempting sweets and high-fat foods out of your home entirely.

- **PLAN AIDS TO HEALTHY EATING.** Make it easy to eat what you should. Instead of "grazing" through the kitchen when you get home from work, have a lettuce salad or precut vegetables ready. Leave fresh fruit in plain sight, or carry an apple with you for the trip home. In essence, create your own low-fat environment.

- **KEEP A FOOD RECORD.** Each time you eat, record it in a notebook or diary, and at the end of the day, add up the total calories you have consumed. You'll get a psychological boost from seeing how well you are sticking to a meal plan that is helping you both to control your diabetes and to lose weight.

Low-Carbohydrate Diets and Diabetes

Most people who have tried to lose weight know what a struggle it can be. It's only natural to be tempted to try some of the latest diets that promise quick results. Many of these diets promote a lower- or low-carbohydrate intake along with a higher protein intake. These diets recommend replacing carbohydrate foods, such as bread, pasta, fruit, and milk, with protein and fat. The proponents of these plans claim that eating carbohydrates results in excess insulin production, which, in turn, causes calories to be stored as fat. Therefore, they argue, by limiting carbohydrate intake, less insulin is produced and more fat calories will be burned. Some of these low-carb, high-protein plans allow essentially unlimited intakes of protein and fat, claiming that only calories from carbs "count." Remember, though, that *all* calories count, not just carbohydrate calories.

Low-carb, high-protein eating plans *do* work—people who follow these diets lose weight and often report less hunger and fewer cravings. But while these diets do seem to work in the short term, the concern is that following them over the long term may result in adverse health effects, such as heart disease, some types of cancer, osteoporosis, gout, and kidney damage. Another important issue surrounding any type of "fad" diet is that most people can only follow them for a short time without getting tired of them. While a daily breakfast of eggs and bacon sounds delicious initially, down the road you'll probably get tired of it and start to crave cereal and fruit. Remember that your eating plan should be a way of life, not something that you follow for a few weeks or months. In addition, eating plans such as the low-carb, high-protein diet are deficient in important nutrients such as vitamins, minerals, and fiber—you can't meet your nutrient requirements by eating only foods that contain protein and fat.

The American Diabetes Association does not recommend that people with diabetes follow low-carb eating plans, but if you truly feel you'd like to try such a diet, discuss it first with your healthcare team. It's often possible to modify low-carb and other "fad" diets to make them safer and more healthful for you.

Physical Activity—The Other Half of the Equation

Physical activity is also important for managing diabetes. Physical activity can increase your body's sensitivity to insulin, and if you are trying to lose weight, physical activity can help you burn excess calories. But to develop healthy thinking about activity, you should first squelch a few myths. For example, "no pain, no gain" implies that for activity to be effective, you must endure pain. This simply isn't true. Your physical activity program should make you feel good, not uncomfortable.

Another myth is that all the activity has to be done at one time. Again, this isn't true. To become fit, you need to accumulate 30 minutes of physical activity nearly every day of the week. You don't have to go to a gym or buy an exercise bike: all physical activities count—from dancing and washing the car to vacuuming the house and raking leaves. However, for physical activity to contribute to weight maintenance, you need to increase the 30 minutes to 60 minutes. The important message here is to start with 5 to 10 minutes and gradually work up to 30 minutes. When you achieve that goal, work on gradually increasing activities to 60 minutes nearly every day of the week.

A third myth is that exercise alone will lead to weight loss. Studies have repeatedly shown that just being more physically active has at most a very small effect on weight loss. This finding is not unexpected, given that approximately 70 miles of walking is required to burn about five pounds of fat. To lose weight, you must cut back on calories consumed. What physical activity does do, however, is to contribute significantly to the *maintenance* of weight loss. Increased physical activity also decreases the risk of heart and vessel disease and death from cardiovascular disease, even in the absence of weight loss. What all of the research findings indicate is that physical activity should be increased to improve health, regardless of its impact on weight. Chapters 9 and 10 discuss how to incorporate physical activity and exercise programs into your diabetes management program.

Burning Calories with Activity

The total amount of calories you can burn with physical activity depends on your weight and on how long and hard you exercise. Table 8-7 gives you an idea of how many calories you can burn with various activities.

However, you also burn extra calories simply by adopting a more active lifestyle. Here are some ways to put more activity into your day:

TABLE 8-7　Calories Expended per Hour of Physical Activity

Activities	Calories per Hour*
Sitting quietly	80
Standing quietly	95
Light activity	240
Office work	
Cleaning house	
Playing golf	
Moderate activity	370
Walking briskly (3.5 miles per hour)	
Gardening	
Bicycling (5.5 miles per hour)	
Strenuous activity	580
Jogging (9 minutes per mile)	
Swimming	
Very strenuous activity	740
Running (7 minutes per mile)	
Racquetball	
Skiing	

* This chart is based on calories burned by a healthy 140-pound person. If you weigh more than 140 pounds, you will probably burn more calories per hour. If you weigh less, you will probably burn fewer calories per hour.

- **Do errands on foot.** Walk to the grocery store or post office.
- **Walk the dog.** Your "best friend" can be a valuable exercise partner.
- **Rely less on mechanical devices.** Use a push lawnmower rather than riding. Also, rely less on other people; deliver your own messages at work.
- **Use the worst parking spaces.** Park your car at the far end of the shopping mall; use the lot farthest from your office or work.
- **Use the stairs.** Stair climbing is a top-notch calorie burner.
- **Redefine housework and yard work.** Rather than thinking of these

as dreary chores, consider them a chance to burn calories. Vacuuming and raking never looked so good!

Physical Activity Tips

Before you begin a program of physical activity, set realistic goals for yourself. But keep setting new goals as you achieve the previous ones. To keep making progress, try the following:

- **MAKE A COMMITMENT AND KEEP IT.** Make the commitment to physical activity just as you would any other important appointment. Physical activity will soon become a habit.

- **GET A PEDOMETER.** This is a small counter that keeps track of how many steps you take. Wear it every day. Start by trying to add an extra 2,000 steps per day. The goal is to eventually accumulate 10,000 steps per day.

- **GET A TRAINING PARTNER.** We all have days when we are tempted to skip our workout. A partner helps you stay on schedule.

- **DO DIFFERENT TYPES OF ACTIVITIES.** Doing the same thing every time can become boring. Alternate the type of activities you do. You might ride a bicycle one day, walk the next, and swim another day.

- **REWARD YOURSELF.** Reward yourself with a small treat when you reach a goal—a new book or CD or a new pair of sneakers. Every extra activity counts toward a healthy lifestyle.

Commitment Matters

Knowing you should lose weight is a good start on the road to better health. The next step is commitment—deciding on a course of action and sticking to it until you reach your goal. But the most important step is understanding yourself. By understanding yourself, you can develop the "healthy thinking" that is important to a successful lifestyle program. Here are some key elements in that thinking:

Recognize your importance. Everyone makes a contribution to society, whether large or small. You are important to your family, your friends, your employer, your community—and most importantly to yourself. In managing your weight, do it for those who care about you. But most of all, do it for yourself!

Take control. Perhaps you have allowed your family to set your schedule, leaving little time for physical activity. They need to know that for the sake of your well-being, things will have to change. Life's pressures can also take a toll on your time—work schedules, community activities, and other obligations. You should identify and take control of these pressures rather than letting them control you.

Be objective and realistic. No one is asking you to run a marathon or lose 50 pounds in a week or even a year. Instead, set reasonable goals. Walk four blocks a day during the first week of your activity program—or as many as you feel comfortable walking.

Stress the positive. Look for positive ways to keep your commitment high. For example, *accept life's flaws.* Rather than abandoning your activity plan because you didn't exercise for three days in a row, learn from your failings and continue your program with confidence. *See things as they really are:* a single setback should not doom your activity program. Again, keep your eyes on your long-term goal. Rather than thinking that physical activities take too much of your time, see it as time to yourself that will make you look better, feel better, and get greater enjoyment out of your life.

The Solution of the Two-Part Equation

Research shows that despite some people's best efforts, they will not be successful at losing much weight. The good news is that you can still improve your blood glucose levels and decrease your risks for complications by being more physically active, following your eating plan, taking your medications consistently, and checking your blood glucose frequently to keep track of your results and make adjustments as needed. That, after all, is what it's all about—becoming healthier, not just focusing on your weight. It's been said before, but because it is so important, here again is a checklist to help you stay true to your goals:

- **Consult your healthcare providers.** They can help you set overall realistic lifestyle goals and provide support and guidance to help you achieve them.

- **Establish an eating plan.** Your dietitian can help. And remember, this is your blueprint for a lifetime of healthy eating. Above all, watch portion size: use measuring cups, spoons, and scales or visualize the correct sizes.

- **Set realistic goals.** Set goals you can control and meet. Write them down in a notebook. Include weekly activity goals or goals for high-fiber foods to add to your eating pattern and high-fat foods to resist. Avoid goals like "I will lose two pounds this week." You can't necessarily control that, given the many factors that influence weight from day to day. Instead, choose something like "I will calculate the total calories I eat each day."

- **Keep a food and blood glucose chart.** A spiral notebook will do. Keep track of what you eat each day, along with your blood glucose checks. It's a good idea to plan a weekly weigh-in and record your weight. Plot your weight each week on a simple chart. Be sure to contact your healthcare providers if your blood glucose levels are getting lower and a medication adjustment is needed.

- **Establish an activity plan.** A good way to begin is to walk 5 to 10 minutes each day. Build up to 30 minutes of activities that you enjoy.

- **Get support.** Enlist the support of family and friends. It's great to have encouragement!

CHAPTER 9

Physical Activity and Fitness Basics

Your body is made for movement—arms that bend, legs that run, and a heart that beats every second of the day. It only makes sense that if you are designed for movement, it's good practice to move regularly! Indeed, physical activity is good for everyone. It helps tone and strengthen muscles. It also gives your heart and lungs a workout, helping them be more efficient both at rest and during physical activities. As your fitness improves, your body can transport oxygen more efficiently, which increases your stamina and endurance. You will have more energy for greater productivity at work and reserve energy for the leisure-time activities you enjoy each day. The information in the next few pages will discuss the basics of physical activity and fitness for people with type 1 and type 2 diabetes. Chapter 10 will cover additional information specifically for people with type 1 diabetes.

The Effect of Physical Activity on Blood Glucose

Being physically active involves using muscles, particularly the large skeletal muscles of your arms and legs. Insulin plays a key role when you exercise because it enables the body's cells to use blood glucose for energy. Besides insulin, other hormones, such as glucagon, are involved in balancing glucose levels during exercise. These hormones tell the liver to release more or less glucose, as needed, for fuel. They also trigger the breakdown of fat stores into a form of fuel called *free fatty acids.*

Muscles generally use these two fuels—glucose and free fatty acids—to get the energy they need to work. Here's how the body normally burns fuel during exercise:

Phase 1.   During the first short bursts of activity, the muscles use their own stored glucose *(glycogen)* first.

Phase 2.   As you continue to exercise, the body uses glucose that is stored in the liver *(glycogen);* this glucose is transported through the bloodstream to the muscles for fuel. This replenishes blood glucose.

Phase 3.   After 15 to 20 minutes, the body begins to burn more fat stores for energy. Although glucose is still being used, it is no longer the primary source of fuel. Now free fatty acids are the preferred fuel for energy.

The change in balance among glucose, fat, insulin, and other hormones during physical activity affects blood glucose levels. Understanding how blood glucose levels can change with physical activity or exercise will help you live safely with an active lifestyle.

Why Physical Activity Is Important for Your Health

It is clear that physical activity is important for everyone's health, but why is it especially important if you have diabetes? One reason is its helpful effect on blood glucose levels. Physical activity lowers blood glucose levels by improving the body's ability to use both glucose and insulin. It does this by activating cell glucose transporters that allow the entry of glucose into cells. Physical activity also helps reverse the resistance to insulin that is often a result of being inactive or overweight. People who take diabetes pills often find they need less medication as they perform regular physical activity. The same is true for people who take insulin; the dose may need to be adjusted to prevent low blood glucose.

Physical activity improves your fitness, whether or not you have diabetes, and being fit decreases your risk of all chronic diseases, especially heart disease. In a very encouraging study, researchers from the Cooper Institute in Texas followed over 21,000 men for an average of eight years. Before the study began, the amount of body fat and level of physical fitness were measured for each participant. Fitness was measured by determining how long the subjects could exercise comfortably on a treadmill. The researchers discovered that regardless of the amount of their body fat, men who were physically fit dramatically decreased their risk of all chronic diseases. The men who were fit, even if they had the most fat, had the same lower risk of having a chronic disease as those who were fit and had the least amount of fat. And men who were fit but had the most fat had a much lower risk than men with the least amount of fat who were unfit. They did the same study with women, and found exactly the same thing. In the first study, they separated out the men with diabetes and found that just as in men in general, men with diabetes who were fit dramatically decreased their risk of coronary heart disease and death from all chronic disease, regardless of their body fatness. These studies support the importance of physical activity and fitness not only to improve weight control but also to decrease the risk of heart disease and other chronic diseases, regardless of body weight. Many studies confirm that physical activity improves blood pressure, strengthens the heart, and lowers risk factors for heart disease. The good news is that the same types of physical activities that improve the body's insulin resistance also decrease these other health risks. In addition to improving mild to moderate high blood pressure, physical activity has a positive effect on blood fats. It helps lower LDL ("bad") cholesterol, which forms plaque that obstructs blood vessels, lowers triglyceride levels, and raises HDL ("good") cholesterol, which protects against heart disease.

Physical activity helps you control your weight and tone your muscles. Although physical activity without changes in eating habits rarely leads to weight loss, it is essential for *maintaining* weight loss. And people who engage in regular physical activity do not generally regain the weight they lost. Also, physical activity during weight loss helps ensure that the weight lost is fat, and not lean body tissue such as muscle, or "water weight," which often occurs from dieting alone.

Regular physical activity also helps *prevent* type 2 diabetes. Accumulating 30 minutes of activity such as walking, biking, or swimming nearly every day of the week, or a total of 150 minutes in a week, has repeatedly been shown to prevent or delay the onset of type 2 diabetes. If you know anyone at risk for diabetes—people who have a family history of diabetes, are overweight, or have problems with blood fats or blood pressure—encourage them to make regular physical activity a high priority.

Physical activity is also a means of dealing with life's everyday stresses. It aids in relieving depression and building self-confidence. Teamed with a healthy eating plan, regular physical activity helps boost energy levels and helps you be more relaxed and feel less fatigued. The result is that you look better, feel better, and have a strategy to keep your diabetes in better control.

Strength Training

Research has shown that everyone, old and young, benefits immensely from activity. In fact, as we age we actually benefit more from regular physical activities. A decrease in skeletal muscle and an increase in body fatness is the primary change in body composition that accompanies aging. Muscle loss and weakness often limits the activities of daily living for many older individuals. Strength training is therefore of importance—any device that provides resistance and stresses muscles can be used. Small hand weights are inexpensive and are available at stores that supply exercise equipment. Many people use specially made large rubber bands for resistance training. Simple weight-lifting devices include Velcro-strapped wrist and ankle bags filled with sand; heavy household objects, such as plastic milk jugs filled with water or gravel; and food cans of various sizes. Benefits of strength training include increased muscle strength and size, improved bone health, increased energy requirements, and increased ability to participate in physical activity.

Creating Your Physical Activity Program

What makes a good activity program? There is no single program that is right for every person with diabetes. You need to develop a program based on your lifestyle, interests, and physical abilities. Ask your doctor or health-care provider if a specialist such as a *clinical exercise physiologist* or a *physical therapist* is part of your diabetes team, or if he or she can refer you to an exercise specialist. Exercise physiologists and physical therapists have clinical training to know how the body responds to exercise. If an exercise specialist is not available, your doctor or another member of your diabetes team can help you get started. Together, you can create a program that fits your lifestyle and medical needs.

Begin by choosing an activity that fits your fitness level and interest, one that you can do on a regular basis and enjoy. Walking, running, bicycling, tennis, cross-country skiing, dancing, stationary cycling, swimming and water exercise, chair exercises, tai chi, and yoga are good activities. There are also common activities (often called "activities of daily living") that contribute to overall physical fitness. Taking stairs instead of an elevator, parking farther from work, getting off the bus a stop earlier, and gardening are all activities that contribute to fitness.

How Often? How Long? How Hard?

To help you get started, there are some very general guidelines for physical activity. But your guidelines will be based on your personal goals and making small improvements over what you are currently doing. The recommendations also vary slightly depending on whether your priority is to improve your blood glucose control or to control your weight or both.

How Often?

Be physically active as often as possible. If your goal is for improved blood glucose control, aim for three to four times a week. If your goal is for weight loss, aim for four to five times a week.

How Long?

Start with smaller amounts of time at the beginning. Even 5 to 10 minutes can work. Then add a few minutes each week until you reach your goals. For improved blood glucose control, build up to 20 to 30 minutes per session. For weight loss, building up to 45 to 60 minutes a session is even better.

If you can't get all of your exercise in at one time, you can break it into smaller sessions. For example, if you want to spend 40 minutes exercising but just don't have that amount of time all at once, try 20 minutes earlier in the day and 20 minutes later. While this method may take you longer to reach your goals, it is better than not being able to reach them at all!

How Hard?

You should always feel comfortable while doing physical activities. Aim for a workload or pace you can handle—one that is not too hard but not too easy. The "talk test" can be your guide. You should always be able to talk while exercising; if you can't, you are working too hard. On the other hand, if you can sing, you may not be working hard enough. But regardless, if you do not feel well or feel pain—stop!

Allow time to warm up and cool down. The best way to warm up muscles is to start doing your activity slowly and at a low intensity for about five minutes. Then increase the intensity of your exercise. Cool down by ending your session with five minutes of slower exercise. This gives your heart a chance to adjust. Avoid stretching at the beginning of your exercise session as you may pull or strain a muscle. Instead, do some gentle stretching after your muscles have been warmed up.

The best time to do activities is the time that best fits in your schedule! It will help if you schedule your exercise just like you would any other appointment on your calendar. Plan to drive to the health club instead of letting yourself drive past it. Plan ahead to take a walk so that it gets done. With a little planning, you will be sure to fit exercise into your life.

Starting Safely

Before starting a program of physical activity, talk with your healthcare provider. You may need medical evaluations for your heart, eyes, feet, or blood pressure. This is important if you are over 35 years old or have had diabetes for 20 years or more. You may need more information as to what is safe and what is *not* safe for you to do. Your healthcare provider can help you design your physical activity plan and make sure your diabetes does not stop you from doing it! The following guidelines can help you get off to a safe start.

- Start your physical activity program gradually and set realistic goals. One of the reasons people often stop exercising is that they do too much too soon. Your body needs time to adapt to new activities, and you need time to adapt to fitting exercise into your schedule.

- Wear a medical identification bracelet or carry another form of identification that says you have diabetes. The identification should include your name, address, phone number, healthcare provider's name and phone number, type and dose of insulin (if you take insulin), and other medications you use. This will let other people know how to assist you if you get into difficulty.

- Check the safety of your equipment—whether it is your bicycle, treadmill, or *even your shoes*. Start with a good fit for your walking shoes. Watch the laces and double tie them if necessary. Small pebbles or other foreign objects in your sneakers can cause blisters or other foot problems. You should also wear socks made of material that wicks moisture away from the skin, and without seams or binding elastics.

- Carry a blood glucose meter with you if you're planning a long period of activity, especially if you are taking diabetes medication that puts you at risk for having your blood glucose level drop too low. These medications include:

Insulin (any kind)
Glyburide (DiaBeta, Micronase, Glynase)
Glipizide (Glucotrol)
Glipizide "GITS" (Glucotrol XL)
Glimepiride (Amaryl)
Repaglinide (Prandin)
Nateglinide (Starlix)
Metformin and glyburide (Glucovance)
Metformin and glipizide (Metaglip)
Exenatide (Byetta)
Pramlintide (Symlin)

When taken alone, some medicines are less likely to cause low blood glucose as a side effect. But be aware that many people need to take more than one type of diabetes medication. The following medications are not as likely to place you at risk for low blood glucose:

Metformin (Glucophage, Glucophage XR)
Pioglitazone (Actos)
Acarbose (Precose)
Rosiglitazone (Avandia)
Miglitol (Glycet)

And, of course, if you are not taking any diabetes medications but controlling your diabetes only by modifying your lifestyle, you are not likely to have a low blood glucose level.

Sometimes low blood glucose occurs during physical activity, despite your best efforts. Always be prepared to treat such a situation by carrying some form of carbohydrate, such as packets of granulated sugar, glucose tablets, cake icing, or LifeSavers. If your activities involve other people, tell them about the risk of low blood glucose and what they should do to help.

■ If possible, exercise with someone else, such as a family member or friend. Not only can a friend help you in case your blood sugar goes low, he or she can keep you motivated, especially when you don't feel like exercising. If you do exercise alone, always tell someone where you'll be going—the route you'll be walking or biking or the gym where you'll be exercising.

■ Drink plenty of water or other noncaffeinated, nonsugared beverages before starting. This is especially important in warm weather and if you plan to exercise for an extended period of time.

Risks for High and Low Blood Glucose

Your healthcare providers will also help you determine if you are at risk for high or low blood glucose during physical activity and how to prevent it. Generally, this is more of a problem for people who have type 1 diabetes, but people with type 2 diabetes who take insulin or any of the diabetes pills listed in the first group above may also be at risk. If you take insulin and are concerned about low blood glucose during physical activity, the risks, prevention, and treatment are discussed in more detail in Chapter 10. It is a good idea for everyone to be aware of the risks, but, more importantly, to know what to do if your blood glucose is high or low during or after exercise. Checking your blood glucose is the *only* way to know the effect of physical activity on your blood glucose.

High Blood Glucose

If you check your blood glucose around the time that you are doing physical activity, you may have some higher values than you are used to seeing. Sometimes this is just because you are checking your blood glucose at a different time of the day than you usually do. The result could still be influenced by the food you have eaten or the way your medications are working. Maybe the results you'll get are the usual blood glucose results for you. Either way, keep track of this information and talk to your healthcare team about what is happening.

Usually you will see blood glucose levels drop with physical activity. So if you start with a reading that is higher, be assured that when you check it again at the end of your activity, you should see a lower blood glucose.

This change depends on how much you did and how hard you did it. If you don't see a drop, or in some cases see a slight increase in your number, don't be discouraged. The work you did still counts, and continued exercise will help your body use insulin better over time.

If you have type 2 diabetes and your blood glucose is over 400 mg/dl, you should not exercise and should contact your diabetes team. If you have type 1 diabetes, more specific information is provided in Chapter 10.

Low Blood Glucose

Hypoglycemia, low blood glucose, is a concern if you are taking insulin or any of the diabetes pills listed earlier in this chapter, that can cause blood glucose to drop too low. If you take insulin, your blood glucose reading when you finish your physical activity should be above 110 mg/dl. If you use any of the diabetes pills that can drop your blood glucose level, your reading when you finish your physical activity should be above 90 mg/dl. However, if your readings are lower, you may be able to prevent these lows from occurring by:

- exercising after a meal
- eating an extra snack before you exercise (see the list of options)
- talking to your healthcare provider about the possibilities of making a change in medications

As things change with your diabetes, you may also have to change some of the activities that are part of your daily routine. Make sure you always know how your diabetes medications work and if you need to plan to prevent low blood glucose from occurring.

Snacks (15 Carbs)

Each of the foods in this list contain about 15 grams of carbohydrate and 60 to 80 calories per serving. Items marked with one asterisk (*) have one serving of fat; items marked with two asterisks (**) have two.

Bread (1 1-oz. slice)   Bagel (½ of a 2-oz. bagel)
Pita (½ of a 6-inch pita)   Bread sticks (2)
English muffin (½)   Unsweetened cereal (¾ cup)

Sugar-frosted cereal (½ cup)

Granola, low-fat (¼ cup)

Rice cakes/Popcorn cakes (2)

Pretzels (2 rods or 3/4 oz.)

Tortilla chips (6–12 or 1 oz.)**

Popcorn (3 cups air-popped or
low-fat microwave)

Melba toast (4 slices)

Goldfish (43)

Snack chips, fat-free
(tortilla, potato) 15–20

Ak-Mak (10 crackers, 2 oz.)

Saltine-type crackers (6)

Crackers, round butter type (6)*

Sandwich cracker with cheese or
peanut butter (3)*

Mini Stoned Wheat Thins (14)

Gingersnaps (3)

Graham crackers (3 squares)

Granola bar (1)*

Animal crackers (8)

Vanilla wafers (5)*

Fig Newtons (2)

Rice Krispie Treat (1)

Choice DM bar (1)

Glucerna Snack Bar (1)

Fresh fruit—small apple, orange,
banana

Grapes (17)

Raisins (2 tbsp.)

Fruit juice bar, frozen, 100% juice
(1 3 oz. bar)

Yogurt, frozen, low-fat
(½ cup)

Ice cream, light (½ cup)*

No-sugar-added fudgesicle (2)

Light-style yogurt (6 oz.)

Go-Gurt (1 2.25-oz. tube)

Tips for Staying Active

- Choose at least two different kinds of activity to prevent boredom.

- Try something new, such as ballroom dancing or a spinning class at the local Y.

- Join a walking or running club. Not only will you make new friends, they'll keep you going when you feel like giving up.

- Use a pedometer. Put it on in the morning and see how many steps you take in an average day—then try to increase that number each week until you reach your personal fitness goal.

- Exercise with a family member, friend, or neighbor.

- Keep track of your progress. Just as you record your blood glucose levels and food intake, recording the type and duration of activity can be helpful and will reinforce how hard you've been working.

- Enlist the support of your family and friends. Explain the role of activity in diabetes control. Make sure you set aside time in your day or evening to fit this in, and that family and friends understand that this is "your time."

- Start out gradually. Nothing can get you off track like sore muscles or having to gasp for breath.

- Figure out the best time for exercise. Some people prefer to exercise first thing in the morning, while others prefer to be active after work. The best time to exercise is when it's best for you!

- Ask your healthcare team for help and support.

Physical Activity—A "Magic Bullet"

Increasing your physical activity is one of the most helpful lifestyle changes you can make. Physical activity reduces insulin resistance and improves the body's ability to handle glucose. Importantly, insulin action improves with physical activity even without weight loss. Physical activity also lowers the level of fat in your blood, helps you lose weight if you need to, lowers stress, and increases your energy level.

Making changes to long-standing habits can be hard. Start with something small. When you are successful, add another small step. You don't need to join a health club or work out, but you do need to commit yourself to regular physical activity nearly every day of the week. Walking is a great way to start. You may start with a daily 5-minute walk around the block, and gradually build up to 30 minutes or longer.

Regular physical activity lowers the risk of heart disease, stroke, diabetes, osteoporosis, fractures, and gallbladder disease. It's clearly the closest thing we have to being a magic bullet! Remember to find activities that you enjoy, start slowly, and enjoy your success. The first step is up to you!

CHAPTER 10

Exercising Safely with Type 1 Diabetes

If you have type 1 diabetes, taking insulin, following a meal plan, and being physically active are part of a delicate balancing act, all working together to keep your blood glucose on track. Adjusting for physical activity or exercise can be one of the more difficult challenges that people with type 1 diabetes face. Therefore, it's important for you to know how physical activity affects your blood glucose. That knowledge will give you a better idea of how to balance insulin and food around the times you are physically active.

Check Your Blood Glucose

Checking your blood glucose is the *only* way to evaluate the effect of exercise or physical activity on blood glucose. You cannot depend on your body to tell you by how you feel whether or not your blood glucose level is too high or too low. Start by checking it before exercising, taking into consideration the timing and quantity of your last meal or snack. Then check your blood glucose after exercising. This will give you an idea of how much your blood glucose changes when you are active. Your blood glucose at the end of the activity should be above 110 mg/dl. This would mean that you are less likely to have a blood glucose level that drops too low during activity, and are also less likely to have the glucose drop too low immediately after that activity because of depletion of all your stores of glucose in the muscle (discussed in the next section). It is a good idea, when exercising, to keep your glucose meter with you, especially when you are changing or increasing activities.

Low Blood Glucose (Hypoglycemia)

One of the beneficial effects of physical activity is that it lowers blood glucose. There can be times, however, when it lowers blood glucose levels too much. This is a common concern for people who take insulin. The problem is caused by *too much* insulin in the blood during exercise. For exercise to lower the blood glucose level, some insulin must be present. However, exercise can lower the glucose beyond what the insulin alone would have done.

When you are active, therefore, the usual amount of insulin that you might take is more than your body actually needs. If you do take this amount, the insulin excess erroneously tells the liver to slow the release of glucose. At the same time, the muscles increase their use of glucose. The result: the level of blood glucose falls quickly, causing low blood glucose, or *hypoglycemia*.

It may surprise you to learn that low blood glucose can occur *after* exercise. Or you may have wondered why you have had a low blood glucose reaction after exercise. When you exercise, you use glucose that was stored in your muscles and liver, called *glycogen*. After exercising, your body not only is more sensitive to insulin but also has to replace glycogen stores. Glucose is removed from the blood to replenish these glycogen stores, and this can cause blood glucose to drop too low. This drop in the glucose level some time after the exercise is over is called the lag effect. Depending on what type of exercise you did and for how long, it can take up to 24 to 48 hours to replenish glycogen. For instance, if you were skiing, biking, or doing yard work or gardening all day, you may find that you have hypoglycemia during the night or even the next day. It is important, then, to check your blood glucose *before* you exercise, but equally important to continue checking your blood glucose *after* physical activity or exercise.

Hypoglycemia can also occur *during* physical activity. This usually happens because your blood glucose level was too low at the beginning to provide you with enough fuel. Once you begin exercising, blood glucose drops very fast and becomes too low. If in doubt, eat a food containing 15 grams of carbohydrate either before or every 45 to 60 minutes during exercise. After a few sessions, you will learn how much and how often you need to eat.

Guidelines and Precautions

To prevent hypoglycemia there are two primary ways to adjust your treatment program—through changes in insulin dose and carbohydrate intake. Adjusting your insulin before you exercise will help prevent hypoglycemia during or after activity. Generally, this should be your first step. There will be times when you also need additional carbohydrate. Good rules of thumb are the following:

- If your exercise is planned, you can decrease the insulin that will be acting during the activity.

- If your exercise is unplanned, you may need to eat additional carbohydrate either before or after the activity. If the activity is longer than an hour, you may need an additional source of carbohydrate during the activity as well.

- If weight control is your goal, plan your exercise so that you can limit the amount of extra food needed to keep your blood glucose from dropping too low. Doing physical activity 30 minutes to two hours after meals is often the best time.

Adjusting Your Insulin

Insulin adjustments should be considered when the activity you are planning to engage in is occurring at the peak action of any of your insulins, is of long duration—more than two hours, is of high intensity, or if you are exercising to promote weight management. The insulins you may consider adjusting are either the rapid-acting, short-acting, or intermediate-acting insulins. Glargine or ultralente are not adjusted for exercise. The following insulins acting during physical activity can be adjusted. Listed below are the different types of insulin and their peak action times:

- Rapid-acting insulin (lispro, aspart, or glulisine): 1/2 to 3 hours
- Short-acting insulin (regular): 1 to 5 hours
- Intermediate-acting insulin (NPH/lente): 4 to 15 hours

The intensity and duration of the activity are factors to consider when you decide how much to decrease insulin. An example of moderate-intensity activity is a brisk walk; that means walking a mile in 15 to 20 minutes. Running is an example of a high-intensity or vigorous activity. The following are terms for the duration of the activity:

- Short = less than 30 minutes
- Intermediate = 30 to 60 minutes
- Long = 60 minutes or more

Insulin adjustments can only be made when exercise is planned. If you are not sure how much to reduce your insulin dose, you can generally start by reducing your insulin that is acting during the exercise time period by 1 to 2 units or 10 percent of your total insulin dose. Table 10-1, Guidelines for Reducing Insulin with Exercise, provides starting guidelines for reducing insulin doses based on exercise intensity and the duration of activity. It is important to remember that everyone responds slightly differently to exercise, and blood glucose checks are therefore essential to determine what is right for you. Your exercise program may require more individualized insulin adjustments, and your healthcare team can assist you in determining these adjustments.

If your blood glucose is less than 110 mg/dl after exercise, eat a snack immediately to prevent a low blood glucose reaction. The snacks listed in Chapter 9 are good choices. By using information from your blood glucose checks before and after exercising, you can see whether you need to make

TABLE 10-1	Guidelines for Reducing Insulin with Exercise	
Amount to Decrease Peaking Insulin	Intensity of Exercise	Duration of Exercise
0%–10%	Low, moderate, or high	Short (less than 30 minutes)
5%–20%	Low	Intermediate to long (30 to 60 min.)
10%–30%	Moderate	Intermediate (30 to 60 min.)
20%–40%	Moderate	Long (longer than 60 min.)
20%–40%	High	Intermediate (30 to 60 min.)
30%–50%	High	Long (longer than 60 min.)

additional changes next time you exercise. For example, if your blood glucose is less than 110 mg/dl after exercising, you may need to reduce your insulin further the next time you exercise.

Adjusting Carbohydrate

During physical activity your muscles use more glucose for energy than when your body is at rest. Sometimes you need extra carbohydrate to maintain the balance between glucose needed for energy while exercising, glucose available from food, and the action pattern of the insulin you have taken. Extra carbohydrate must often be consumed before exercise to prevent low blood glucose, especially if you are not able to decrease your insulin dose.

You may need an extra 10 to 15 grams of glucose for every hour of moderate-intensity exercise, and about double that for an hour of high-intensity exercise. The following are adjustments for carbohydrate before and during exercise.

■ A carbohydrate snack (15 grams of carb) should be eaten 15 to 30 minutes before exercise.

- Eat an extra 15 to 30 grams of carbohydrate for each 30 to 60 minutes you plan to exercise.

Checking your blood glucose before and after exercising provides your best guide to whether you need to add carbohydrate, adjust insulin, or do both when you exercise. Keeping good written records that include your blood glucose level, insulin dose, amount of carbohydrate eaten, and details of physical activity can help you learn from your experiences.

Preventing Hypoglycemia After Exercise

Checking your blood glucose after exercise helps you determine whether you are still at risk for a low blood glucose. Sometimes you may need to continue checking your glucose for up to two to four hours after exercise. Exercise may even cause your blood glucose to drop for the next 24 hours following the activity. As noted previously, this is known as the lag effect of exercise. If a low blood glucose reaction occurs after your exercise session, you may need to eat additional carbohydrate or decrease your insulin dose even more before your next session. Table 10-2 contains general guidelines for insulin and carbohydrate adjustments to help you avoid hypoglycemia after exercise.

High Blood Glucose (Hyperglycemia)

What happens if there is *not enough* insulin circulating in the blood during exercise? Without enough insulin, glucose can't get into the cells to provide them with energy, so it begins to build up in the bloodstream. The liver senses that the cells are "starved" for glucose and mistakenly begins to release more glucose into the bloodstream. But there wasn't enough insulin to take care of the glucose present in the first place. Now there's even more glucose. The result: the muscles don't get any glucose and the level of blood glucose increases. With insufficient insulin, with or without exercise, ketones are often produced in the urine, signifying the metabolism or burning of fat for energy because of the lack of insulin and the inability to make use

TABLE 10-2	Guidelines for Adjustments in Carbohydrate and Insulin Based on Blood Glucose After Exercise	
If Your Blood Glucose After Exercise Is:	**Guidelines**
Less than 110 mg/dl	Snack immediately: • 15 g carbohydrate if no meal or snack is planned for 30 to 60 minutes • 30 g carbohydrate if no meal or snack is planned for more than 1 hour • Reduce insulin further next time you exercise • If at bedtime, eat 30 g carbohydrate
Between 111 and 160 mg/dl	Insulin dose is correct for exercise • Continue with your exercise program • Continue monitoring glucose after exercise
Greater than 161 mg/dl	No need to reduce insulin • Assess impact of last meal or snack • Continue monitoring blood glucose after exercise

of glucose. This is not a good situation for someone who is planning to exercise, so if your insulin is insufficient, particularly if you are spilling ketones, you should not exercise until the situation is corrected. In summary, it is important to keep blood glucose in the normal range during exercise, which requires the right amount of insulin—not too little and not too much.

But there is another occasion when exercise raises the blood glucose level instead of lowering it. In fact, it is more likely the reason for high blood glucose after exercise than insufficient insulin. You risk this effect if you engage in activities of a high intensity, such as exercise or sports of repeated short bouts, especially if you become breathless. For example, after weight lifting or power activities, a game of singles tennis, or track events, it would not be surprising to find glucose levels higher than before you started. Whenever you exercise, your body tries to ensure that there is enough glucose for fuel. So glucagon and other hormones cause the liver to release glucose. Your body doesn't know exactly how much glucose you need, but to be sure you have enough, it may release more glucose than is needed. This occurs in everyone doing high-intensity activities, but if you have diabetes, your blood glucose levels may rise and stay higher longer than in someone who does not have diabetes. A common problem often follows. Individuals check and, finding their blood glucose to be high, decide to take additional insulin. The combination of extra insulin and the naturally dropping blood glucose levels after exercise can then cause too *low* a blood glucose level. This low blood glucose can happen several hours after the exercise or even the next day. The best solution is not to take the extra insulin but allow the body to naturally lower blood glucose. This becomes more of a medical concern when blood glucose levels are already high because of a lack of insulin. Without the right amount of insulin, blood glucose cannot enter the muscle cells and blood glucose levels can go higher with physical activity. Because of this concern, you should follow the blood glucose guidelines provided in Table 10-3.

Precautions

There are times when you need to be especially careful if you plan to exercise. Below are some reminders.

- *When your insulin is working the hardest.* If you take insulin, you know it lowers your blood glucose. Exercise also lowers blood glucose. When exercise and insulin are working together, your blood glucose may drop too low. Learn to adjust your insulin or eat extra carbohydrate at these times.

- *When blood glucose is high.* If your diabetes has been poorly controlled for a period of time because of lack of insulin, exercise will not lower your blood glucose. Fortunately, this doesn't happen very often these days. It might be a concern at the time of diagnosis, when, not realizing you have diabetes, your blood glucose levels might have been ele-

TABLE 10-3	When It's Okay to Exercise with Diabetes
Type 1	If fasting blood glucose is 250 mg/dl or higher, check for ketones; if positive for ketones, DO NOT exercise.
	If blood glucose is between 251 and 300 mg/dl, and negative for ketones, it is okay to exercise.
	If blood glucose is over 300 mg/dl, and negative for ketones, exercise with *extreme caution.*
	Check blood glucose 10 to 15 minutes into exercise to make sure it is dropping. Make sure you drink plenty of water to stay hydrated.
Children with type 1	Follow the guidelines above—except that it is okay to exercise with blood glucose levels up to 400 mg/dl
Type 2	Can exercise with blood glucose levels up to 400 mg/dl (regardless of whether or not using insulin)

vated for several days, or during illness, such as the flu. It is usually recommended that you not exercise with high blood glucose, especially with ketones, and if you are not feeling well. Call your healthcare providers instead, and work to lower your blood glucose to the proper level.

■ *When exercising during the evening.* You are at greater risk of low blood glucose levels overnight if you exercise late in the evening. It is important to have a bedtime snack if you exercise after your evening meal, or to know how to adjust insulin at these times. If possible, complete exercise two hours before bedtime.

- *Avoid alcohol before or immediately after exercise.* Alcohol without food intake can lead to hypoglycemia, and adding exercise increases the risk.

- *Avoid hot tubs, saunas, and steam tables directly after exercise.* These cause one to maintain an increased heart rate and may lower your blood glucose.

So Why Exercise?

Making insulin adjustments, gauging your carbohydrate intake, and frequently monitoring your blood glucose may seem like a lot of work in order to exercise safely with diabetes. However, being physically active is a key step in helping you manage your diabetes. A regular exercise program can bring dramatic results. It can lower blood glucose levels and decrease your risk of heart disease. An exercise program should be individually tailored for you and designed to compliment your lifestyle and help you achieve your desired goals. Discuss your exercise program with your clinical exercise physiologist, physical therapist, diabetes educator, or doctor to determine the type of adjustments you need to make. It's equally important to meet with your healthcare team if you're currently not exercising but want to start. It may not always be easy; in fact, it can seem like a lot of work—but it's extremely important and will pay off in very big ways.

CHAPTER 11

Successfully Making Lifestyle Changes

Taking charge of your diabetes means that you need to make some lifestyle changes. This may mean making changes in some of your food choices or in how much you eat, or it may mean becoming more physically active, or it may mean you need to take medications such as pills or even insulin. At this point you may be thinking, Wow, there was a lot of information about lifestyle changes in the last seven chapters—where do I begin? Fortunately, some recently published research helps answer that confusion. One study identified food habits that were related to blood glucose control in people with diabetes. And another study compared structured physical activity programs with home-based physical activities and found you don't need to belong to a health club or go to a gym to achieve successful results from physical activity. We'll discuss the findings of these studies later in this chapter.

Stages for Successful Lifestyle Changes

It's not surprising that some individuals find it hard to make lifestyle changes with regard to such important things as eating and physical activity. To better understand and help, researchers have studied how people make changes. They discovered that individuals make changes in stages, which researchers call stages of change. As you read the next paragraphs, try to decide which stage best describes you at this time.

How Ready Are You to Make Changes?

Many individuals begin in the *precontemplation* stage, during which their attitude toward lifestyle change is described as "Never." That means they have no intention of changing behavior no matter what anyone says or advises. Usually this is because they are unaware they have a problem. If you are a precontemplator, perhaps someone important to you bought this book for you, and you are only reading it to humor them. That's great because this is the first step. The researchers found that what helped individuals move from this stage to the next was receiving information that convinced them that it was important for them to make changes.

The next step is *contemplation*. In this stage individuals are aware that they have a problem and are seriously thinking about change "Someday." However, no commitment to take action in the near future has been made.

Or are you in the *preparation* stage, which is the stage of decision making described as "Soon"? In this stage, commitment to take action within the next 30 days has been made, and individuals are already trying to make small behavioral changes.

The goal is to help you get to the *action* stage, or "Now." This is the stage in which you change behaviors that you have determined are important for you to change. Maybe you decide you will eat breakfast every day. Or that you will check your blood glucose level once a day. Or maybe you decide you will walk for ten minutes four days a week. Or you might decide that you will take the medication your doctor said was important for you every day.

After you have maintained a change for six months, you are in the *maintenance* stage, described as "Forever." But researchers also discovered that people move back and forth between stages. This is called *relapse*. Relapse is natural and to be expected. The goal is to make the periods of relapse shorter and shorter and further and further apart—to stabilize behavior change and to avoid relapse.

So think about what stage you might be in, and answer the following questions:

- Have you been thinking about making some food and/or physical activity changes to improve blood glucose control?
- What changes are you willing to make?
- What will help you make these changes?
- What can your family and friends or healthcare providers do to help you?

What Will Help You Make Changes?

If you have decided that you are ready to make some changes, there are some strategies that will help you do this. When people with diabetes hold two important beliefs, they are more likely to make changes and to begin taking charge of their diabetes—the first belief is that diabetes is serious, and the second is that their own actions can make a difference. However, you also must have confidence in your ability to make and maintain a change. Education and practice can increase your level of confidence and belief that you can take charge!

Support from family and friends can also be of assistance. The secret is to find the right balance. The right amount of support can help you make and continue lifestyle changes, but more than what you want can negatively affect your ability to make and continue change. Family members can care too much or care too little. It is commom to find that individuals with diabetes sometimes have arguments with family and friends over what they eat and how they manage other aspects of diabetes. And it's just as common for family and friends to be viewed as the "diabetes police." Share your feelings and frustrations with family and friends so they'll know if they are helping or hindering you as you try to do the best you can to manage your diabetes.

There are some other strategies you can use to maintain change. Not surprisingly, people who have been successful at making changes have said that the technique that helped them the most was *self-monitoring*. This means keeping records of food, physical activity, and blood glucose. These people also admitted they didn't like doing it, that it was boring and tedious, but to help them make changes, record keeping was essential. Keeping records helped them be aware of what they were doing and decide what needed to be changed. As they made changes, they liked writing them down so they could see what they had done. If you decide you need to make some changes in your eating and physical activity habits, you will find that keeping food, physical activity, and blood glucose records will help you. By keeping records, you and your healthcare team can make decisions about your diabetes care. Keeping diaries is doubly beneficial—they help you make changes, and they help you and your team evaluate whether the changes you make are beneficial or whether other changes are needed.

When making changes in eating, *environmental control* can also help. Identify factors in your environment that trigger eating. For example, you may identify certain times of the day that are a problem for you. Many individuals report a difficult time for them to control eating is from 4:30 P.M. on. Behavioral specialists speculate that this is because the structure of your day breaks down at this time. You may have been busy at work, school, or home, but now you are done with your scheduled activities. In order to relax, you may start eating. These specialists suggest that you need to make plans for what you will do after 4:30 and throughout the evening. Otherwise, it is just too easy to watch TV and snack. Taking a class, walking the dog (or walking yourself), reading, or phoning a friend are all activities you might consider. Eating at specific times, avoiding buying foods that are difficult to control eating, and setting aside a time and place for physical activities are other helpful strategies.

What Interferes with Making Changes?

Most people living with diabetes go through times when they feel *stress*. This is a normal feeling and no doubt happens to you as well. Sometimes it's caused by the day-to-day frustrations of diabetes, which at times can be confusing, aggravating, and burdensome. At other times your feelings can include anger ("Why me? This isn't fair!"), fear ("What is going to happen to me?"), guilt ("Did I do something wrong? Did I eat too many sweets?"), depression ("I feel so alone"), and even denial ("If I just ignore diabetes, it will go away"). Such thoughts and feelings are common and normal among people with diabetes—and can even help you move from the precontemplation phase to taking action. Talk to people you care about and who care about you concerning what is bothering you. Share your feelings with your healthcare team, especially the behavioral specialist. Join a diabetes support group. Or just find some time during the day for some quiet relaxation.

Stressful situations that arise in everyone's life can cause you to stop being involved in your diabetes care. Stress can also directly affect your blood glucose level, making it even more frustrating to have to deal with both your stressful problem and your diabetes management. Learning relaxation skills has helped many individuals through periods of stress. Some people find meditation to be helpful, while others practice yoga or deep-breathing techniques. Make sure you have some quiet time to yourself every day, even a short while, to help you relax, unwind, and refresh.

You've heard it before, but it's worthwhile repeating: participating in physical activities can be a great way to overcome stress. Researchers have found over and over again that people who engage in regular physical activities handle stress better. Just taking the time to care for yourself and having a few minutes alone to think through whatever is bothering you and causing you stress can sometimes be helpful. But many individuals find physical activity helps them relax and handle life better. This may be a direct effect of the exercise-induced production of substances called endorphins, and an indirect effect of exercise forcing one to get away from daily stresses, even for a short period.

Eating Habits That Work—Start with Carbohydrate Counting

Researchers interviewed people with type 2 diabetes to see what eating habits were important. Out of this research came the 12 Do's for Basic Eating Practices. Not surprisingly, 6 of the 12 were related to carbohydrate, highlighting the importance of beginning lifestyle food changes by learning about carbohydrate counting. In Chapter 4 we said it was important to learn what foods contain carbohydrate, and to know what the portion sizes are for one carbohydrate choice, or serving, and how many carbohydrate servings to select for your meals and your snacks.

Here are some do's related to carbohydrate counting:

- Limit foods high in sugar, such as regular soft drinks and desserts.
- Limit portion sizes; that is, eat your agreed-upon number of carbohydrate servings in the right portion sizes.
- Eat low-fat foods for breakfast, such as cold cereal, oatmeal, whole-wheat bread, and fruit.
- Eat two vegetables for dinner, or a combination of one vegetable and salad at the main meal of the day.

In Chapter 6, we discussed the importance of being careful to limit total fat, and saturated fat as well. So once you've learned about carbohydrate counting, learn about fats. Here are the do's related to fats:

- Reduce your intake of high-fat foods such as potato chips, whole milk, pizza, chocolate, and fried foods.
- Choose low-fat foods such as broiled or baked main courses, salads, vegetables, and low-fat dressings.
- Eat low-fat foods for lunch such as vegetables, salads, fruit, tuna, chicken, low-fat lunch meats, and low-fat cheeses and dressings.

There were also two do's in the meal-planning category:

- Eat regularly. This means eating three meals a day, making time in your schedule for eating, and not skipping meals.
- Plan meals by using a shopping list, planning a weekly menu, and taking meals to work or on trips.

And not surprisingly, the three biggest *challenges* came from the dining out category:

- Eating at buffet, fast-food, and large chain restaurants: these restaurants feature large portion sizes and high-fat foods and have a limited selection of vegetables.
- Choosing high-fat or high-carbohydrate menu selections, such as fried foods, high-fat meats, sauces, pasta, bread, and gravy.

- Eating high-fat sources of protein such as prime fat meats, fried meats or fish, and processed meats.

Physical Activities—Just Go Ahead and Do It!

It's clear that planning for meals is important. But is it also important to have structure for physical activity? Interestingly, the answer is no. For example, researchers compared on-site supervised exercise programs with a comparable program of home-based activities. During the first six months two groups did the same number of minutes of physical activity per week. However, at 15 months, those who exercised at home did more minutes of activity and had lost more weight than those who exercised on site. Two other studies also showed that participants who exercised at home did just as well as those who attended structured exercise programs. So, contrary to the findings related to food choices, structured physical activity does not appear to improve short-term or long-term results. In fact, less-structured physical activity seems to lead to better long-term success. With less structure comes a reduction in exercise-related demands and barriers, such as travel time, health club dues, or embarrassment about weight or shape. The answer to what works for physical activity is everything. Do whatever is convenient for you, and do it when it is convenient. The message is—it's important, just do it!

Everyone is different, though. You may find that planning or scheduling exercise is a big help. Many people find that noting their exercise session in their calendar, appointment book, or PDA reminds them that they need to fit it in.

Some Additional Ideas to Help Make Changes Easier

1. It's important to realize that you can't make too many changes at one time, especially if you're new to diabetes. Focus on changing one behavior, and then move on when you're confident you've mastered it.
2. You need to set specific, realistic goals for yourself. So rather than say-

ing "I'm going to lose a lot of weight," break it down and instead say "I'm going to work on losing five to ten pounds over the next two months by decreasing food portions and walking five times a week."

3. Reward yourself for changing a behavior or accomplishing a goal—go away for the weekend, buy a new CD or something else you've been wanting, or do something with friends.

4. Seek support from your healthcare team—don't hesitate to ask questions of your healthcare provider, dietitian, or diabetes educator.

5. Getting your family involved, too, with helping you change behaviors—make it a family affair. Cook healthy meals for the whole family; take walks after dinner; explain to them some of the things you've learned about nutrition and the need for regular physical activity.

Good News and the Bottom Line

The good news is that there is much you can do to overcome difficult feelings and to harness the power of your thoughts and emotions to help you manage your diabetes more easily and effectively. Perhaps the first step is learning more about diabetes and how you can take charge and manage it well. Knowing that your diabetes control won't be perfect all the time can help you overcome some of your guilt or frustrations—everyone has "bad" days. Understand that each person with diabetes has different goals and targets—and celebrate your achievements as you get closer to your own goals. Make sure you work with your healthcare team on a plan for self-management that is clear and reasonable. If you feel constantly overwhelmed or anxious about having diabetes, ask your healthcare provider for a referral to a mental health specialist. If you are confused, don't be shy—ask questions. Perhaps reading this book will help answer some of these questions as well. The bottom line in making change is for you to believe that even though change may seem difficult, the result—a healthier you now and in the future—is definitely worth it!

PART THREE

Monitoring and Treating Diabetes with Medications

CHAPTER 12

Glucose Monitoring

When you have diabetes, your body's metabolism is no longer on "automatic." Without help, it can no longer keep your blood glucose in normal range. That's where *you* play a key role—stepping in to make decisions about your diabetes management. To do this, you need to know your blood glucose levels. This is accomplished by checking (some refer to it as testing) your blood glucose on a regular schedule. Thus, your overall diabetes treatment plan involves checking your blood glucose (sometimes referred to as self-monitoring of blood glucose, or SMBG) as well as figuring out how food, physical activity, and medication affect your blood glucose levels. By putting all these pieces together, you will be able to better understand and manage your diabetes. Throughout this book, when we speak of "checking" your blood glucose, we are talking about the regular blood glucose checks that you do each day. When we refer to "monitoring," we are talking about staying in tune with every aspect of your diabetes treatment program (blood glucose checks, medication, food, physical activity) to make sure that all of the pieces are working together and that your blood glucose stays in your target range.

You stand to gain many benefits from monitoring your diabetes program. It will help keep your blood glucose in control, which in turn will allow you to feel better, avoid complications, and have more energy to carry out your daily activities with enthusiasm. If you monitor your diabetes carefully, your life, both at home and at work, will be interrupted by fewer problems related to diabetes.

Two Ways to Evaluate Your Blood Glucose Control

Checking your blood glucose at home helps you know day to day how well your treatment program is working. It provides the feedback to help you determine whether changes are needed in your meal plan, physical activity program, or medications. The pattern of your blood glucose levels helps you and your healthcare provider make better treatment decisions.

In addition to regular blood glucose checks, there is an extremely important blood glucose measurement called hemoglobin A1C—referred to commonly as A1C. An A1C is a laboratory test that evaluates overall control and helps you and your healthcare provider know how well your diabetes treatment plan is working.

The blood glucose checks that you do each day and the A1C cannot be substituted for each other. They reflect different measurements of diabetes treatment, and thus they complement each other.

The Importance of Checking and Monitoring— The Evidence

Research involving more than 1,400 people in the United States and Canada shows that people with diabetes can cut their risk of long-term problems by reducing their A1C as much as possible. This landmark study, called the Diabetes Control and Complications Trial (DCCT), took ten years and was completed in 1993. A key finding of the study is that individuals who use insulin treatment programs that provide insulin in a pattern that mimics normal insulin production (called *intensive therapy* in that study, and *physiologic replacement therapy* by many people now), which allows them to achieve lower A1C values, are much less likely to experience complications than people who use more conventional, less natural insulin replacement programs. The study also showed that if the people using "intensive therapy" had complications when they began the treatment, the complications didn't progress as quickly, particularly once the intensive therapy had been used for some time. These complications include eye disease, kidney disease, and painful nerve damage. In fact, the DCCT showed that people who reduce their A1C can cut their risk of complications by 50 percent or more!

Another study, called the United Kingdom Prospective Diabetes Study (UKPDS), showed similar results in people with type 2 diabetes. The UKPDS recruited over 5,000 individuals newly diagnosed with type 2 diabetes from medical centers in the United Kingdom and followed them from 10 to 11 years. It showed that individuals with type 2 diabetes who achieved lower A1C values, in this case using oral antidiabetes medications, were less likely to experience complications than people who did not lower their A1C levels. Aggressive treatment of even mild-to-moderate hypertension was also beneficial in preventing complications.

Measuring A1C and blood glucose checks are tools for diabetes control. Doing both will help you be healthier today—and tomorrow.

Checking Your Blood for Glucose

Checking your blood glucose values is your best tool for diabetes control. You check your blood glucose with a small device called a *glucose meter*. There are many different models on the market, and your healthcare providers can help you decide which one will work best for you. A small needle called a *lancet* is used to get a drop of blood from your finger, arm, or other site. The blood is placed on a special strip, which is put into the meter. The meter "reads" the strip and gives you a blood glucose reading.

Blood glucose levels are constantly changing. By checking your blood glucose several times over the course of the day, you can get a better sense of the pattern of your glucose. Knowing the factors that influence glucose levels can be crucial to understanding the pattern. For instance, an increase in blood glucose can be the result of insufficient insulin or diabetes medication, too much food, too little activity, or increases in *stress hormones*, released during times of stress, illness, or infection. Too low a blood glucose can result from too much insulin or diabetes medication, not enough food, unusual amounts of physical activity, and skipped or delayed meals. In addition, errors in using your meter may result in high or low blood glucose readings. That's why it's important to be sure you know how to use your glucose meter appropriately. Your healthcare team should instruct you on the proper technique for using your type of meter.

There is no such thing as a good or bad blood glucose number. A blood glucose number is just a number—but an important one, because it provides you with information. The numbers allow you to learn what causes your blood glucose to go too high or too low. If you choose to eat a different food or more food than usual, you will learn by checking your blood glucose what effect the food has. If you start a physical activity program, you will be able to see how it changes your blood glucose. Blood glucose checking also helps you determine whether the emotions you may be having are the result of high or low blood glucose levels.

Keep a Logbook

To use the results of your blood glucose checks, it is important that you keep a record of your blood glucose numbers in a logbook. Ask your healthcare providers for one if you do not already have one. Most blood glucose meter companies can provide you with a small logbook that you can keep in your meter case. Figure 12-1 is an example of a diabetes-monitoring log, with information recorded for two days.

Figure 12-1   Simple Glucose Log

Date	Breakfast	Lunch	Supper	Bedtime	Medications	Comments
2/20	165		140		Glyburide, 5 mg at breakfast	Walked after lunch
2/21	123	92		254	Same	Dined out at supper

You may be wondering why you should keep a logbook at all when most meters today have a memory to store blood glucose results. Although meters with memories can be useful, most of them cannot record variations in your daily schedule such as physical activity or snacking, and they don't help you see patterns in your blood glucose levels. They provide only part of the data needed. Handwritten logs allow you to record variations in the timing of your daily activities, which will help you to better understand your blood glucose patterns. If you don't like the idea of using handwritten logs, consider using a computerized logbook. Some of these computerized logs can be downloaded into a PDA or handheld computer for convenience.

A log should have space to record blood glucose results—both before and after meals, as well as in the middle of the night. You should be able to read across a row and see a number of values for various times of the day. But most important, you should be able to scan down a column and see the values for a particular time of day for a number of days running. A separate section should be used to record insulin doses or medications. It will be important for you to note when your glucose is above or below target range. A useful tip is to circle glucose readings that are above or below your target range. Use a red pen to circle high readings, and a blue pen to circle low readings.

A "comment" section is used to record events that affect control, such as an illness or unplanned physical activity. Although the comments need to be brief, they should be written so that you can look back at them later and use the information to interpret glucose patterns. There really isn't room in logs to keep detailed food information, although some have room to record the amount of carbohydrate you consume. Many people find it helpful to record only the number of carbohydrate servings or choices eaten at various times throughout the day, especially if it differs from the number usually eaten. Others find a notation such as "overate" or "light lunch" to be helpful. Keep in mind that more detailed food records are important to keep if you are trying to lose weight, for example, or are fine-tuning your insulin-to-carb ratio (see Chapter 5). An example of a more detailed glucose log is provided in Figure 12-2. *Be sure to bring your log with you to all of your medical appointments.*

Figure 12-2 Detailed Glucose Log

Glucose-Monitoring Results

Date 20__	Before Breakfast	Before Lunch	Before Supper	Bedtime	Other

Insulin Doses

Before Breakfast		Before Lunch		Before Supper		Bedtime		Comments
Reg/ Rap	Long/ Inter	Reg/ Rap	Long/ Inter	Reg/ Rap	Long/ Inter	Reg/ Rap	Long/ Inter	

KEY: *Reg* = regular; *Rap* = rapid; *Inter* = intermediate insulin: NPH or lente; *Long* = Long-acting insulin: ultralente, glargine
In Comments section, record variations in activity, food consumption, and timing.

Understanding What Blood Glucose Levels Mean

There are a few things you need to know in order to understand what your blood glucose numbers mean.

- Your target blood glucose range. For most people, the target is 90 to 130 before meals. Ask your healthcare provider what your target should be.
- The right procedure for checking your blood glucose.
- When to check your blood glucose. (Will you be checking before meals only, or perhaps sometimes after meals as well?)
- How often to check your blood glucose.
- How to look for patterns in the blood glucose numbers you've written in your log. For example, look at all your blood glucose numbers before breakfast and ask yourself if there is a pattern. Are the blood glucose levels higher than your target? Are they lower? Once you see a pattern, ask yourself what might be causing the blood glucose to be too high or too low. If you know the cause, change it. If you don't, call your healthcare providers. Ask them to help you better understand how to make sense of your blood glucose numbers.

What Should Your Blood Glucose Numbers Be?

Discuss your target glucose range with your healthcare providers. Many people aim for blood glucose between 90 and 130 mg/dl (milligrams per deciliter) before meals and less than 160 mg/dl two to three hours after the meal. Your target may be different, so be sure you know what yours is. When your blood glucose levels aren't in the target range, you should work with your healthcare providers to make changes in your diabetes plan. These changes might involve adjusting your eating pattern, your physical activity program, the type of diabetes medication you take, or the amount. Eventually you will learn how to make these changes yourself.

How Do I Know If I'm Doing Blood Glucose Checks Correctly?

It is important that you check your blood glucose accurately. Be sure to demonstrate how to use your meter for your healthcare providers. They can correct any errors. If you think your meter is not working right, call the customer service phone number on the back of the meter for advice.

Tips on getting accurate blood glucose results from finger checks

To get an accurate blood glucose result, you need to be sure

- to store your strips in a cool, dry place at room temperature
- your test strips haven't expired; check the expiration date
- the meter has been coded properly and matches the strips you are using
- you have a clean finger
- you have an adequate drop of blood

How to get a good drop of blood from a finger

Before pricking your finger,

- wash your hands with warm water
- shake your hands below your waist
- squeeze or "milk" your finger a few times

If you are using a site other than a finger, such as a forearm, make sure you are doing the procedure properly and that your meter is made to test at sites other than a finger.

Alternate-Site Testing Meters

Some glucose meters allow you to check your blood glucose from a site other than your fingertips. Sites include the upper arm, the forearm, the base of the thumb, and the thigh. Alternate site testing is a useful option for those who find that their fingers are too sensitive or become too painful, or for those who may have difficulty getting sufficient blood—due to calluses, for example. However, alternate site testing does have a few limitations: since blood glucose levels in the finger change more quickly than levels in other parts of the body, results from alternate sites can differ from those of your fingers. This is a concern if you are hypoglycemic and don't realize it. Talk with your healthcare team if you're interested in trying one of these meters. Below are a few things to consider:

- Be sure that your meter is designed to do alternate site testing (not all are).
- Remember that checking your blood glucose at a site other than your fingertip may give you a different result than you would get with a finger check when glucose levels are changing rapidly, such as after a meal or during or after exercise.
- Do not check your blood glucose at an alternate site if you
  - think your blood glucose may be low (hypoglycemia)
  - you do not feel symptoms when your blood glucose is low
  - the site results do not agree with the symptoms you are experiencing

Instead, use your fingertip in these cases.

Your diabetes educator can show you how to properly use your alternate site testing meter.

How to Store and Dispose of Waste

- store supplies in a dry, cool place; avoid extremes in temperature
- keep strips in their original container

- dispose of lancets in a puncture-proof plastic container or in a metal coffee can
- seal the container with tape when nearly full and discard according to local guidelines for contaminated waste products

When Should You Check Your Blood for Glucose?

Ask your healthcare providers when it is best for you to check your blood glucose. You may want to check at different times of the day to get an idea of how well your treatment program is working.

Generally, the best times to check are before breakfast, before lunch, before dinner, and at bedtime. Sometimes it is helpful to check blood glucose two hours after the start of your meal, to see the effect of food on your blood glucose levels.

For people taking insulin, checking at all these times helps determine how the various doses of insulin are working; for people using pills to treat their diabetes, the pattern of glucose levels revealed by checks can help your healthcare provider decide which pill is best for you—as they often work differently at different times of the day—and whether the pill or pills are working properly.

If You Check Your Blood Glucose Levels

Before breakfast—this result tells you what happened during the evening and night. Remember that for people with type 2 diabetes, glucose is frequently elevated in the morning because the liver releases too much glucose overnight. People assume that means they ate too much the evening before, but this may not be the case. The food you ate at dinner or bedtime should be used or stored in three to four hours if adequate insulin is available.

- Checking your blood glucose before breakfast tells you if you have taken the right dose of insulin or oral medication the night before.

- If you manage your diabetes by lifestyle (nutrition and physical activity) alone, the prebreakfast blood glucose indicates whether the insulin supplied by your body is sufficient overnight.

Two to three hours after the start of a meal—this result tells you how the carbohydrate you ate at the meal affected your blood glucose level.

- If you take a rapid-acting insulin, checking your blood glucose three hours after you eat tells you if you took the right amount of rapid acting insulin at mealtime. Your healthcare team should give you an idea as to what blood glucose values to aim for before a meal, one hour after a meal, and three hours after a meal.

- If you manage your diabetes by lifestyle alone or with diabetes pills, checking your blood glucose two hours after a meal shows whether the insulin supplied by your body is sufficient to lower blood glucose levels that naturally rise after eating. Your blood glucose should be less than 160 mg/dl two hours after the meal.

Before lunch or dinner—this result tells you if you have enough insulin throughout the day. Your body needs insulin throughout the day and night for many different body processes to work correctly.

- If you take insulin, this result tells you how well your insulin is working. If the blood glucose before breakfast, at other meals, and at bedtime are all out of range, your basal insulin may need to be adjusted. If your blood glucose is out of range only sometimes, then the rapid-acting or short-acting insulin may need to be adjusted. This will be discussed in more detail in later chapters.

Before bedtime—this result tells you if you have enough insulin for the night.

- If you take insulin or certain diabetes pills, this check will tell you how well the pills or insulin that you took at dinner worked and whether you need a snack at bedtime. If your blood glucose is below 120 mg/dl and you are using lente, NPH, ultralente, or glargine at bedtime, a snack may be recommended. A typical bedtime snack consists of one or two carbohydrate choices (or 15–30 grams of carbohydrate), such as three graham crackers, or even a sandwich. Your healthcare team can help you decide whether you need a snack, and if so, the right amount of carbohydrate to eat.

Your healthcare providers will tell you what times are the most useful for you to check your blood glucose. They will also show you how to use this information with your diabetes treatment program.

Examples of How Often and When to Check Blood Glucose

For people with type 1 diabetes, checking four or more times a day, every day, is recommended. Check blood glucose levels before every meal and at bedtime. Sometimes it is also necessary to check two hours after a meal to see how well rapid-acting insulin taken before the meal is working. A middle-of-the-night check may also be needed if hypoglycemia overnight is suspected.

For people with type 2 diabetes, there is not one specific pattern that is right for all people with type 2 diabetes. Some people may be using insulin programs similar to those used by people with type 1 diabetes, and the same recommendations, listed above, would apply. For those using insulin to supplement their own insulin and not to fully replace the natural insulin patterns throughout the day, the monitoring schedule will be determined by the specific insulins that are being used.

In general, it is recommended that everyone do a "block" of glucose checks: check frequently for a few days in a row, at a frequency that your healthcare team suggests—maybe once a month or up to once a week, depending on your needs. This block of checks would consist of a check four times a day, usually for three to four days in a row. Between blocks, check less frequently, maybe varying the times among the pre-meal and post-meal times. This pattern of checking is applicable for people with type 2 diabetes who are using insulin but are not using the "intensive" or physiologic programs (who are, for example, using bedtime or twice-daily insulin only), or even using pills, and want to periodically see how their medications are controlling their glucose levels throughout the day. This pattern of checking is helpful if you want to know whether the medication you take covers the amount of food you eat, or to determine whether you are eating the right amount of carbohydrate.

For people with type 2 diabetes whose blood glucose levels are in control and stable—usually treated with diabetes pills—checking before meals twice a day every day may be recommended. On one day, check before breakfast and supper; the next day, check before lunch and bedtime.

When to Check Your Glucose More Often

There are times when you will want to check your blood glucose more often than usual. You may think of other times as well as the following:

- when changes are made in your treatment program—such as medication doses, meal plan, or activity
- when low or high blood glucose levels are present
- during periods of stress, illness, or surgery
- when you are pregnant
- when taking new medications, like steroids

Checking for Ketones

At certain times, it is very important to test for substances, called ketones. Ketones are acid substances made when the body has to burn fat rather than glucose for energy or fuel. This happens when there is not enough insulin to help the body use glucose for energy. Since the body is unable to use glucose, it starts to burn fatty acids, which leads to the production of ketones. The ketones build up and make the blood more acidic, which can result in a condition known as *diabetic ketoacidosis*. The body considers ketones to be like poison and tries to dispose of them as quickly as possible through the urine and through the lungs when you breathe out. In fact, a sign that you might be producing ketones is a fruity smell to your breath. A special kind of urine test strips can detect the presence of ketones and will give someone an idea of how high his or her ketone level may be. Ketones along with a high blood glucose level can make you very sick and cause a medical emergency.

Ketone testing should be done by people with type 1 diabetes when their blood glucose is greater than 250 mg/dl. People with type 2 diabetes who are using insulin, particularly if they are on multiple daily insulin injections, are sick or under stress, and who have blood glucose levels over 300 mg/dl should also test for ketones. All pregnant women with any type of diabetes should check for ketones when their blood glucose levels are high.

Ketones may also result from weight loss. In this case, your body has enough insulin, but because of decreased food intake it uses fatty acids for fuel. Because there is enough insulin, blood glucose levels are normal. Ketones are dangerous to people with diabetes when there are HIGH blood glucose levels along with the ketones. If your blood glucose level is over 250 mg/dl and you are spilling ketones in your urine, you need to contact your doctor, as you may need additional insulin. In the meantime:

- Drink plenty of water or sugar-free beverages to "flush out" the ketones.
- Continue checking your blood glucose every three to four hours, checking for ketones if your blood glucose is over 250.
- Do not exercise if your blood glucose is greater than 250 and ketones are present.
- If you are ill, have recently had surgery, or are under a large amount of stress, use the sick-day rules that your healthcare team has given you. Also, see Chapter 19 for more sick-day guidelines.

On rare occasions, if someone is sick and has not been eating much for a few days, he or she may have ketoacidosis with lower blood glucose. As a general rule, if you have diabetes, are sick, and have not been eating for a day or so, even if you do not see any obvious problems with your glucose levels, you should check with your healthcare provider.

How to Check for Ketones

The most common way to check for ketones is with the use of urine ketone strips, available in foil-wrapped packets or vials that can be purchased at your drugstore without a prescription. Common product names are Ketostix and Chemstrip K. The test result may be negative or show small, moderate, or large numbers of ketones. Ketone strips that measure blood ketones are also available. Follow the manufacturer's guidelines and procedures when testing for ketones. Ketone strips do expire, just like the strips for your glucose meter, so be sure to check the expiration date before using them.

New Types of Monitors

It is now possible to do continuous blood glucose monitoring to determine 24-hour blood glucose patterns and to detect unrecognized low blood glucose. One such system consists of a sensor, inserted just under the skin, that records glucose levels in the fluid beneath the skin for up to 72 hours and can give valuable information as to a person's overall blood glucose patterns.

Another device is worn on the wrist and can provide up to six glucose readings each hour for a maximum of 13 hours. It works through a process called *reverse iontophoresis*, in which a low-level electric current passes through intact skin and extracts glucose molecules. Neither of these monitors can presently replace regular blood glucose checks, but in the future, as these monitors improve, they will have the ability to provide you with important continuous information about your blood glucose levels.

The A1C Test

The A1C, a lab test usually done in your provider's office, is also an essential part of your treatment. The A1C provides a measure of your average glucose control over a period of time. This average is referred to by a percent such as six percent, seven percent, eight percent, nine percent, or higher. The number reflects the average of your blood glucose levels, day and night, for two to three months. Checking your blood glucose provides an instantaneous snapshot. It tells you where your glucose is at a moment in time. The A1C tells you the average over a longer time; it tells you the trend, or in what direction the glucose level is moving, and whether it is moving up or down rapidly with a lot of force or just drifting gently. The A1C provides the longer view. During the two to three months that the A1C measures, you may have had some very high blood glucose levels and some very low levels that you needed to treat at the time or make adjustments for, but overall, if your A1C is in your target range, then your treatment plan is probably working. Your healthcare provider will let you know what your target A1C number is; for most people it is less than seven percent.

How Does the A1C Work?

The A1C test is the most accurate and meaningful test for determining *overall* diabetes control. It provides information that helps you and your healthcare team assess your average blood glucose level over a period of approximately 8 to 12 weeks. The basis for the test lies in the way blood glucose interacts with hemoglobin, a substance that carries oxygen from the lungs to all parts of the body. Hemoglobin is found in the red cells of the blood, which have a life span of about four months. Your body constantly creates new red blood cells as old cells die. When new cells are created, glucose binds to the protein on them through a process called *glycosylation*. When blood glucose levels are elevated, more glucose is glycosylated, or "attached," to hemoglobin. This glucose attaches slowly and, when measured by the A1C test, can tell you, on average, what the blood glucose level has been over the past two to three months. The test does not tell you what happens on a day-to-day basis—that's where checking your blood glucose comes in. So, used in conjunction with your blood glucose checks, the A1C test provides essential information on your treatment program.

Some conditions cause inaccurate results, such as anemia and kidney and liver disease. Consult with your healthcare providers if you have concerns about the accuracy of your test results. Nevertheless, the A1C test is a powerful tool! Many studies have shown a relationship between A1C levels and the risk of developing complications.

How Often Should You Have an A1C Test?

Everyone with diabetes, whether type 1 or type 2, needs to know what his or her A1C level is, as well as his or her individual A1C goal. As part of routine care, Joslin Diabetes Center recommends that an A1C be measured two to four times a year for people with type 1 diabetes, and at least twice a year for those with type 2 diabetes, though more frequent testing is helpful to provide feedback to you and to your healthcare providers.

Typically, to have your A1C level measured, you visit your healthcare provider or a lab. However, there are now kits available for performing A1C tests at home. With all but one of the available tests, you place a drop of blood on a test strip and send the sample to a lab. One system allows you to test your A1C at home and also provides results without having to mail in a sample. Ask your healthcare providers about the use of A1C kits, and make sure that if you use the home kit, you do it correctly. Most important, discuss the results of these tests with your healthcare providers.

What Should Your A1C Be?

For people without diabetes, the normal A1C range is between 4 and 6 percent. Joslin Diabetes Center and the American Diabetes Association suggest that the target goal for people with diabetes is an A1C of less than 7 percent, and that there is need to take action if the A1C is greater than 7 percent. Talk with your doctor to determine what a realistic A1C goal is for you. Remember: the higher your A1C, the higher your risk of developing complications. If your A1C is higher than your target, you need more information to decide what kind of changes you should make in your diabetes treatment program.

This additional information will come from checking your blood glucose. If your A1C is above your target, it tells you that changes need to be made, but it doesn't tell you what changes would be useful. Blood glucose checking is the tool that allows you to learn more about how various foods, physical activity, and medications affect your blood glucose on a daily basis so that you can make needed adjustments. Each blood glucose value is like a piece to a puzzle. The more pieces of the puzzle you have, the clearer the big picture is.

Fructosamine Tests

In addition to self-monitoring blood glucose checks and A1C tests, the *fructosamine test* may be recommended by your doctor at certain times. The main difference between this test and an A1C is that it can detect overall changes in blood glucose control over a shorter time than the A1C test. Fructosamine levels indicate the level of blood glucose control over the past two to three weeks. So when changes are being made in your diabetes treatment plan, this test quickly reveals how the changes are working and whether other changes should be considered. This test may be ordered and performed by your healthcare provider.

Checking Versus Monitoring

As we pointed out at the beginning of this chapter, there is a difference between "checking" and "monitoring." *Checking* is the measurement of blood glucose. You can also "check" an A1C test. *Monitoring* is the plan for using this information to treat your diabetes effectively. People with diabetes may do a lot of checking, but if they don't understand or know what to do with the results, then they are not monitoring their diabetes. It is important that you understand what to do with the results—how to interpret them, what action you should take, and when to call for help. If you are not sure how to interpret your blood glucose readings or what action to take after checking it, be sure you discuss this with your healthcare providers at your next opportunity.

CHAPTER 13

Diabetes Pills

Many people with diabetes need medications to bring their blood glucose into good control. Depending on your body's needs, your doctor may have prescribed medications to help manage your blood glucose. Fortunately, there are many different types of diabetes medications available today to treat type 2 diabetes. Among them are *oral glucose-lowering medications*, also referred to as *oral antidiabetes medications*, or "diabetes pills," which are used in combination with meal plans and physical activity to lower blood glucose as well as in combination with each other and with insulin. Diabetes pills are only prescribed for people with type 2 diabetes. If you have type 1, these pills will not be part of your treatment.

When Are Diabetes Pills Needed?

If type 2 diabetes is diagnosed early, the ability of the beta cells in the pancreas to secrete insulin is still fairly good and the degree of insulin resistance may not be that great, so that changing eating habits and being more active, with a focus on losing weight, may be sufficient to bring glucose levels into control. Unfortunately, many individuals have high blood glucose levels for many years before they are diagnosed with type 2 diabetes. By this time, the beta cells in the pancreas are not able to produce as much insulin and the insulin resistance may be more severe. If this is your situation, it may mean that your treatment program will start with lifestyle strategies—meal planning and physical activity—but will also include diabetes pills. Lifestyle strategies are essential and effective throughout the course of diabetes, but as time passes, both diabetes pills and insulin are often needed to achieve target goals.

The goal of treatment is to achieve normal glucose levels to maintain good health and avoid the complications of diabetes. For many individuals diabetes pills, either alone or combined with each other or with insulin, are needed to achieve normal glucose levels. This does not mean that you have done anything wrong, and it does *not* mean you or your diet "failed." Rather, it is the result of the natural course of diabetes over time, whereby the beta cells fail to make enough insulin.

It is also not true that if you need to take medications (or more medications), your diabetes is getting worse. Nor is it true that if you need insulin, your diabetes has become a more serious disease. Over time, your body changes, and the progression of diabetes usually leads to the need for pills, and perhaps eventually insulin. It is not worse, nor is it unexpected—it is just the progression of time and the diabetes. The goal of treatment is to help your body use the insulin it is still able to make or, when necessary, to replace insulin. Whatever medication is needed to do this should be used. The normal progression described above is different from your diabetes actually getting worse. Your diabetes gets worse if you do not do what is necessary to return your blood glucose level to as normal a level as possible. Early treatment with medications helps prevent complications. It is also not true that if you take pills or insulin, you don't need to follow a meal plan. All of the medications work better if you also pay attention to what you eat and get regular physical activity.

Who Can Take Diabetes Pills?

Diabetes pills aren't for everyone with diabetes. They are effective only if your pancreas is still capable of producing insulin. This means that some people—those with type 1 diabetes and those with type 2 diabetes whose bodies have lost the ability to produce insulin—cannot use them.

The good news is that there are a number of new diabetes pills that have different sites of action. Remember that type 2 diabetes is caused by insulin resistance that can be present throughout the body, particularly in the liver, and the inability of the pancreas to make enough insulin to overcome that resistance. Therefore, diabetes pills that work on each of these problems can be combined. And for some individuals with type 2 diabetes, diabetes pills are even combined with insulin. This is done if the pancreas's ability to make insulin is reduced so much that additional supplements of insulin are needed. Overall, the goal is either to help your body use its own insulin more effectively or to give it extra if needed.

How Do Diabetes Pills Work?

Before the 1990s, therapy was limited to diabetes pills called *sulfonylureas* and insulin combined with lifestyle changes. The sulfonylureas work mainly to increase the amount of insulin made by the pancreas, and thus the insulin level was the only thing that could be targeted with treatments. But since that time, new classes of diabetes pills have become available that target the different steps in the metabolism of glucose in your body that can lead to the development of type 2 diabetes.

Describing how the pills work will take us through the major steps in the metabolism of glucose. Let's start with the beta cells of the pancreas, which produce the insulin. One of the defects that can cause type 2 diabetes is a reduced ability to make and release insulin. Even when the pancreas can make large amounts of insulin to try to overcome this insulin resistance, because the body doesn't use insulin effectively, the increased amount is not sufficient to keep blood glucose levels normal. The beta cells thus produce a relative *insufficiency* of insulin. They begin to slow down. Then, over time, the pancreas produces still less insulin, and the deficiency becomes even more pronounced.

Another part of the abnormal production of insulin, typically seen early in the course of type 2 diabetes, is a reduction in the amount of insulin secreted right after eating. Normally the pancreas releases a short, rapidly peaking burst of insulin immediately after eating. This "first phase" of insulin release lasts about 15 minutes or so and keeps glucose from rising rapidly after food is eaten. The first phase of insulin release is then followed by a second, delayed, and more prolonged phase of insulin release. This is the insulin that handles most of the food consumed in a meal.

When a person has type 2 diabetes, his or her beta cells don't respond well to the rise in glucose levels immediately after starting to eat food, so that the first-phase (after food is eaten) release of insulin is delayed, blunted, or even missing. In fact, a rise in glucose levels right after eating in someone who may be at risk for developing diabetes may be an early sign that diabetes is beginning.

Thus, there is a group of pills that increase the ability of the pancreas to make insulin work to restore both that first immediate phase of insulin secretion, as well as the longer second phase of insulin release. Thus, there are pills specifically designed to work best on increasing that immediate release of insulin, while others are designed to work more effectively on the longer, second phase.

Another problem that causes type 2 diabetes occurs throughout the cells of the body, when the muscle, fat, and liver cells have a decreased sensitivity to the actions of insulin. This is the "insulin resistance" we have referred to. There are other diabetes pills that work to improve insulin action by overcoming that resistance, allowing the glucose that is circulating in the bloodstream to more effectively enter the cells to be used for energy. The situation is of particular concern in the liver, which stores glucose. When insulin resistance is present in the liver, the liver may release too much glucose back into the bloodstream. This often happens overnight and causes blood glucose levels to be elevated in the morning. There are thus diabetes pills that reduce insulin resistance throughout the body. And there are pills that work on muscle and fat, making the body more sensitive to the effect of insulin—these are often referred to as insulin sensitizers—as well as pills that work in a similar manner on the liver to reduce the amount of glucose it produces.

One final type of medicine is available. Say a person cannot produce that first phase of insulin release right after eating has started, but can still make the second, later phase; if the absorption of carbohydrate could be slowed, the incoming glucose could be matched with the later insulin secretion. There are some diabetes pills that can delay carbohydrate absorption from the intestine, accomplishing this.

Types of Diabetes Pills

There are different classes of diabetes pills, each working in a different way, that accomplish the tasks discussed above. Your healthcare provider will determine which pill or combination of pills will work best for you. However, you should know some important facts about the diabetes pills you are taking. You need to know

- the name of your pills
- the dose you should take
- when to take it
- what to do if you forget a dose

You should also know how your pills work, and be aware of potential side effects.

Table 13-1 lists the classes of diabetes pills currently available, their brand and generic names, how they are taken, how they work, and important characteristics for you to know if you use these medications.

TABLE 13-1	Diabetes Pills		
Diabetes Pills	**How to Take**	**How They Work**	**Characteristics**
Sulfonylureas Amaryl (glimepiride) Diabeta, Micronase (glyburide*) Glucotrol, Glucotrol XL, (glipizide*) Glynase (micronized glyburide)	Take before a meal	Stimulate your pancreas to release more insulin both right after a meal and then over many hours	Combine well with other groups of diabetes pills Because they cause more insulin to be made, they can lead to blood glucose levels that may be too low
			continued on next page

* Generic available

TABLE 13-1 **Diabetes Pills** *(continued)*

Diabetes Pills	How to Take	How They Work	Characteristics
Meglitinides Prandin (repaglinide) **D-Phenylalanine Derivatives** Starlix (nateglinide)	Both should be taken with meals; if you skip a meal, skip the dose	Stimulate your pancreas to release more insulin right after a meal	Work quickly when taken with meals to reduce high blood glucose levels Less likely than sulfonylureas to cause low blood glucose
Biguanides Gluocophage Riomet (metformin liquid) GlucophageXR (metformin extended release) Fortamet (metformin extended release) Glumetza (metformin extended release)	Glucophage and Riomet: usually taken twice a day, with breakfast and the evening meal GlucophageXR, Glumetza, and Fortamet: once a day, with the evening meal	Reduce the amount of glucose your liver releases between meals	Do not cause weight gain and may promote small amount of weight loss; do not cause low blood glucose; may reduce cholesterol and triglycerides
Thiazolidinediones Actos (pioglitazone); Avandia (rosiglitazone)	Usually taken once a day; take at the same time each day	Make your body more sensitive to the effects of insulin	Increase the amount of glucose taken up by muscle cells and keep your liver from overproducing glucose; may improve blood fat levels
Alpha-glucosidase Inhibitors Precose (acarbose); Glycet (miglitol)	Take with first bite of the meal; if not eating, do not take	Slow the absorption of carbohydrate into your bloodstream after eating	Taken with meals, thus limiting the rise of blood glucose that can occur after meals; do not cause low blood glucose

continued on next page

Diabetes Pills	How to Take	How They Work	Characteristics
Combination Pills Avandamet (rosiglitazone and metformin) Glucovance (glyburide and metformin) Metaglip (glipizide and metformin)	Check with your doctor—usually taken once a day	Combine the actions of each pill	May decrease the number of pills you need to take (Some combination tablets may lead to low blood glucose levels if one of the included medications has this effect)

How to Take Diabetes Pills

Here are some important tips to follow, regardless of what diabetes pill or pills you take:

- Follow your meal plan and physical activity program. They are essential for your diabetes pills to work most effectively.

- Take the right dose.

- Take it at the right time. Most pills are to be taken before a meal or with the first bite of a meal. Glucotrol is the only exception—it works best when taken 30 minutes before a meal.

- If you miss a dose, write it in your logbook so that you will know why your blood glucose was high later. DO NOT take an extra dose unless your doctor has told you to do so.

- Do not change how many pills you take without asking your doctor. Your risk of side effects can increase.

- Check your blood glucose at the times specified by your healthcare providers. If your blood glucose or hemoglobin A1C is within target, the dose is working. If not, check whether you have been eating the right amount and types of food or whether you have forgotten to take the right amount of diabetes pills. If your blood glucose remains high for more than a week, contact your healthcare provider. A change in dosage may be needed.

- Do not take any pills that are past the expiration date.

- If you are pregnant or are planning to be, talk to your doctor to discuss a change in your diabetes medication. Diabetes pills should be discontinued before becoming pregnant. Insulin may need to be substituted for the diabetes pills.

- Always inform all your healthcare providers about all the medications you are on. While most medications interact safely with diabetes pills, some can interfere with how your diabetes pills work. A change in the dose of your diabetes pill may be needed.

- Call your healthcare provider if your blood glucose levels are consistently low. If there is an increase in your activity level or a reduction in your weight or calorie intake, pill dosage may need to be changed.

Side Effects

Because the various diabetes pills work differently, the side effects are also different. Some of these are listed below. Note that many are common symptoms with many possible causes, so it is usually best to check with your healthcare provider before assuming that your medication is to blame for side effects.

Special Circumstances

There are special considerations with many of the diabetes pills. Summarized below are important tips to follow when using some of the pills currently on the market.

Actos, Avandia. To determine whether your liver is affected by the pills, your doctor will check your liver functions before you begin taking Avandia or Actos, and periodically thereafter. It is important to contact your doctor if you have the following symptoms: nausea, vomiting, fatigue, loss of appetite, or dark urine. Avandia and Actos may increase the risk of pregnancy in some premenopausal women unless adequate contraception is used. Discuss birth control methods with your healthcare provider.

TABLE 13-2   Side Effects of Diabetes Pills

Generic Name (Brand Name)	Main Side Effects	How to Prevent or Reduce the Side Effects
Glyburide (Diabeta) Glyburide (Micronase) Glyburide (GlynasePres Tab) Glipizide (Glucotrol) Glipizide GITS (Glucotrol XL) Glimepiride (Amaryl)	Low blood glucose Occasional skin rash; irritability Upset stomach	Follow your meal plan and activity program. Call your healthcare provider if your blood glucose levels are consistently low. If there is an increase in your activity level or a reduction in your weight or calorie intake, the dose may need to be changed.
Nateglinide (Starlix) Repaglinide (Prandin)	Effects of pills diminish quickly and they must be taken with each meal; may cause low blood glucose	Follow your meal plan and activity program, and call your healthcare provider if either changes.
Metformin (Glucophage)	Can cause appetite loss, nausea, abdominal pain, vomiting, mild diarrhea, and upset stomach (usually only within the first 1–2 weeks of starting) Hypoglycemia is not likely to occur when metformin is taken alone. In rare cases, lactic acidosis may occur in people with abnormal kidney or liver function	As above. Always tell people who may be treating your liver or kidney problems or performing tests or medical procedures on you that you take metformin, as it might need to be stopped if liver or kidney complications occur (see below).

continued on next page

TABLE 13-2   Side Effects of Diabetes Pills *(continued)*

Generic Name (Brand Name)	Main Side Effects	How to Prevent or Reduce the Side Effects
Pioglitazone (Actos) Rosiglitazone (Avandia)	May cause swelling (edema) or fluid retention, small amounts of weight gain, headache, backache, fatigue, and, rarely, shortness of breath May worsen heart failure	Talk with your healthcare provider and have your liver function tests done the recommended intervals. Contact your healthcare provider if you have the following symptoms: nausea, vomiting, fatigue, loss of appetite, shortness of breath, severe edema, or dark urine.
Acarbose (Precose) Miglitol (Glycet)	Gas, diarrhea, stomach upset, abdominal pain	Side effects should disappear over a few weeks. If not, call your healthcare provider.

Glucophage. Take with meals, once, twice, or up to three times a day. There are situations in which it is important to temporarily stop taking Glucophage, because it may affect your kidneys or liver function. Your doctor may have you stop taking Glucophage when you are severely ill, such as when you lose a lot of body fluid, or when you are going to have any surgery or special X-ray procedures that require an injection of iodine contrast dye.

Glucotrol. Take 30 minutes before mealtime. (Extended-release formulations can be taken with the meal.)

Prandin. Take it just before mealtime or up to 30 minutes before. If you skip a meal, skip your dose. If you add a meal, add a dose before that meal.

Precose. If used alone, Precose will not cause low blood glucose. However, low blood glucose can occur when Precose is combined with sulfonylurea pills, Prandin, or insulin. When low blood glucose does occur, treat it with 3 to 4 glucose tabs, glucose gel, or 10 to 12 ounces of milk rather than sucrose (table sugar), because Precose slows the absorption of sugar.

Combination Therapy

Knowing that type 2 diabetes is caused by multiple defects that lead to high blood glucose levels, you can see why a combination of diabetes pills may often be needed. Some healthcare providers may start by prescribing the combination pills listed in Table 13-1. Or your doctor may start with one type of diabetes pill, and if your blood glucose goals are not met, rather than increase the dose of that pill, add a second one. Still other doctors will ask you to start with a combination of diabetes pills that are not already combined.

Remember, the goal is to help you achieve an A1C level of less than 7 percent. Most pills will lower the A1C about 1 percent—some less, and some more. However, if you have made all the lifestyle changes you can make and your A1C is still 9 percent, for example, it is unlikely that one medication alone will successfully lower your A1C. In this case, your doctor may start with one type of diabetes pill but quickly add another if your glucose goals aren't met. Or your doctor may decide to start your treatment program with a combination of diabetes pills. On the other hand, if your A1C is 8 percent, you may be able to meet your target goals with one pill and lifestyle changes.

When A1C levels are nearer to 10 percent, your doctor may suggest the use of three diabetes pills. The disadvantages to this approach are the expense and the potential for side effects. Your doctor may therefore recommend adding insulin to your treatment program. An injection of insulin may be given at night and diabetes pills used during the day.

Incretin Mimetics

As this book went to press, the first of a new class of diabetes medications received FDA approval for use and was being introduced into the market. The medication group, known as the **incretin mimetics** or just **incretins**, help stimulate the pancreas to make more insulin. However, unlike the medications discussed above, these may better coordinate the balance between the incoming glucose from meals and the amount of insulin that is secreted. Some of these medications may also help reduce the appetite. One group, a synthetic version of the naturally occurring hormone GLP-1, has to be injected, although long-acting formulations are being worked on so that the injections may not have to be frequent.

The first specific medication in the new class, exenatide (Byetta), has just been approved for use. This medication comes in a pre-filled pen device and is injected twice daily, usually before breakfast and dinner.

Exenatide is recommended for use by people with type 2 diabetes who are taking metformin or a sulfonylurea or a combination of the two and are not achieving adequate glucose control. The most common side effect has been nausea. Exenatide should not be used by anyone with severe kidney or gastrointestinal problems and it is not approved by the FDA for use in children.

Other New Treatments on the Horizon

Other medicines are being developed that work to increase the secretion of insulin by mechanisms similar to the incretins and are likely to be available in the near future. One such group, the DPP-IV inhibitors, may be given in pill form. Although easier to take than the injected GLP-1 inhibitors described above, this group seems not to have the effect of reducing appetite.

Another new group of medications is similar to the **thiazolidinediones** (Actos, Avandia) in their effect on glucose. However, they may also have the added beneficial effect of improving the lipids (blood fats). At present, this group of medications is referred to as Dual PPARs.

Actual medication types with brand names exist for some of these new treatments, but because FDA approval is pending, we cannot provide specific information. Joslin's website (www.joslin.org) will provide further information if and when these medications become available.

You can see that there are a lot of treatment options available today, with more on the horizon. Type 2 diabetes requires aggressive, multicomponent treatments to reduce the risk of complications. And always remember, diabetes pills work better when you also follow your eating and physical activity programs.

CHAPTER 14

Insulin Basics

Scientists tend to use the word *breakthrough* sparingly, saving it for the most remarkable advances. But the discovery of insulin in the past century can be categorized as a breakthrough—one of the greatest medical achievements of all time. Insulin has saved and improved the lives of millions of people with diabetes who cannot produce enough insulin to meet their body's needs. If you are among that group, insulin is prescribed to help restore and maintain normal blood glucose levels. Used in conjunction with meal planning and physical activity, insulin can improve the quality of your life immeasurably.

The Story of Insulin

Insulin is a hormone manufactured by the beta cells in the islets of Langerhans in the pancreas. Insulin *treatment* has only been available since shortly after its discovery in 1921. Before then, many people died from diabetes, or, if they had type 2 diabetes, they lived for a number of years but functioned very poorly. But thanks to the efforts of two Canadian doctors, Frederick Banting and Charles Best, insulin was extracted from the pancreases of animals and injected into other animals that had diabetes, with dramatically successful results. Within a year, insulin was being used to treat humans.

Over the years, several changes have occurred in the way insulin is manufactured. It was initially extracted from cattle or pig pancreases, and was often a mixture of the two. For most users, animal-based insulin was quite acceptable. But some people experienced side effects from these early insulins because of impurities, and allergies because the insulin was from animals. These allergic responses could vary from a slight redness and itching to considerable swelling and pain at the injection site. Most users' immune systems perceived the insulin as a foreign substance, and their bodies responded by making antibodies to counteract it. Some people who had this reaction developed resistance to the action of insulin and required unusually large doses of it. However, for most, the antibodies could affect how effective the insulin was, causing its action to be less predictable. Over time, manufacturers were able to develop ways to remove most of the impurities from animal insulin. Highly purified animal insulin became available, and side effects were significantly reduced.

In the early 1980s, scientists revolutionized the production of insulin further by developing synthetic *human insulin*. Because it is produced through genetic engineering and is not taken from animals, it is identical to insulin produced by the human body. This makes its structure identical to that which a person's own pancreas would make if it could. In addition, concern had been expressed that there could be a shortage of animal-source insulin if an alternative were not available. The development of human insulin guaranteed there would be sufficient insulin supplies to all in need of it.

Insulin analogs are the most recent advance in the manufacturing of insulin, and these allow the design of insulin-replacement treatment programs that come very close to mimicking the normal patterns of insulin secretion in someone who does not have diabetes.

Insulin Therapy

Because the goal of insulin therapy is to mimic how the body would naturally produce insulin, it is useful to think about how normal insulin secretion occurs. Before you had diabetes, your blood glucose levels were maintained within the normal range by a slow, continuous secretion of natural insulin from the pancreas into the blood—this continuous secretion is called the *basal* insulin supply. It kept your glucose level within the normal range of approximately 70 to 140 mg/dl (or 70 to 100 mg/dl before a meal). And when you needed extra insulin, such as at meals, the pancreas provided additional bursts. This extra insulin, when given as an injection, is often referred to as a *bolus* of insulin. Through this coordination of basal and bolus insulin secretion, insulin levels in your blood were regulated automatically.

Now that you have diabetes, the match between injected insulin and your body's needs is not as finely tuned as it was when your pancreas was working normally. With injected insulin, your insulin needs may not always coincide with the pattern or the amount of the injection.

The difficulty of matching injected insulin with your body's needs is caused by many factors, such as the type of insulin, the injection site, the depth of the injection, and even the temperature of the skin and the surrounding air. Variations in your meals—including the time at which you eat and the amount and type of food eaten—also contribute to a mismatch. Changes in physical activity and other events in your life—stress, illness, infections—have an impact on your body's need for insulin as well.

Despite these difficulties, the key to insulin therapy is to design treatments that replace insulin in a manner that resembles the way the body normally produces it. The goal is to keep your blood glucose levels as close to normal as possible, over the course of the day and night. Throughout the decades since the discovery of insulin, much of the effort in insulin-production technology has been to develop newer insulins that could accomplish this more effectively. Fortunately, today we have more insulin options and ways of delivering the insulin—including *insulin pumps*—than ever before. You and your healthcare providers can develop a daily insulin plan that fits your meal plan and activity patterns. However, you must be an active participant.

- The first step is that you must communicate with your healthcare providers so that they understand what your usual eating and activity patterns are. This is essential for them in developing an insulin plan for you.

- The second step requires that you actively check your blood glucose, record the numbers in your logbook with other important information, and discuss it with your healthcare provider or diabetes team. This information is also essential in developing the insulin plan.

- Once you have an insulin plan, you must continue to check your glucose and make adjustments in insulin doses to accommodate daily variations in life events that can affect glucose levels, such as the food you eat and your physical activity.

Facts About Insulin

To manage your diabetes effectively, you need to understand some basic facts about insulin:

- Insulin must be injected—it cannot be taken orally (by mouth) because it is digested in the stomach juices, which destroy its effectiveness.

- Insulin is measured in *units*, often designated by the letter *U*. Most insulin used today is *U-100*, which designates a concentration of 100 units of insulin per milliliter (ml) of volume. In the past, concentrations such as U-40 were used. The difference between these insulins is one of concentration, not strength of the unit—a unit is always a unit. People living in or traveling to other countries may find another strength of insulin called U-40. If you have to use U-40 insulin, you must use U-40 syringes, and not your usual U-100 syringes. U-500 is available for people with extreme insulin resistance. At the other end of the spectrum, some children may require very small amounts of insulin. Insulin can be diluted to U-10, U-25, or U-50 by using a diluting fluid obtained from the insulin manufacturer. Table 14-1 can be used as a guide if you are in a location where the insulin does not match your syringe. However, you should obtain the correct syringe as soon as possible to reduce the chance of dosing errors.

- The proper syringe must be used to measure the correct dose. For example, a U-100 syringe must be used to measure units of U-100 insulin.

- If you take 30 units or less of insulin at a time, you can use the $^3/_{10}$-cc syringe. The $^1/_2$-cc syringe may be used if you take 50 units or less, and the 1-cc syringe is designed for those needing up to 100 units of insulin. If your insulin needs have been increasing, you might want to buy syringes that give you an opportunity to increase your dose if needed. Using a syringe that more closely matches your insulin dose helps you more accurately draw up your insulin.

- If you change the syringe you use, check dosage lines carefully. In some syringes, one line is equal to one unit of insulin, but in others, each line is equal to two units of insulin.

- There are different *types* of insulin: rapid-acting, short-acting, intermediate-acting, long-acting peaking, and long-acting peakless. These types of insulin vary in three important ways, all related to *time:*
  - *Onset*—how quickly the insulin starts to work
  - *Peak activity*—when the insulin works the hardest
  - *Duration*—how long the insulin continues to work

TABLE 14-1	Use of Syringes That Do Not Match the Insulin Being Used	
If your insulin is:	And your syringe size is:	Then if you draw up one unit of liquid in the syringe, it contains (units) of insulin
U-100	U-40	2.5
U-100	U-80	1.25
U-500	U-100	.5
U-40	U-100	.4
U-80	U-100	.8
U-40	U-80	.5

- Different companies make different brands of insulin. Always use the same brand and type of insulin that your healthcare provider has prescribed.

Types of Insulin

When insulin was first made available, only one type existed. It was short-acting (called regular), working over a brief period of time without much variation. The standard treatment was to take several injections a day. Later, other types became available that provided longer duration of action. The modern equivalent of these longer-acting insulins is what we call intermediate-acting insulins (NPH and lente), which were designed in hopes of decreasing the number of daily injections. This goal may not always have been wise medically, but the development of these newer insulins has led to the modern array of insulins that do allow more accurate mimicking of natural patterns of insulin action than in earlier years. Among today's insulins, the major difference is the timing of their action.

Please note that the times listed in the following discussion of each of the insulins are *ranges*. Timing actually varies from person to person. Table 14-2 summarizes the onset, peak activity, and duration of the insulins commonly used today.

Figure 14-1 depicts when the different types of insulin are at their peak and how long they last (duration). You can refer to it as you read the following insulin descriptions.

Figure 14-1   Insulin Action Chart

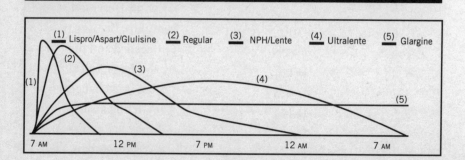

TABLE 14-2	Onset, Peak, and Effective Duration of Current Insulins		
	Onset	Peak	Effective Duration
Rapid-acting aspart (Novolog) lispro (Humalog) gluisine (Apidra)	10 to 30 minutes	½ to 3 hours	3 to 5 hours
Short-acting Regular	30 to 60 minutes	1 to 5 hours	8 hours
Intermediate-acting NPH Lente	 1 to 4 hours 1 to 4 hours	 4 to 12 hours 4 to 15 hours	 14 to 26 hours 16 to 26 hours
Long-acting, peaking Ultralente	4 to 6 hours	8 to 30 hours	24 to 36 hours
Long-acting, peakless glargine (Lantus)	1 to 2 hours	Flat, basal-like	24 hours

Rapid-Acting Insulin

There are now three FDA-approved rapid-acting insulins:

- lispro (Humalog)
- aspart (Novolog)
- glulisine (Apidra)

These are rapid-acting analog insulins, made by changing one amino acid in their chemical structure. Analog insulins are in a clear solution; they begin to work about 10 to 30 minutes after they are injected, peak in about an hour, and continue to work for about 3, possibly up to 5, hours. All rapid-acting insulins should be injected immediately before a meal. In fact, meals should NOT be delayed if you have injected one of these insulins. Because these insulins leave the bloodstream quickly, snacks are not needed and there is less chance of low blood glucose several hours after a meal. They are all quite similar in their activity. However, you should not use them interchangeably unless advised to do so by your doctor. Sometimes rapid-acting insulins may be given *after* meals for some children, because what they are going to eat is often difficult to predict before meals. People who have *gastroparesis,* a type of diabetic neuropathy that affects the digestive system, may also benefit from taking rapid-acting insulin after a meal rather than before.

Short-Acting Insulin

The common form of short-acting insulin is called *regular* (Humulin R and Novolin R), and it also comes in a clear solution. It usually begins working 30 to 60 minutes after being injected. It works hardest 1 to 5 hours after the injection and is completely gone after 6 to 8 hours. The larger the dose of regular insulin, the longer the duration of action.

The peak of regular insulin occurs about 3 hours after injection, which is somewhat later than the half-hour to one-and-a-half-hour time frame during which glucose rises after eating. Because of its delay in onset and late peak after the meal, regular insulin should be injected at least 30 minutes before a meal. To prevent low blood glucose levels when it peaks, snacks are often needed.

Intermediate-Acting Insulin

The intermediate-acting insulins are *NPH* (Humulin N and Novolin N) and *lente* (Humulin L, Novolin L). They begin to work within 1 to 4 hours after injection, reach their peak in 4 to 15 hours, and may continue to work for up to 14 to 26 hours after injection. NPH stands for neutral protamine hagedorn. Protamine is a protein that when added to regular insulin delays the insulin's absorption from under the skin, making it work over a longer period of time. Hagedorn is the name of the person who developed this type of insulin. *Lente* means "slow" and is made by adding zinc to regular insulin, which forms crystals that slow the rate of its absorption into the bloodstream, prolonging its action. Both NPH and lente have a cloudy appearance.

Long-Acting Peaking Insulin

Ultralente (Humulin U) is a long-acting insulin that doesn't begin working until 4 to 6 hours after injection. It has a relatively low, prolonged peak, which occurs 8 to 30 hours after injection, and continues to work for up to 24 to 36 hours. While it does have a peak, its peak is quite blunt and, when given before breakfast and before dinner, can produce a basal effect. Ultralente, which is also made by adding zinc to prolong its activity, is a cloudy solution. Ultralente, which is considered a long-acting insulin, may be absorbed at different rates in different people. For some people, therefore, ultralente functions as intermediate-acting insulin, while for others it is long-acting.

Long-Acting Peakless Insulin

Efforts to develop insulin analogs that mimic natural insulin action patterns have produced a more effective basal insulin, glargine, that is essentially peakless. It's release pattern from the injection site is smooth and continuous, lasting up to 24 hours. And although it provides a long-lasting effect, insulin glargine's onset is relatively rapid. The good news is that it has a flat action profile that effectively mimics the basal effect of natural insulin. Another advantage of glargine is that it can lower fasting (morning) glucose levels without causing overnight low blood glucose.

Insulin glargine is the only insulin used to provide a basal insulin supply, either intermediate-acting or long-acting, that is clear in appearance. However, insulin glargine must NOT be mixed with any other type of insulin. Because insulin glargine has no peak, injections of rapid-acting insulin must be given before all meals, and sometimes before snacks, to provide bolus coverage for food intake. Both types of insulin are clear in appearance, so it is very important that you choose the correct dose from the correct vial. (Insulin glargine comes in a bottle with a different shape and a different-color cap in order to prevent confusion.)

Insulin glargine can be injected at any time during the day, as long as it's the same time each day. Usually, however, it is given at bedtime. Insulin glargine is used as part of a treatment program aimed at mimicking normal insulin action patterns for persons with either type 1 or type 2 diabetes. The duration of action may be shorter in young children, who may require twice-daily injections.

Another long-acting analog with basal action characteristics, called *insulin detemir*, was just approved by the FDA as this book went to press. It should be on the market by the time this book is available. Its action profile is slightly shorter but more predictable than glargine. Differences in usage will likely be determined once detemir has been made available and more general usage experience has been gathered.

Fixed Mixtures of Insulin

Premixed insulins are solutions of rapid-acting or short-acting insulin and NPH insulin. They are most commonly used by persons with type 2 diabetes who have difficulty mixing insulin. They may also be convenient for people whose diabetes control is stable with one of these combinations. The disadvantage is that the mixtures have a fixed ratio of the two insulins and daily adjustments are therefore difficult to make. They are usually not recommended for persons who can mix the insulin themselves and for whom flexibility is important. These would include:

- Children and adolescents
- Anyone with type 1 diabetes
- Thin (and thus more insulin-sensitive) people with type 2 diabetes
- Pregnant women

Exceptions to this list would be those who because of poor eyesight or dexterity may be more likely to make errors in preparing their insulin doses.

As of this writing, the following premixed solutions are available in the United States:

- 70/30, regular and NPH: 70% NPH insulin and 30% regular insulin
- 50/50, regular and NPH: 50% NPH insulin and 50% regular insulin
- 75/25, lispro and NPL: 75% insulin lispro protamine suspension (NPH-like) insulin and 25% insulin lispro
- 70/30, aspart and aspart protamine: 70% insulin aspart protamine suspension (NPH-like) and 30% insulin aspart

Future Insulins

The next stage of insulin development seems to be focused on how insulin is delivered. Inhaled insulins are actively being developed. While delivery of insulin by methods other than injection may have appeal, it remains to be seen how these newer products will be used in treatment.

Insulin Injections Using Syringes

To take insulin, you need to learn how to measure and inject a proper dose. Insulin is injected by means of syringes, insulin pens, and insulin pumps (discussed in Chapter 16). It is injected into subcutaneous fat, the fatty tissue just beneath the skin and above the layer of muscle. Disposable syringes and needles are commonly used. The disposable plastic syringes cannot be boiled to sterilize and usually come with preattached needles that are extremely fine, ranging in gauge from 29 to 31. The higher the gauge number, the thinner the needle.

Injection Techniques

Proper technique is important. Insulin injection techniques are illustrated in Figures 14-2 and 14-3.

The following tips will help make injecting insulin easier:

- To avoid infection, be sure the skin at or around the injection site is clean. Wipe your skin with an alcohol swab or wash the area with soap and water.

- Pinch some skin and tissue firmly, but not too tightly, between the thumb and one finger of one hand, holding the syringe like a pencil in the other hand. A good amount of skin and tissue beneath the skin should be included in this grasp so that the injection will be well beneath the surface of the skin.

- Push the needle straight into the skin (at a 90-degree angle) and push the plunger down. Let go of the pinch and pull the needle out.

Figure 14-2

Single Dose

1. Wipe off top of bottle with alcohol swab (cotton and alcohol).

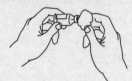

2. Roll bottle upside down and sideways between hands. Clear insulins do not need to be rolled.

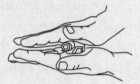

3. Pull plunger of syringe to number of units of insulin you should inject.

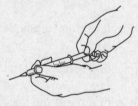

4. Put needle through top of insulin bottle and push plunger down. This puts air into the bottle of insulin.

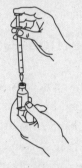

5. With needle still in bottle, turn bottle upside down.

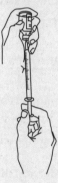

- If injecting an arm, the grasp can be simulated by pushing your arm against a solid object, such as the top of a chair or the edge of a door, to push up the skin.

- Do not be concerned if a small amount of blood appears after the needle is withdrawn. Simply press the spot gently and briefly with cotton.

- Air bubbles can be avoided by rolling the bottle of cloudy insulin gently between the palms of the hands for mixing. Do not shake the in-

6. Pull plunger halfway down to fill the syringe with insulin. Check syringe for bubbles. If you do not see bubbles, push plunger to number of units of insulin you should inject. Remove needle from bottle.

If you see air bubbles, push all of the insulin back into the bottle. Then do Step 5 and Step 6 again.

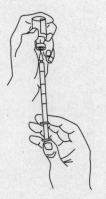

8. Pinch skin, pick up syringe like a pencil, and push needle straight into skin. Push plunger down.

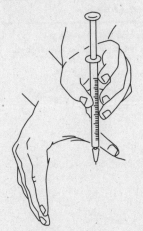

9. Let go of skin and pull needle from skin.

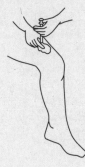

7. Wipe skin with alcohol swab.

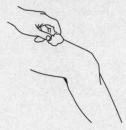

sulin bottle to mix (clear insulin does not need to be mixed). An air bubble is nothing to worry about because insulin is injected into fatty tissue, not into a vein. However, air bubbles can reduce the quantity of insulin injected.

■ Insulin should be injected into subcutaneous fatty tissues. If insulin is injected too deeply and into muscle or a blood vessel, it is absorbed more rapidly. If the injection is too superficial, absorption will be slower and less predictable and could result in high blood glucose.

Figure 14-3

Mixed Dose

1. Wipe off top of bottles with alcohol swab (cotton and alcohol).

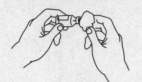

2. Roll cloudy bottle between hands.

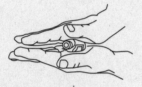

3. Pull plunger of syringe to number of units of cloudy insulin you should inject.

4. Put needle through top of cloudy insulin bottle. Keeping bottle upright on table, push plunger down, putting air into bottle. Take needle out. Syringe should be empty.

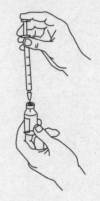

5. Pull plunger of syringe to number of units of clear insulin you should inject.

The following are guidelines for mixing insulin:

- Wipe off the tops of bottles of insulin with an alcohol swab.
- If using NPH or lente, roll the cloudy bottle of insulin between the hands, then inject air first into the cloudy bottle, then into the clear one.
- Draw the clear insulin into the syringe first. (Remember, the clear insulin glargine cannot be mixed with other insulins.)
- Be sure to eliminate all air bubbles in the syringe before injecting.

6. Put needle through top of clear insulin bottle. keep bottle upright on table. Push plunger down.

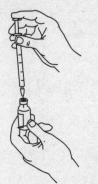

8. Pull plunger out about 10 units past the number of units of clear insulin you should inject. Check insulin in syringe for bubbles. If you do not see bubbles, push plunger to number of units of clear insulin you should inject. Remove needle from bottle.

If you see bubbles, push all of the insulin back into the bottle. Then do Steps 5–8 again.

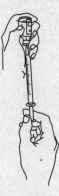

7. Leave needle in clear bottle and turn bottle upside down.

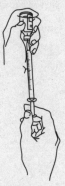

(Continued)

- It is important to inject a mixture within 5 minutes if you are mixing.
  - Insulin lispro, insulin aspart, and insulin glulisine start to bind to the longer-acting insulin after they have been mixed in a syringe for 5 minutes. These mixtures should not be held for longer than 5 minutes.
  - Syringe can be prefilled. However, because regular insulin begins to bind to the longer-acting insulin after it has been mixed for 5 minutes, it is important to be consistent with the use of premixed insulin. The binding goes on for 24 hours, during which time the insulin's action is unpredictable. If you are pre-

Figure 14-3 *(continued)*

9. Turn cloudy bottle upside down. Put needle through top of bottle.

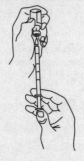

10. Pull plunger slowly to the number of total units of clear and cloudy insulins you should inject. Remove needle from bottle.

11. Wipe skin with alcohol swab or wash the area with soap and water.

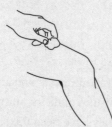

12. Pinch skin, pick up syringe like a pencil, and push needle straight into skin. Push plunger down.

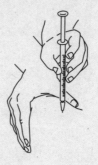

13. Let go of skin and pull needle from skin.

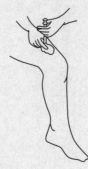

filling syringes, always wait 24 hours after mixing before injecting that insulin.

- Do not mix glargine in the same syringe with any other insulin.
- Refrigerated premixtures of regular and NPH insulin are stable for up to 21 days. Store syringes with needles pointing up, so suspended particles do not clog the needles.

- 75/25 insulin should not be prefilled.
- Do not premix and store regular and lente, or regular and ultralente.
- A prefilled syringe should be rolled between the hands before injecting.

Insulin Injections with Insulin Pens

Insulin pens provide a simple and convenient way to inject insulin, and their use is becoming increasingly popular. Disposable insulin pens are now available. Insulin pens are convenient, particularly when eating out or traveling, accurate, and helpful if you are on multidose insulin regimens. They are especially convenient for taking a mealtime insulin dose.

The insulin pen has two parts—the pen, which holds insulin, and the needle. Because the pens already contain insulin, the needles don't have to be used to puncture the rubber tops on insulin bottles, so they can be even finer than the needles used with syringes.

However, the pens can inject from only one cartridge of insulin. They can therefore be used to inject only one type of insulin or a premixed insulin. If you need two types of insulin, you must take two insulin pen injections. Nevertheless, because of the convenience and finer-gauge needles, many people still prefer this approach.

Pens are relatively simple to use. In general, they include a means by which to select the number of units of insulin (usually in the form of a dial) and a simple injection mechanism for pushing the insulin through the needle. Your healthcare providers can show you the different insulin pens that are available and demonstrate how to use them.

Injection Sites

Injections are given in places on your body where you have fatty tissue, including your abdomen, the top of the thigh, the back of the arm, and the hip and buttock area. An injection that contains one type of insulin is called a *single dose*. An injection of two insulins given in the same syringe at the same time is called a *mixed dose*.

Figure 14-4   Injection Sites

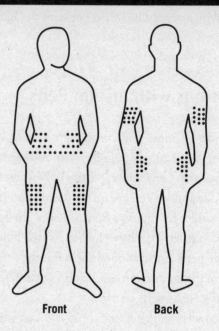

Front   Back

It is important to change, or rotate, the sites where you inject insulin. Repeated injections at the same site can cause fat to accumulate over time. Your skin can become bumpy, lumpy, or thickened, and your insulin will not be absorbed properly. The accumulation of fat reduces and delays the absorption of insulin. Sites are shown in Figure 14-4.

The speed at which insulin is absorbed into your body is different depending on where you inject it. Insulin is more rapidly absorbed by the abdomen, followed by the outer part of your upper arm, then the outer part of your thigh. It is absorbed most slowly from the hips and buttocks. (If your blood glucose is low, it is best to inject insulin into the thigh or buttocks and eat soon after.) An exception to this ranking of sites by absorption occurs with insulin glargine, as no significant differences in absorption between sites have been observed with its use.

For your body to absorb the insulin you inject in the same way each time, it may be helpful to rotate sites in a set pattern. Here are two rotation patterns for you to follow. Choose one that works for you.

Option 1: Choose a particular site for a particular injection time. For example, you may inject your morning insulin in your abdomen, your lunch insulin in your arm, and your dinner insulin in your thigh.

Option 2: Choose a site, such as the abdomen, and inject there for one month. Then move to a new site.

Tips for Injecting Insulin

- STOMACH: Stay at least two inches away from the navel or any scars you may already have when using the abdomen for injections.

- THIGH: Inject at least four inches, or about one hand's width, above the knee and at least four inches down from the top of the leg. The best area on the leg is the top and outer area of the thigh. Do not inject insulin into your inner thigh because of the number of blood vessels and nerves in this area.

- ARM: Inject into fatty tissue in the back of the arm between the shoulder and the elbow.

- BUTTOCK: Inject into the hip or "wallet area" and not into the lower buttock area.

- When rotating sites within one injection area, keep injections about an inch (or two fingers' width) apart.

- Do not inject into scar tissue or areas with broken vessels or varicose veins. Scar tissue may interfere with absorption.

- Massage or exercise that occurs immediately after the injection may speed absorption because of the increased circulation to the injection site. If you plan on strenuous physical activity shortly after injecting insulin, don't inject in an area affected by the exercise. For example, if you plan to play tennis, don't inject into your racket arm. If you plan to jog or run, don't inject into your thighs.

■   When using an insulin pen, inject straight in and be sure to hold the pen in place for a few seconds after the insulin is delivered to ensure that no insulin leaks out.

Taking Care of Insulin and Syringes

How Insulin Should Be Stored

Although manufacturers recommend storing your insulin in the refrigerator, injecting cold insulin can sometimes make the injection more painful. To counter that, you can store the bottle of insulin you are using at room temperature (59 to 86 degrees Fahrenheit) for about one month. Do not keep bottles in a hot place, such as near a heater or in direct sunlight. Also, do not keep them near ice or in places where the insulin may freeze.

If you buy more than one bottle at a time, store the extra bottles in the refrigerator. Then take a bottle out as necessary ahead of time so it is ready for your next injection. Unopened bottles are good until the expiration date on the box or bottle.

Do NOT use insulin after it has been kept at room temperature for longer than a month. Also, do not use insulin after the expiration date printed on the bottle. Examine the bottle closely to make sure the insulin looks normal before you draw it into the syringe. Insulin aspart, lispro, regular, and glargine should be clear and not cloudy. Check for particles or discoloration of the insulin. NPH, ultralente, and lente should not be "frosted" or have crystals in the insulin or on the insides of the bottle, or small particles or clumps in the insulin. If you find any of these in your insulin, do NOT use it. Return unopened bottles to the pharmacy for exchange or refund.

Syringes

Most people use plastic syringes, which are made to be used once and then thrown away. Some people use a syringe two to three times. If you reuse a syringe, follow these steps:

1. Flush the syringe with air to prevent the needle from clogging.
2. Do not wipe the needle with alcohol. This removes the Teflon coating.
3. Recap the needle when not in use.
4. Store the syringe at room temperature.
5. Keep the outside of the syringe clean and dry.
6. Throw the syringe away if the needle is bent or dull or if it has come in contact with any surface other than skin or the top of the insulin bottle.
7. Discard if the calibration lines are difficult to read from wear.
8. Be sure to check your skin around injection sites for unusual redness or signs of infection.
9. Never share syringes.
10. An insulin pen should never be stored with the needle still attached, as this can lead to insulin leakage and air in the cartridge.

How to Dispose of Syringes and Pen Needles

It is a good safety practice, and good for the environment, to dispose of syringes and lancets properly. The following are guidelines for proper disposal:

■ Dispose immediately after use into a heavy-duty, nonbreakable container—one that cannot be punctured—such as a coffee can or detergent container.

■ To decrease the chance that another person will use your syringe after you dispose of it, separate the plunger from the barrel. Do NOT recap, bend, or break needles.

■ When your disposal container is nearly full, it should be covered, taped, and labeled "contaminated." Dispose according to local and state medical waste rules. Each city and town has its own rules for throwing away used needles. Check with yours about throwing away your needles. If your town doesn't have specific rules, check with a local hospital. Do NOT put in recycle bins.

Insulin—A Wonderful Medication

Many people have difficulty accepting the fact that insulin must be injected. Physicians even use the possibility of insulin injections to threaten people with diabetes: "If you don't [fill in the blank with whatever is not being done], we will have to start insulin." It is thought of as a last resort: "We have tried *everything* that is available to control your diabetes. There is nothing else left. We *have* to start insulin."

Thinking of insulin in such a negative way is unfortunate. Insulin is an effective therapy for treating diabetes and preventing complications. If you have type 1 diabetes, you need it to survive. If you have type 2 diabetes, when your body is unable to make sufficient insulin, you need it to maintain good health. Healthcare providers should therefore really be saying: "Aren't we fortunate that we have insulin to treat you with now that other methods are no longer sufficient!" Remember, it doesn't mean your diabetes is worse—your body just needs some extra help from injected insulin. Almost everyone feels better after starting insulin. Indeed, it is very good news that insulin is available to control diabetes.

Authors' Note: As this book was going to print, we were notified that Eli Lilly would be removing the human insulins Lente and Ultralente from the market, as well as their purified animal-based versions of Regular and NPH. The reasons for taking these off the market include a decline in demand along with the increased availability of faster-acting human analog insulins. It is estimated that less than 2 percent of the 3.5 million people using insulin in the United States have been using the four insulins being discontinued.

It is not possible at this point to delete every reference to these two insulins (Lente and Ultralente) in the Joslin Guide, but please be aware that as of the end of 2005 they will no longer be available. In all cases, if you are using these insulins you should contact your healthcare providers for guidance. If you are using human Lente, you may be able to switch to human NPH without much difficulty, although it might be a good time to review your insulin program to make sure it is working as well as possible. If you are using Ultralente, you will need to adjust your insulin program, and may use this as an opportunity to change to one of the peakless basal insulins, glargine or detemir.

CHAPTER 15

Physiologic Insulin Treatment

For decades, *conventional insulin treatment* has been the usual program for people who need insulin. With this approach, the insulin regimen is decided first, and the person with diabetes has to eat and live according to the time actions of the injected insulins. Basically, people using this treatment program must live the same every day. *Physiologic insulin therapy*, however, operates from a different assumption—that your daily activity level, eating style, and metabolism are not always the same and that therefore insulin doses also need to change from one day to the next.

The goal of insulin therapy is to mimic the way the normal pancreas would respond to the body's need for insulin, and physiologic insulin therapy is an attempt to mimic normality as closely as possible. The term *physiologic* means that the program works similarly to the way the body would if it could. Physiologic insulin replacement programs have also been referred to as "intensive" insulin therapy, but the term *intensive* tends to put some people off. We now prefer physiologic. Achieving physiologic insulin replacement requires more frequent checks of your blood glucose, and more adjustments in your insulin dose or food intake than less physiologic programs. Other insulin program options are available but don't usually provide the flexibility that most individuals with diabetes need or desire.

Choosing an Insulin Program

In recent years, with better blood glucose monitoring and insulin injection tools, people have come to realize that conventional versus intensive therapy is not an either-or proposition. There is really a spectrum of degrees by which programs mimic natural, or physiologic, insulin patterns. Today, because of the range of insulin types available, many insulin programs can be developed for people with diabetes. The goal is to develop a program that works for you and keeps your blood glucose in excellent control. Ultimately, you should select the degree to which you need to be "physiologic" with your insulin treatment based on a review with your healthcare provider of the following issues:

■ **YOUR MEDICAL NEEDS.** The less able your pancreas is to secrete insulin, the more physiologic your replacement program should be. Certainly, people with type 1 diabetes would benefit from it, and many with long-standing, insulin-requiring type 2 diabetes would benefit from a more physiologic program.

■ **EXTRA WORK.** Are you willing and do you have the ability to do the extra work and perform the extra injections and monitoring needed to increase the physiologic nature of your treatment program?

■ **YOUR WILLINGNESS TO MAKE DECISIONS.** A physiologic insulin program requires not only that you do more blood glucose checks, but also that you use the information to make decisions about your insulin doses and food choices. How comfortable do you feel about learning to assess your diabetes control, looking at factors such as your insulin dose, food intake, activity, and timing and making these decisions on a daily basis?

■ **YOUR LIFESTYLE.** How much flexibility do you need or want in daily routines of eating, activity, and timing? If you have a relatively predictable life, with a fairly consistent daily schedule and activity level, a program that is less physiologic may provide you with adequate control. But if your lifestyle is more variable and not as predictable, a physiologic insulin program is likely to be better for you.

■ **SAFETY.** Some people have difficulties caused by wide swings in glucose levels. The more physiologic the replacement program, the more chance there is that they can control these wide swings more successfully.

As you read the following descriptions of insulin program options, think about which one would be best for your lifestyle and discuss it with your healthcare provider.

Initial Insulin Program for Type 2 Diabetes: One Late-Day Injection

Once it is determined that insulin therapy is needed for someone with type 2 diabetes, the decision must be made as to the design of the initial program. Often, an early sign that insulin is needed is the inability to make insulin in the quantity necessary to maintain glucose control throughout the day. A key indication of this is a rising fasting (first thing in the morning, before eating) glucose level—some people can still make enough insulin during the daytime, but nighttime becomes a problem. An important question for your healthcare provider is whether you can still manage to make enough insulin during the day so that you just need an insulin injection at night to help cover that morning level, or whether you need more than one daily injection, to cover the full 24-hour day.

For those who struggle with a high morning glucose level, the most common first step toward insulin therapy is the use of a late-day insulin injection, usually in combination with daytime diabetes pills. While these people are in the early stages of the decline of their pancreas's ability to make insulin, they still have insulin resistance and would thus be helped by pills. In this stage, mealtime insulin secretion remains sufficient to prevent a rise between a pre-meal glucose level and a post-meal level from being more than about 50 to 60 mg/dl.

Key reasons to use late-day insulin therapy:

- Maximized oral medication treatment
- A1C levels not at target
- Fasting glucose elevated (approximately 200 mg/dl or greater) but glucose levels often a bit better later in the day

For many years, a typical late-day insulin program used bedtime intermediate insulin (NPH or lente). The long-acting peaking insulin, ultralente, was another option. Alternatively, for people who have lots of insulin resistance and showed very high glucose levels following the larger evening meal, predinner premixed insulin could also be used. The clinical objective was to lower fasting glucose levels.

The newer, long-acting nonpeaking insulin analogs are changing things. Glargine (Lantus) and detemir (Levemir) are now other options. Glargine has often been used as the initial late-day therapy, given at bedtime. It is less likely to cause low blood glucose levels during the night than intermediate insulin, which can peak during that time. Yet it is usually very effective at controlling the fasting glucose elevations.

Longer-acting nonpeaking insulins provide basal insulin coverage for most of the day, and thus provide some additional insulin during the daytime, which is often beneficial. Individuals needing bedtime insulin treatment may have the most difficulty with controlling the fasting glucose level, but they may also often experience a less obvious reduction in the ability to secrete insulin throughout the daytime. However, if the fasting glucose is elevated but glucose levels drop later in the daytime, particularly when glargine is being used, then intermediate insulin at bedtime or premixed insulin at suppertime would be an alternative.

Of course, this approach would not work for people with type 1 diabetes, who are unable to make insulin day and night. They need a full-day insulin coverage program.

More Conventional, Multiple Fixed-Dose Insulin Replacement Programs

A program of two to three daily injections with the insulin dose remaining the same has traditionally been referred to as a conventional insulin replacement program. The insulins used may be mixtures of rapid or short-acting insulin with intermediate insulin, prepared by the individual or obtained as a premixed preparation. Doses are adjusted only for significant variations in food consumption, activity, or event timing. A set dose of insulin is injected according to anticipated insulin needs, and to keep everything in balance, regular eating habits and predictable levels of activity are required.

Is this possible? To some extent, and for some people, yes. Some people are able to maintain a predictable lifestyle. If so, a conventional insulin program can give good to excellent control of blood glucose. Achieving success requires that everything that happens to your body—your eating habits, activity level, and metabolism—is similar from day to day. The obvious disadvantage to this approach is lack of flexibility.

A discussion of how to make a decision as to what type of insulin program would be right for someone with type 2 diabetes can be found later in this chapter.

More Physiologic Conventional Insulin Programs

As stated earlier, the decision to use or not use a physiologic program is not an all-or-nothing issue. Conventional programs can be made more physiologic. Many refer to these programs as *intensified conventional insulin programs*. These treatments also use two to three daily injections, but, in contrast to some of the more physiologic insulin programs, they do not include an injection before every meal—lunchtime injections are usually not part of the program. However, they do begin to allow you to make daily decisions about your treatment. Adjustment guidelines for rapid-acting insulin doses given at meals—breakfast and dinner—are developed. If you plan to eat more or less than you usually do, you adjust the mealtime dose based on the adjustment guidelines. You may also adjust for activity variations, and be able to accommodate schedule changes, like a later dinner or sleeping in on a weekend.

Physiologic Insulin Programs

With physiologic insulin programs that are closest to natural insulin patterns, bolus (mealtime) and basal (background) insulins are used to mimic normal release of insulin from the pancreas.

Rapid-acting insulin or, occasionally, short-acting regular insulin is given before meals. These insulin doses are adjusted based on eating plans for carbohydrate-containing foods, activity changes, and glucose levels. They may also be altered for significant timing variations, but often these programs are more forgiving of variations in the timing of eating. Making these adjustments requires you to check your blood glucose frequently and vary your insulin doses accordingly.

In addition, some form of basal insulin, such as insulin glargine and, when available, other true basal insulins, is used. Multiple doses of intermediate-acting or ultralente given one or two times a day have also been used. Externally worn insulin pumps are another option. Pumps administer bolus doses of rapid-acting insulin before meals and provide a slow infusion of the same insulin to produce a basal effect. Pump therapy is discussed in Chapter 16.

Probably everyone who uses insulin could benefit from physiologic insulin therapy, particularly in light of the research findings of the DCCT, described earlier, which concluded that people with diabetes who keep their blood glucose levels as close to normal as possible dramatically reduce their risk of developing complications. In addition to providing insulin in a more natural pattern both day and night, physiologic insulin programs mimic two other important characteristics of a normal pancreas—the ability to sense blood glucose levels, and to respond with the right amount of insulin. The difference is that you have to check your blood glucose and "think" for your pancreas in order to decide what the right amount of insulin may be.

What Type of Insulin Therapy Is Best for You?

If you have type 2 diabetes, conventional therapy, with fewer daily dose adjustments and injections, which less closely mimics natural patterns, may be effective for you, particularly if your pancreas can still secrete insulin. However, such programs often do not work as well as they should, possibly because the body's cells have developed resistance to the action of the insulin. In such cases, the purpose of treatment is to provide the extra insulin the body needs to make up for this resistance. While you may ultimately benefit from a physiologic insulin program, if you are new to diabetes, you may just be trying to get the basics down. You may want to use one of the more conventional approaches before advancing to a more physiologic program.

If you have type 1 diabetes, you should definitely consider a physiologic insulin program. The only time a conventional insulin program is likely to work well for you is in the early stages of type 1 diabetes or during the remission ("honeymoon") stage, when your body is still able to secrete some of its own insulin. But eventually your body loses the ability to secrete insulin, and a physiologic insulin program more closely imitates the way a normal pancreas secretes insulin.

If you have an unpredictable lifestyle, regardless of the type of diabetes you have, you will benefit from a physiologic insulin program. Perhaps you change work shifts frequently or travel extensively, especially internationally. Or maybe your activity levels change hour by hour, or day by day. If so, you require a treatment program that is more adaptable to your changing routine.

Starting a Physiologic Insulin Program

The advantage of the basal/bolus approach using rapid-acting insulins such as lispro, aspart, and glulisine is that it allows for more frequent adjustments and therefore gives you maximum flexibility of lifestyle while maintaining your targeted glucose goals. Doses are adjusted based on anticipated carbohydrate intake, activity, and blood glucose levels.

Basal and bolus insulin needs each account for about one-half of your insulin requirements. If you are lean, your healthcare provider may start you with 0.3 to 0.5 units of insulin per kilogram (kg) of body weight per day. Half of this dose is basal insulin and half bolus insulin. Basal insulin is provided by a long-acting insulin. Today insulin glargine is commonly used; and detemir, recently released, is also likely to be widely prescribed. The basal insulin glargine is injected once a day. It can be given at any time during the day, but once that time has been decided on, it should be given consistently at that time. Bedtime is often convenient, although some individuals prefer breakfast, lunch, or even dinner. Detemir is also usually used once daily, either at dinner or bedtime. If the pre-dinner glucose target cannot be achieved, however, twice-daily detemir (morning and evening) is suggested. Generally, mixing detemir with other insulins is not recommended.

Glargine can NOT be mixed with other insulins and so must be injected separately. Glargine works well because it has a smoother action pattern than ultralente or the intermediate insulins. It has also proved to be effective in controlling morning (fasting) glucose levels and in reducing the risk of low blood glucose overnight. However, some individuals may use NPH or ultralente given twice a day for their basal insulin. The disadvantage of these insulins is that they have a peak and therefore don't provide the smooth action of true basal insulin.

Basal insulin doses are more important for initial control since they are responsible for overnight and fasting (morning) glucose levels. Therefore, when a new program is being started, these doses are usually adjusted first, followed by adjustments in bolus insulin doses. Fasting blood glucose and pre-meal blood checks are used to adjust basal insulin doses.

The second part of these programs is the rapid-acting insulin that is given at mealtimes based on planned carbohydrate intake. The calculation of the quantity of insulin needed to cover meals is often determined using the *insulin-to-carbohydrate ratio*, described in detail in Chapter 5. When beginning this type of insulin program, the bolus (mealtime) dose may be divided so that, of the insulin that is to be given as rapid-acting before meals, 40 percent is given at breakfast, 30 percent at lunch, and 30 percent at dinner. Insulin-to-carbohydrate ratios are used to fine-tune these doses. For convenience, the bolus insulin can be given by means of an insulin pen. While some individuals may use regular insulin for a bolus dose, its disadvantage is that it peaks after the post-meal glucose peak. The peak of the rapid-acting insulins is more likely to coincide with post-meal glucose peaks.

Figure 15-1 is a drawing of the effects of an insulin program made up of a mealtime rapid-acting insulin and one injection of glargine at bedtime.

To adjust bolus insulin doses, blood glucose is checked before a meal

Figure 15-1

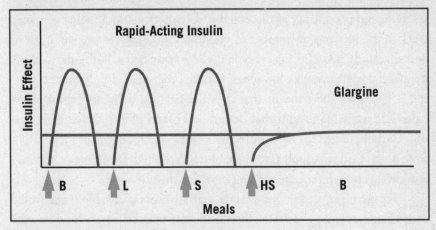

B=Breakfast; L=Lunch; S=Supper (dinner); HS=Bedtime

and two hours after the start of the meal. An appropriate blood glucose at this point would be 40 to 80 mg/dl above the glucose before the meal.

Correction or *sensitivity factors* can be used to further adjust mealtime insulin doses for a high or low blood glucose level. They are also described in detail in Chapter 5. However, it should be noted that physiologic insulin programs involve more than "fix the insulin dose" or "chase the numbers." There can be many reasons for blood glucose variability, and incorrect insulin doses are not the cause of all ills. For example, too low a blood glucose level can cause a *rebound hyperglycemia*. Seeing that your blood glucose is high may cause you to think you need to add more insulin, when in this case you may actually need less insulin. High and low blood glucose adjustments are discussed in the next chapters. To understand and interpret the factors affecting your glucose levels, blood glucose checks and record keeping are essential. Your logbook can provide clues to many factors that influence glucose control. If you feel puzzled about your glucose check results, be sure to bring your logbook to your next medical visit for discussion.

Insulin-to-Carbohydrate Ratios

Carbohydrate counting, as discussed in Chapters 4 and 5, helps you keep track of the servings or number of grams of carbohydrate you eat at meals and snacks. It is useful for everyone who has diabetes, but is particularly helpful if you are using a physiologic insulin program. Carbohydrate counting is based on the concept that it is the balance between carbohydrate eaten and available insulin that determines blood glucose levels after eating. Carbohydrates do have differing effects on blood glucose levels, but from a practical standpoint, counting total carbohydrate grams or servings is accurate enough for determining mealtime insulin doses.

For example, you might assume that a teaspoon of table sugar would make blood glucose rise faster than a slice of bread. In fact, however, the bread contributes about 15 grams of carbohydrate, while a level teaspoon of sugar contributes only 4 grams. The bread will therefore have about three times the effect on blood glucose as the table sugar. Of course, even though equal amounts of carbohydrate respond in about the same way if the two foods have equal amounts of carbohydrate, not all carbohydrates are equally healthy.

In order to determine what your bolus dose should be, it is helpful to have an insulin-to-carbohydrate ratio. This ratio tells you how much carbohydrate a dose of rapid-acting insulin, such as lispro, aspart, or glulisine, or short-acting, such as regular, will cover. The ratio is related to your degree of insulin sensitivity, and it varies from person to person. Your ratio may also be slightly different at different times of the day. For example, you may find you need more insulin for the same amount of carbohydrate you eat at breakfast compared to that same amount at lunch or dinner. Please refer to Chapter 5 for guidance on how to calculate your insulin-to-carbohydrate ratio and your sensitivity factor.

Starting an Insulin Program if You Have Type 2 Diabetes

People with type 2 diabetes who need insulin may start with one late-day injection, as discussed earlier, particularly if fasting glucose levels are elevated. Alternatively, full-day coverage may be needed from the start. So a key decision for you and your healthcare provider, once it is determined that insulin is needed, is whether to start with the once-daily late-day approach, or the full, multidose program. If you check your glucose levels at various times during the day, including pre- and post-mealtimes, and keep good records of the results, you will be providing the information that is needed to help you and your healthcare provider make the best possible decision about the initial insulin program.

If the late-day program is selected, intermediate-acting insulin or insulin glargine can be given at bedtime, or a fixed-mixture insulin such as 75/25 or 70/30 may be given at dinner, along with some or all of the daytime diabetes pills. Taking insulin later in the day helps control fasting blood glucose levels, while diabetes pills add to glucose control throughout the day. The late-day insulin dose often begins with 10 to 20 units and is then adjusted upward as needed based on your fasting blood glucose levels. A full, multidose insulin program is needed when your blood glucose levels remain above target throughout the day, especially if your blood glucose is high after meals. At this point, a conventional, an intensified conventional, or a physiologic insulin program is started.

A conventional insulin program may consist of mixed insulins, such as rapid-acting (lispro, aspart, or glulisine) or regular insulin and NPH, at breakfast and dinner—a premixed insulin may also be used. Another option is to move the NPH to bedtime and take only rapid-acting or regular insulin before dinner. Your healthcare provider may start with 0.5 to 0.7 units of insulin per kilogram of body weight per day. Two thirds of the total daily insulin is injected in the morning, and one third at night. Within each time (morning and evening), one third is rapid-acting or regular insulin, and the remainder intermediate-acting insulin. However, most individuals who are insulin resistant eventually require 1.0 to 1.2 units of insulin per kilogram of body weight per day.

Figures 15-2 and 15-3

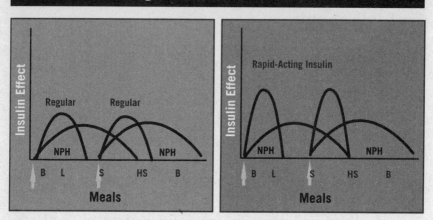

B = Breakfast; L = Lunch; S = Supper (dinner); HS = Bedtime

Figures 15-4 and 15-5

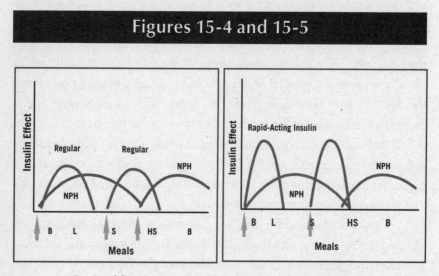

B = Breakfast; L = Lunch; S = Supper (dinner); HS = Bedtime

Figures 15-2 and 15-3 are drawings illustrating a conventional insulin program with either rapid-acting or regular insulin mixed with NPH injected before breakfast and dinner. Figures 15-4 and 15-5 are drawings of a conventional insulin program with either a rapid-acting or regular insulin mixed with NPH injected before breakfast, a rapid-acting or regular insulin injected at dinner, and NPH injected at bedtime.

Intensifying a Conventional Program

The next step occurs when a conventional insulin program is intensified. With this type of program adjustment, scales, called *algorithms,* for rapid-acting (lispro, aspart, or glulisine) or regular insulin are used. These algorithms are developed for you by your physician and tell you how to adjust your insulin depending on your blood glucose levels. The mealtime insulin doses for breakfast and dinner are adjusted according to actual glucose levels and according to planned food and activity and their timing. Compared with a fixed-dose program (which uses the same doses every day), this program is more effective and flexible because of the frequent blood glucose checks. However, your sliding scale is based on the assumption that you're eating a fixed amount of carbohydrate at each of your meals. The scale has a correction, or sensitivity factor built in to "correct" for high blood glucose readings. If you eat more carbohydrate at a meal, your post-meal blood glucose will likely be high. Some people who use a sliding scale and eat more carb on certain occasions, such as when dining out, may take more insulin than their usual dose. For example, for every additional 15 grams of carb eaten at a meal, a person may take one additional unit of insulin. Your healthcare team can help you determine how to safely take more insulin for extra carb eaten.

Generally, insulin doses should not be adjusted by more than two units at a time, and changes should not be made too often without a review by your healthcare provider. This program is similar to a physiologic insulin program. However, a true physiologic program requires rapid-acting or regular insulin doses with every meal, along with basal insulin or insulin pump therapy. Figure 15-6 is an example of an insulin algorithm that uses insulin doses before each meal.

Thus, to put this sequence into perspective, the first step in intensifying a conventional program might begin with bedtime insulin. Then, "conventional" therapy with two or three daily injections may come next. That can be intensified (made more physiologic) by using adjustable doses of rapid- or short-acting insulin (algorithms). A true physiologic insulin replacement program would use adjustable doses of rapid-acting insulin before *each* meal, with a basal insulin as background. Determining the doses of rapid insulin by an algorithm allows one to respond to the blood glucose

Figure 15-6

Insulin Dose Schedule For: _____

Date: _____ Patient Number: _____

SHORT (Regular) OR RAPID-ACTING INSULIN (Lispro / Aspart / Glulisine):

Blood Glucose	Breakfast	Lunch	Supper	Bedtime Snack
0–50	2	1	0	0
51–100	4	3	3	0
101–150	7	5	5	0
151–200	8	5	6	0
201–250	9	6	7	2
251–300	10	8	8	3
300–400	12	9	10	4
Over 400	14	10	12	5

Intermediate- or Long-Acting Insulin (NPH / Lente / Insulin Glargine or Detemir):   18

The above figure represents an insulin adjustment algorithm for a peakless insulin (detemir or glargine) program. (Similar algorithms are used for other intensive insulin programs.) Eighteen units of glargine are given at bedtime, while the blood glucose check results at the time of the injection determine the premeal regular or rapid-acting insulin dose.

level that was present at the time the insulin dose was taken, usually before meals. A further step is to use carbohydrate counting, which allows adjustments to be based on both the glucose level and the anticipated food intake.

Recently, a new medication, pramlintide (Symlin), has been introduced. This injectable medication, given with meals but separately from insulin, can help stabilize glucose patterns and reduce insulin doses for those having significant difficulty managing blood glucose levels with the usual insulin treatment techniques.

Before you decide which of these insulin programs is best for you, there is one more alternative. You may want to look into the advantages and disadvantages of insulin pumps. Pumps are discussed in the next chapter.

Remember, the overall goal is to work with your healthcare team to find an insulin program that works best for you. There are pros and cons to every program—the key is to choose one that will help you control your blood glucose and minimize your risk of complications. Your healthcare team is available to support you in whichever method you choose.

CHAPTER 16

Insulin Pumps

One of the major advances in diabetes treatment in recent years has been the evolution in insulin pump therapy. Insulin pumps are worn outside the body and release insulin into body tissues by way of tubing and a needle. The person using the pump must determine the proper insulin dose by checking his or her blood glucose, like someone on a physiologic insulin program does. Insulin pumps use only rapid-acting insulin, and doses are adjusted based on blood checks and determined using carbohydrate counting. The primary benefit of an insulin pump is that it permits the user a more flexible lifestyle than someone using injections.

Insulin pumps, however, require the greatest involvement of the person with diabetes and require mastery of blood glucose monitoring, carbohydrate counting, and adjustment of insulin for changes in activity, illness, and low or high blood glucose. Insulin pumps also require mastery of the mechanics of pump use. Pumps must be worn at all times. Stopping insulin delivery for more than one or two hours without substitute injections puts the user at risk for hyperglycemia (high blood glucose) and ketoacidosis.

How Do Insulin Pumps Work?

Insulin pumps are small mechanical devices, typically the size of a beeper or small cell phone. Insulin is contained in a reservoir, or syringe, inside the pump. The disposable insulin reservoir is regularly filled by the user and can hold up to 300 units of insulin. It is connected to plastic tubing called an *infusion set*. Infusion sets are changed every two to three days. Today's most common infusion sets use a guide needle for subcutaneous insertion, but only a soft, flexible *cannula* actually remains under the skin. The most common site for insertion of the infusion set is the abdomen, although the hip and thigh areas may also be used. Most infusion sets have a "quick release" feature that allows the user to easily disconnect from the pump for showering, exercise, or intimate moments.

Pumps deliver insulin similarly to physiologic insulin programs—in basal and bolus amounts. *Basal insulin* is delivered at a slow, continuous rate and is designed to mimic the basal insulin released by the pancreas normally. Basal insulin controls blood glucose in the fasting or pre-meal state. Basal rates, measured in *units per hour,* reflect the number of units of insulin infused over a one-hour period. They can typically vary from less than 0.4 units per hour to as much as 2 units per hour or more. Basal rates are typically programmed in 0.05-unit increases per hour. Pumps can be programmed to vary the basal insulin infusion rate for various time intervals over 24 hours. Typically, users require from two to four rates a day; it is unusual to require more than six or eight. For example, many adults and adolescents (but not children) require slightly more insulin at the end of the sleep cycle. This is a time when blood glucose tends to increase naturally and is called the *dawn phenomenon.* The pump can be programmed to cover the rise in blood glucose at this time.

Bolus insulin doses are larger bursts of insulin used to cover food and to correct high blood glucose. Bolus doses can be determined using insulin-to-carbohydrate ratios and sensitivity factors (see Chapter 5). They can be fine-tuned to 0.1 unit, and some pumps have features that can alter the way a bolus is delivered. For example, a *combination (dual) wave* or an *extended (square) wave* bolus may be used to cover foods that are higher in fat (high-fat foods may slow the digestion of a meal), or meals eaten over an extended period of time. An extended bolus can be programmed to deliver insulin over a designated period of time instead of all at once. This feature is useful when a person is eating over a long time, such as at a wedding.

Pumps release insulin into the body continuously, so people must check their blood glucose often to ensure the pump is being used safely and effectively. Only with frequent blood checks can a proper decision be made about the flow of insulin. Pumps may also be used with pramlintide (Symlin) injection therapy. Researchers are trying to develop an automatic pump that would be implanted in the body. Ideally, this system would measure the blood glucose level by itself and then inject the correct amount of insulin automatically. The user would not have to do regular blood checks or make adjustments to the pump.

Injections or Pump?

If you decide on physiologic insulin therapy, you have two basic options: multiple daily injections or the insulin pump. At first glance, the pump may look easier to use. But there are several factors to consider.

- Compared with a syringe or insulin pen, the pump is part of a more complex system, and it requires more frequent blood glucose checks. However, newer insulin pumps are easier to use than ever before. But because insulin is continuously infused into the body with the pump, if proper precautions are not taken, the risks of using a pump can be greater than those associated with injections.

- Finances may be a consideration as well. Some insurance plans will not cover some or any of the costs of pump therapy.

- Having adequate support from family or someone close who can help and provide support is a great benefit.

- You'll need to work very closely with your healthcare team to learn about the pump and fine-tune your basal and bolus doses. It's important that you have a diabetes team with whom you feel comfortable.

■ Be prepared to spend time "testing" basal and bolus doses, as well as keeping detailed records of your blood glucose levels, food intake, and activity. If you're not willing or make this commitment, a pump may not be the best choice for you.

The decision to use pump therapy should not be made lightly. Yet for people who decide to use a pump and do everything necessary to manage this approach, successful control usually results. Pumps come the closest to mimicking normal insulin patterns, so they can come close to providing normal blood glucose levels.

Too many people, however, make the mistake of thinking that a pump will allow them to abandon the other parts of their diabetes program, such as meal planning and physical activity. This is not true. They remain an essential part of your program. Although pump users will probably experience fewer high and low blood glucose levels, these will still occur. To successfully use an insulin pump requires extensive education. If you are thinking about it, you need to put some thought into the best time, considering events in your personal life, to begin the training for pump therapy. You must be committed to the time investment required to safely and successfully begin this new therapy.

Potential Problems with Pump Therapy

There are two main potential problems with pump therapy—infusion-site infections and unexplained hyperglycemia leading to diabetic ketoacidosis. With proper education, these risks can be virtually eliminated.

To prevent skin infections at the infusion site, the following guidelines should be followed:

■ Infusion sets should be changed every two to three days. The new set should be placed at least one inch from the previous site.

■ Hands should be washed and a clean working area used for the pump supplies when changing an insulin cartridge or infusion set.

- For most pump users, soap and water can be used to clean the skin prior to inserting an infusion set. For individuals who are prone to skin infections, an antiseptic cleanser should be used.

- Wipe the skin with an adhering agent with antibiotic properties such as IV Prep before inserting the infusion set.

- Infusion sets should feel comfortable at all times. If pain, discomfort, redness, warmth, or swelling occurs, the infusion set should be removed immediately and insulin taken by injection. If the area appears to be infected, a topical antibiotic should be applied. If there is no improvement in 24 hours, call your healthcare provider.

The second risk is ketoacidosis. Diabetic ketoacidosis (DKA) is discussed in more detail in Chapter 19. Since pumps use primarily rapid-acting (rarely regular) insulin alone, even a short interruption in delivery may lead to elevated blood glucose and ketoacidosis in a matter of hours. Any glucose reading greater than 250 mg/dl without a known association with food, stress, illness, or insulin omission should be treated promptly. Ketones should be checked in the urine or blood any time there is unexplained high blood glucose. If moderate to large ketones are present, you can assume that for some reason insulin was not delivered properly and supplemental insulin should be taken by injection, not by a pump bolus. Call your healthcare providers for instructions on what the insulin adjustments should be. Blood glucose and ketones should be rechecked every two to three hours and supplemental insulin taken until blood glucose levels are acceptable. If no ketones are present, a pump bolus can be used for the correction dose, but blood glucose should be checked in one to two hours to confirm that the glucose is decreasing and the problem is being resolved.

Sick-Day Pump Adjustment

Sick-day insulin guidelines for pump users are similar to sick-day guidelines for individuals using physiologic insulin programs. Sick days are discussed in Chapter 19. The key point is that you need more insulin during illness. Blood glucose should be checked every two to four hours, and ketones should be checked if your blood glucose is greater than 250 mg/dl. Discuss with your healthcare providers guidelines for adjusting insulin during illness. This is very important, as ketoacidosis can develop very quickly.

Pump Adjustments for Exercise

Because individuals' responses to exercise vary, trial and error is often the best way to determine how best to make changes. The point to remember is that insulin must be decreased to prevent hypoglycemia (low blood glucose). Basal rate adjustments and/or bolus adjustment may be needed depending on the timing of the exercise. The pump can be discontinued for a short time. This is particularly useful for strenuous exercise, contact sports, and water sports.

Keep in mind the lag effect of exercise, whereby hypoglycemia can develop after a prolonged period following exercise. A reduced basal insulin dose may be needed for an extended period.

Additional carbohydrate may be needed in addition to lower insulin doses. Extra carbohydrate combined with a reduction in or temporary suspension of basal infusion may be used for extremely strenuous exercise, for daylong events, or for exercise that has not been planned or compensated for in advance.

Going Off the Pump

You may decide to take a "break" from pump therapy for a number of reasons. Perhaps you'll be traveling for work, or going on vacation. While the pump is actually ideal for these situations, some people find it easier to go back to injections during these times. Or maybe your pump has malfunctioned and you have to send it back to the manufacturer to be repaired or to get a new one. Whatever your reasons, work closely with your healthcare team if you decide to take a "pump vacation." They'll help you determine the type and doses of insulin you'll need to take by injection (your "off pump" doses). The good news is that you can always resume pump therapy when you're ready.

What's Best for You?

There are many ways to use insulin, and you should work with your healthcare providers to identify the best program for you. Remember, the overall goal is to create a dosing schedule that works in concert with your meal plan and activity schedules. Not everyone can manage physiologic insulin programs. But research now demonstrates what diabetes specialists at Joslin Diabetes Center have been saying to their patients for nearly a century—if you keep your blood glucose as close to normal as possible, you can decrease your risk of complications.

If physiologic therapy is the best plan for you, it will take some effort to develop an effective routine. You will have to closely monitor your blood glucose, and you will need to learn carbohydrate counting and use it effectively. In addition, you need the support of a skilled healthcare team. Neither physiologic therapy nor pump therapy is a "solo act," and the information in these chapters covers the details of such programs only broadly. Furthermore, the benefits of physiologic insulin programs may take some time to achieve. In fact, your reward may be what *doesn't* happen. For example, your program may help you prevent a severe insulin reaction (low blood glucose). Or your reward may come even further in the future—the reduced risk of developing complications from diabetes. But whether your rewards come now or in the future, they can be great. And the feeling of success and good health can make all the effort worthwhile.

PART FOUR

Adjusting Your Treatment Program

CHAPTER 17

Adjusting for Low Blood Glucose (Hypoglycemia)

In treating diabetes, we usually think of trying to control *high* blood glucose. But at times, people with diabetes actually have more problems with *low* blood glucose, also called *hypoglycemia*. Low blood glucose is more likely to occur in people who use insulin or diabetes pills that stimulate insulin release, so the guidelines outlined below are more likely to apply to this group.

What Is Low Blood Glucose?

Generally, a blood glucose below 80 mg/dl with or without symptoms, or below 90 mg/dl with symptoms, is considered a *low blood glucose*. However, some people may be aiming for glucose control in which levels below 80 are common and deemed safe. Others may be at risk of significant difficulties from low blood glucose if they see values even higher than 80. Safety is really the key, and you should work with your healthcare team to decide what value should be considered a low glucose value for *you*.

Some people can tell their blood glucose is low simply by the way they feel. Some, however, cannot, and some may be able to determine that their blood glucose is low by how they feel at some times but not at others. Studies have proven that using how you "feel" is not always a reliable means of determining your blood glucose level. Therefore, it is important to confirm your blood glucose level by checking it.

Symptoms of Low Blood Glucose

Low blood glucose can occur suddenly. Early signs include shakiness, nervousness, sweating, dizziness, weakness, irritability, hunger, and heart pounding. Symptoms that develop more slowly include crying, anger, and drowsiness, confusion, staggered gait, inability to complete work, blurred vision, and headache. To others, you may seem to have an unsteady walk, have a glassy look to your eyes, show changes in your behavior, look pale, or seem unable to focus on a conversation.

Whenever you feel any of these problems coming on, you should check your blood immediately. Monitoring your diabetes, and its treatment, including blood glucose checking, is important because some of the symptoms of low blood glucose are similar to symptoms of high blood glucose and symptoms of medical conditions unrelated to diabetes. Also, be aware that some people who have had diabetes for a long time or who control their diabetes very tightly may lose the ability to recognize some of the symptoms. In such cases, extra caution—and monitoring—is very important. People with type 2 diabetes are less likely to experience low blood glucose levels, especially reactions that would cause one to become unconscious.

Once you know that your blood glucose is low, you should begin treatment right away to bring it back up into the normal range. If you allow low blood glucose levels to go untreated, more serious problems may develop—possibly even convulsions or unconsciousness.

Causes of Low Blood Glucose

The most common cause of low blood glucose is delayed or missed meals. Any time you reduce the amount of food you eat, or skip or delay a meal, you will have less glucose in your blood than if you had followed your meal plan. This creates a situation in which your body has too much insulin (either injected as part of your treatment, or stimulated by one of the pills that works to do so) for the amount of glucose in your blood. The insulin works on whatever glucose is already in the blood, causing it to drop to levels that are too low for you.

Another cause of low blood glucose is increased physical activity or unplanned activity without reducing your insulin or eating more carbohydrate. Physical activity lowers the amount of glucose in the blood; the more physical activity you engage in, the lower your blood glucose will drop. If you are taking insulin or pills that stimulate your pancreas to make more insulin, both of which lower blood glucose, increased physical activity on top of your usual dose, or without extra food to compensate, can lead to low blood glucose.

Low blood glucose can also be caused simply by taking too much insulin or too many of the diabetes pills that stimulate the pancreas to make more insulin. With more insulin present in the body than needed, the extra insulin works on the glucose already in the blood, resulting in a blood glucose level that is too low for you. This is called an *insulin reaction* (formerly referred to as *insulin shock*).

How to Manage Low Blood Glucose

First, check your blood with your glucose meter to make sure that your glucose level is indeed low. In fact, always check your blood any time you feel differently from how you normally feel, just to make sure that low blood glucose is not the problem. Why? Because symptoms of other medical conditions are similar to those of low blood glucose. If you determine that your symptoms are indeed the result of low blood glucose, treat IMMEDIATELY. Any food or beverage containing carbohydrate can be used for treatment. A food or beverage that is *only* carbohydrate (see Table 17-1) will more effectively raise your blood glucose and will have fewer calories than a food that contains both carbohydrate and fat, such as a candy bar. Fifteen grams of carbohydrate can raise your blood glucose level about 40 to 50 mg/dl. So if your blood glucose is around 50 mg/dl, 15 grams of carbohydrate has the potential to raise it to about 90 to 100 mg/dl. If your blood glucose is lower than 50 mg/dl, you may need to treat immediately with 30 grams of carbohydrate. However, it is also important not to overreact and overtreat hypoglycemia, which is easy to do. Overtreating can result in *hyperglycemia.*

If you experience low blood glucose because your insulin dose has been too high, your daily dose or dosing plan might need to be adjusted. If you take diabetes pills and have an unexplained episode of low blood glucose, speak to your doctor about possibly reducing your medication. Before adjusting either the dose of insulin or diabetes pills because of a low blood glucose level, however, be sure there are no other obvious reasons for the problem. First, determine whether the low blood glucose level is part of a repeated pattern—for example, you have had lows at about that time of day in the recent past—or whether it is a single episode. Repeated lows suggest that part of your treatment routine—medication, food, and activity pattern—may not be properly balanced. A single event, on the other hand, may suggest that rather than there being a problem with the usual treatment plan, something went awry on one day to cause a problem.

Next, you should try to figure out what might have caused the glucose level to drop to a low range. Think back and try to identify a reason, such as changing the timing of meals, skipping a meal, doing more physical activity than usual (without adding extra carbohydrate or reducing your insulin dose), or inaccurately measuring your insulin dose. Again, think of things that might have been occurring regularly (if you have been having repeated low glucose levels), or some one event (if you had a single low glucose). If none of these seems to be the reason for your low blood glucose, you should probably reduce the particular insulin dose (or dose of diabetes pills) the next day. It is usually better to err on the side of reducing the dose (you can always raise it again) than to have another, possibly serious, hypoglycemic event.

Remember, low blood glucose can be prevented by

- taking the right amount of insulin or diabetes pills at the right time
- eating the usual amount of food at the right time
- planning for extra physical activities

General Guidelines for Treating Low Blood Glucose

- **FOLLOW THE 15-15 RULE.**
  - Eat or drink a food or beverage containing 15 grams of carbohydrate. Table 17-1 lists foods containing 15 grams of carbohydrate. Choose a food that is convenient for you to consume.
  - Wait 15 minutes and recheck your blood glucose. If your blood glucose is below 80 mg/dl, repeat the treatment—eat or drink 15 more grams of carbohydrate.
  - If it is about an hour until your next meal, eat an additional snack with 15 grams of carbohydrate such as 6 saltine crackers or 3 graham cracker squares.

- **RECHECK YOUR BLOOD GLUCOSE IN ABOUT ONE HOUR.** Blood glucose levels begin to fall again in about an hour. If your blood glucose is below 80 mg/dl, treat again.

- **TREAT LOW BLOOD GLUCOSE IMMEDIATELY.** Most people who use insulin occasionally experience mild insulin reactions. Some even have them frequently. Treat insulin reactions promptly to prevent more serious problems.

- **BE PREPARED TO TREAT INSULIN REACTIONS AT HOME OR AWAY.** Carry a readily available carbohydrate such as glucose tablets or soft candies with you at all times (see Table 17-1). Do not eat chocolate or nuts to achieve a fast rise in your blood glucose. These foods contain fat, which takes longer for your body to digest, thus slowing the rise in blood glucose—and they also have more calories.

- **DO NOT PANIC.** Insulin reactions can be frightening. It is important, however, to try to think as clearly as possible. Eat some food or drink a beverage containing carbohydrate and allow it 10 to 15 minutes to act. If necessary, repeat the treatment.

- **CARRY A MEDICAL-ALERT ID TAG.** Always carry some form of identification showing that you have diabetes.

- **CHECK YOUR BLOOD GLUCOSE IF YOU FEEL SYMPTOMS OF LOW BLOOD GLUCOSE BEFORE DRIVING.** If your blood glucose is less than 100 mg/dl, eat 15 grams of carbohydrate before driving. And always keep a source of carbohydrate in your car, such as glucose tablets or juice boxes. People who have had problems with hypoglycemia, particularly if they may not have warning symptoms or have had a reaction while driving in the past, should check their blood glucose before driving regardless of whether they feel symptoms or not.

- **PREPARE FOR LONG DRIVES.** Never drive a car for more than three hours without eating. If you are behind the wheel, be even more sensitive to subtle symptoms that could be a reaction. If you experience an insulin reaction while driving, or even mild symptoms suggestive of one, pull over to the side of the road, check your glucose level, and eat a readily available carbohydrate before resuming your drive.

- **IF YOU DRINK ALCOHOL, DO SO WITH FOOD.** Alcoholic beverages can cause low blood glucose if you take insulin and drink without food. Always be sure to limit the amount of alcohol you drink.

- **ADJUST YOUR INSULIN.** If you use insulin, there are several ways you can adjust for low blood glucose. If the low glucose was severe, with symptoms such as confusion or loss of consciousness, then reduce the insulin acting at that time the next day to avoid another bad event. However, if the glucose was just low and you are not sure whether the cause was a single event that day or a pattern, cautiously wait another day or two before reducing the insulin. In general, guidelines should be given to you by your healthcare providers as to how to handle these situations, because while some providers may want you to self-adjust, others may want you to contact them immediately. Further recommendations are listed later in this chapter; see also Chapter 15 for more information on insulin use.

- **MONITOR OTHER MEDICATIONS.** Some medications can cause low blood glucose. Be sure your healthcare providers know *all* the medications and any type of supplements you are taking.

- **PREPARE FOR LONG-DURATION ACTIVITY.** Speak to your healthcare provider for advice on insulin adjustments and appropriate snacking guidelines if you are planning any all-day activities, such as hiking or skiing. Even people taking only diabetes pills may need some dose adjustments on these days.

- **CALL YOUR HEALTHCARE PROVIDER.** Call your doctor or healthcare provider if you have an insulin reaction and do not know what caused it.

TABLE 17-1   **Carbohydrates for Treating Low Blood Glucose (Hypoglycemia)**

The following foods and drinks contain 15 grams of carbohydrate and can be used for treating low blood glucose:

3 glucose tablets or 4 dextrose tablets

4 ounces (½ cup) orange juice

3 ounces (⅓ cup) regular cranberry or grape juice

4 ounces (½ cup) fruit drinks, such as HiC

5–6 ounces (½ cup) regular soda, such as Coke or Pepsi

3–4 teaspoons of sugar dissolved in water

4 Gummi Savers

4 Star Bursts

2 Chuckles

7–8 jelly beans

3 large marshmallows

1 tablespoon of syrup, such as honey or maple syrup

1 small tube of cake icing (½ ounce tube)

¼ cup dried fruit

2 tablespoons raisins

Guidelines for Adjusting Insulin to Prevent Low Blood Glucose

If you take insulin, there are several adjustments you may make to prevent low blood glucose.

- The changes you make in your insulin dose depend on the kinds of insulin you use, the time of day of injections, and the time of day the insulin reactions happen.

- Determine which of the insulins you use was working during the time of your low blood glucose, and, if more than one, which was probably working the hardest. If you have determined that the low blood glucose was caused by too much insulin, decrease that insulin by 1 to 2 units the next time you inject it. If two or more daily blood glucose levels are low, adjust first the insulin working the hardest when the earliest low glucose occurred. Do not adjust more than one dose or type of insulin at a time.

- If there is no improvement in your blood glucose by the next day, make the same adjustment a second time and call a member of your healthcare team for advice.

- When any change in insulin or pills, or the addition of exenatide or pramlintide treatment, results in a low blood glucose, it doesn't necessarily mean that the change was wrong and should be reversed. Always check with your healthcare provider. The adjustment of another part of your treatment may actually work better.

Children and Hypoglycemia

Hypoglycemia, or low blood glucose, can be a special problem in children with diabetes who use insulin. A young child may not understand what is happening but may behave differently. Parents must check the child's blood glucose if they are not sure. If it is not possible to check the blood glucose, they should assume that it is low and treat the child accordingly.

Issues Specific to Women

Women with diabetes who use insulin can experience more frequent hypoglycemia during menstruation. Changes in hormones at that time may be the reason. Pregnancy is another time when low blood glucose or hypoglycemia can happen frequently.

Additional Problems of Hypoglycemia

There are other problems associated with low blood glucose and special times when you should be on the lookout for symptoms. These problems and occasions are described below.

Hypoglycemic Unawareness

The longer you have diabetes, the more likely *hypoglycemic unawareness* may become a problem for you. It can also be more of a problem if you have just had a hypoglycemic reaction—symptoms of a second reaction following shortly after the first may not be felt as easily. Normally, when blood glucose levels drop, hormones such as glucagon and epinephrine are released, and they cause the liver to release glucose in order to raise blood glucose levels. Hormones that act to raise blood glucose are called *counterregulatory* or *stress hormones*. These hormones are also the cause of many of the symptoms, such as sweating, shakiness, and anxiousness, that people associate with hypoglycemia—particularly early in its course.

In some people with diabetes, the release of these hormones is decreased or absent, which reduces the symptoms of low blood glucose and limits the release of glucose. If you have this problem, it means your blood glucose has to drop lower before you feel symptoms, and this may cause you to delay treatment. Because your body does not respond well to hypoglycemia, it is not unusual for one low blood glucose to be followed by another, the symptoms of which, as noted above, may not be readily felt. The hormones that are supposed to be helping to raise your blood glucose may be blunted during that second reaction, further reducing the symptoms from low blood glucose but not the low blood glucose itself. Studies have shown that careful treatment programs designed to avoid hypoglycemia can restore the counterregulatory response. If you think you have hypoglycemic unawareness, therefore, it is important for you to work with your healthcare providers to design a treatment program that will prevent hypoglycemia. It may be that for a certain period you will need to increase your target glucose goals.

Rebound Hyperglycemia

One of the more confusing results of insulin treatment is *rebound hyperglycemia,* which can follow hypoglycemia. If your glucose level drops either too low—usually below 60 mg/dl or so—or too quickly, it triggers the counterregulatory hormones discussed above, glucagon and epinephrine, to release stored glucose from the liver and muscles into the bloodstream. This rise in glucose is called a *rebound* and can lead to high blood glucose levels. If you recognize the symptoms of low blood glucose and find high blood glucose afterward, you will be aware of the cause. But if you have hypoglycemic unawareness, described above, you may have lost the ability to sense the classic symptoms of low blood glucose. In this case, you may not be aware that the hyperglycemia was actually caused by hypoglycemia. The proper adjustment for hypoglycemia with rebound hyperglycemia is a REDUCTION in insulin dose to eliminate hypoglycemia. In these circumstances, it is important to resist the temptation to increase your insulin dose the next day in response to the hyperglycemia, or even to take more insulin the same day to "chase" the hyperglycemic rebound. Doing so only makes the situation worse.

The effects of the counterregulatory hormones continue even after the low blood glucose has been treated. In fact, your blood glucose may rise to levels as high as 250 to 300 mg/dl or more and remain high for 12 to 24 hours. While rebounds may not last much longer than that, the residual effect of raising the blood glucose level can last as long as 48 hours, eventually resolving itself as the extra glucose in the blood is used up by the cells or returned to the liver for storage. If you try to compensate for high blood glucose during a rebound (by taking extra insulin, eating less food, or increasing exercise), your blood glucose may swing back the other way—dropping too low after the liver has replenished its stores of glucose. During a rebound, therefore, you should continue to eat and exercise as usual. You should not take extra insulin unless the high glucose levels continue for more than three days.

Keep in mind that some of the hyperglycemia following hypoglycemia may result from overtreatment of the low blood glucose. This is another reason to follow the guidelines for treatment listed above.

Rapid Drop in Blood Glucose

You may occasionally experience a rapid drop in blood glucose levels when your insulin is peaking or when you are exercising. In such situations, you may have some of the symptoms of low blood glucose, even though your glucose may be well above 80 mg/dl. By checking your blood, you can determine whether you are experiencing a rapid drop or actual low blood glucose. If you feel signs of low blood glucose but are in doubt about the cause, it is best to eat a carbohydrate serving rather than risk the onset of more serious symptoms. Even if your glucose level is not *too* low, it is a good idea to slow a rapidly dropping blood glucose level.

Low Blood Glucose at Night

When adjusting insulin for high blood glucose, you should never increase your dinner or bedtime dose of long-acting or intermediate-acting insulin without checking your blood glucose between 2 and 3 A.M. Low blood glucose that occurs at night when you are normally asleep is often called *nocturnal hypoglycemia*. It may be caused by too much long-acting (peaking or basal) or intermediate-acting insulin in the dinner or bedtime dose. An advantage of using a long-acting peakless ("basal") insulin such as glargine or detemir is that its smooth action is less likely to cause the blood glucose level to drop too low during the night.

You may be awakened by a low blood glucose level at night, or you may sleep through it. When you awake in the morning, a headache may be the only clue that your glucose dropped during the night. Or you may remember having bad dreams or perspiring. Your bed partner may comment that you were more restless than usual. These are all symptoms of low blood glucose during the night. Your blood glucose levels may have returned to normal by breakfast, or they may be unusually high before breakfast, because of the body's mechanism for correcting low blood glucose. By monitoring your blood glucose in the middle of the night, you can learn if your blood glucose levels are being maintained in the normal range while you are sleeping.

Instructions in the Event of Coma or Convulsions

It is unlikely that you will have a convulsion (seizure) or become unconscious during an insulin reaction. However, these serious symptoms may occur if you do not recognize the early symptoms of low blood glucose—or if you ignore them. In addition, a small percentage of people with diabetes do not experience these early symptoms and are unaware of their low blood glucose until more serious symptoms occur, such as a convulsion.

Family and friends should know that if you are unconscious, you should not be given any liquid or food that requires you to swallow. Sources of sugar such as honey, sugar gels, or icing sugar for cakes can be carefully placed inside your cheek or beside the tongue. However, if you become unconscious or have a convulsion from low blood glucose, the best option is for you to receive an injection of a hormone called *glucagon*. Glucagon is produced in the pancreas, but unlike insulin, which lowers blood glucose, glucagon raises blood glucose by stimulating the liver to release stored glucose into the bloodstream. Glucagon should be injected into your skin (like you inject insulin) by a family member, friend, or healthcare provider, or you should be taken by ambulance to an emergency center or hospital. Glucagon may cause nausea or vomiting, so you should be placed on your side when the injection is given. Under NO circumstances should anyone try to force food or liquid into your mouth.

Once you have been given an injection of glucagon, it takes about 5 to 10 minutes for convulsions to subside or for you to regain consciousness. If your condition does not improve within that time, you should be given a second injection.

If the convulsions do not subside or if you do not regain consciousness, you should immediately be taken to an emergency room for treatment, which often involves injecting a glucose solution into a vein. If there is any doubt about the ability of your family or friends to use glucagon, you should be transported to a nearby emergency room or hospital as quickly as possible.

Also, be aware that people can become comatose for reasons other than a low blood glucose level, such as a heart attack or stroke. If there is any question that something other than hypoglycemia may be the cause, and certainly, as noted above, if glucagon does not work, you should be transported to the nearest emergency room immediately. It is usually advisable to call an ambulance to do this, if possible.

If you have been treated successfully without being moved to an emergency room and your condition has improved, eat a snack. Otherwise you may have another severe reaction a short time later. Always keep glucagon on hand for an emergency. A family member or friend with whom you live should learn how to prepare and inject glucagon if the need arises. You can purchase glucagon at your local pharmacy, but you must first obtain a prescription from your doctor. Glucagon comes in a kit consisting of two items:

- A bottle of glucagon in dry-powder form
- A syringe prefilled with diluting solution

Directions for preparing and injecting the glucagon are included with the kit. Glucagon kits are marked with an expiration date, after which their effectiveness is no longer guaranteed. Check your kit regularly to make certain the date has not expired.

Summary

What to do when you experience the symptoms of low blood glucose

1. Check your blood glucose to confirm that it is low. Your healthcare team should provide you with a particular glucose level and inform

you that if your blood glucose level drops below it, they would consider your blood glucose too low. Your blood glucose check will determine if the level is below that set by your healthcare team. If you cannot check, go to the next step.

2.   If your blood glucose is low, drink or eat 15 grams of carbohydrate, such as: 4 ounces (½ cup) of fruit juice or 6 ounces of regular soda, soft candy such as 2 Chuckles, or 3 to 4 glucose tablets. Be sure to carry one of these items with you at all times.

3.   Wait 10 to 15 minutes. If you still feel the side effects of low blood glucose, check your glucose again. If it's still low, repeat step 2. If your blood glucose continues to be low after a second serving of carbohydrate, call one of your healthcare providers.

4.   If your next meal is more than an hour away, eat a snack. In about an hour, check your blood glucose again.

5.   If you take insulin, and if the low blood glucose event was unexplained, adjust your dose according to the guidelines given to you by your healthcare providers.

6.   If you use diabetes pills, check with your doctor to see whether your medication should be reduced.

7.   Try to figure out why your blood glucose got too low. Talk to your healthcare providers if it happens again or if it was a very severe reaction.

CHAPTER 18

Adjusting for High Blood Glucose (Hyperglycemia)

Despite your best intentions, not every day will go smoothly in your diabetes treatment program. As you monitor your blood glucose, don't be surprised if you occasionally find that your levels are too high or low. This can happen even if your diabetes is well managed. Your goal is to have as few high and low blood glucose episodes as possible and to treat them while the symptoms are mild. By learning the early signs of high and low blood glucose, you can make the proper adjustments before more serious problems develop.

Sometimes your blood glucose may become high, a condition called *hyperglycemia*, even when you are feeling well and taking good care of your diabetes. However, if you have type 1 diabetes and your blood glucose rises very high, with ketones present, you may become sick with an illness called *ketoacidosis*, also referred to as *diabetic ketoacidosis*, or *DKA*. See Chapter 19 for more information on DKA.

What Is High Blood Glucose?

Your blood glucose is generally considered "high" when it is 160 mg/dl or above your individual blood glucose target. When monitoring your blood glucose, you should always record and analyze the results. If your blood glucose is consistently above your target goal, it means that you need to make some changes in your diabetes treatment plan.

Symptoms of High Blood Glucose

Unfortunately, many people do not experience any obvious physical symptoms that alert them that their blood glucose is too high. Not that we would want people to be uncomfortable, of course! However, the problem is that many people have glucose levels that are too high for a long time without having symptoms that tell them there is something wrong and thus spur them to action. On the other hand, some people may experience symptoms; often these are similar to those that led them to discover that they have diabetes, such as thirst, fatigue, frequent urination, or blurred vision. With or without symptoms, the best way to find out whether you have high blood glucose is to check your blood glucose. Depending on symptoms is *not* a reliable way of gauging your blood glucose level. Only by regularly checking your blood glucose and having your A1C measured will you get a good idea of your overall blood glucose levels.

Causes of High Blood Glucose

Your treatment program is based on a balance of medications, food intake, and physical activity. If your blood glucose and A1C are consistently above your target goals, it means you need a change in your treatment program. For people using insulin, the most frequent cause of high blood glucose is insufficient amounts of insulin. This may mean you need to increase your insulin doses or even change your insulin program. If you take a diabetes pill, it may mean you need to combine that pill with another one or with insulin. If you already use pills and insulin, the insulin may need to be adjusted. If you manage your diabetes by lifestyle (meal plan and physical activity) alone, it may mean it is time to add medications to your program. The goal is to have enough insulin to control your blood glucose.

Your blood glucose may also be high because of illness or infection, or because of stressful events in your life. Some medicines and dietary supplements, such as certain vitamins, also cause high blood glucose, so it is important to tell your doctor about any medicine or supplements you are taking. Sometimes the cause of occasional high blood glucose levels is too much food. If you eat too much—more food than is outlined in your meal plan—and don't cover it with the right amount of insulin or diabetes pills, the amount of glucose in your blood will be too high. In particular, the high blood glucose may occur just after meals, and be easily detected unless you check your glucose levels at those times. If your insulin or medications are inadequate to cover the amount of food you eat, your body will not be able to use all of that glucose as a supply of energy or even store it in the liver or muscles for later use. Glucose will remain in the bloodstream, and levels will continue to rise until sufficient insulin is available to help move it into your cells.

Another cause of hyperglycemia may be less physical activity than usual. Physical activity lowers your blood glucose, and if you don't exercise as much as you usually do, your blood glucose may rise.

The bottom line, if your blood glucose is too high, is that you have too little insulin in your bloodstream, your insulin may be working at the wrong times, or your cells may be resisting the actions of insulin. Below are some general guidelines for determining the cause of hyperglycemia.

Adjusting Diabetes Pills

If you have type 2 diabetes, your pancreas may still be able to produce some insulin, but not enough (or it may not be effective enough) to maintain blood glucose within a normal range, even if you are following your meal plan and participate in regular physical activity. In such cases, your doctor may prescribe one or more diabetes pills to boost your body's production of insulin and/or to make your body more sensitive to available insulin. Or maybe your pancreas is just no longer able to produce insulin. If this is the case, you may need to begin taking insulin. For more information, see Chapter 13, Diabetes Pills, and Chapter 14, Insulin Basics. If your blood glucose is running consistently higher than the goal you and your healthcare provider have set, it is important to call your doctor to discuss whether

What Causes a High Blood Glucose?

Too much food	Have you increased your portion sizes?
	Have you changed your eating habits or food choices?
	Have you eaten too many high-fat foods?
Too little physical activity	Have you decreased or eliminated your usual activity?
	Are you doing too little?
Not enough diabetes pills or insulin	Have you been taking the prescribed doses?
	Are you injecting insulin into the same area over and over?
Taking medication at the wrong time	Have you been taking the medication at times other than those recommended by your doctor?
"Bad" or spoiled insulin	Do you have spoiled insulin?
	Does your insulin look different?
	Was your insulin exposed to very hot or cold temperatures?
	Has your insulin expired?
Illness, infection, injury, or surgery	Are you feeling sick?
	Do you have any infections?
Incorrect and/or inaccurate glucose monitoring technique	Is the drop of blood too small?
	Are you using the correct technique?
	Does your meter need to be cleaned?
	Have your strips been exposed to very hot or cold temperatures or not been kept in an airtight, dry container?
	Is your meter calibrated to your current bottle of strips?

you should begin or increase your diabetes pills, or whether, perhaps, you should begin taking insulin or increase your insulin dose. DO NOT change your diabetes medications without talking to your healthcare team, or at least having instructions from them on how to do so on your own. However, you may want to perform more blood glucose checks at various times during the day—before meals, one to two hours after meals, and at bedtime. The pattern of glucose levels can help your healthcare team decide how to adjust your medications.

The need for more diabetes pills or insulin over time is a normal, expected change in the treatment of your diabetes and is a result of the natural progression of type 2 diabetes. Over time your beta cells become less able to make enough insulin, and the treatment must keep up with this change. To keep these cells working longer and more efficiently, do whatever is required to keep your blood glucose normal.

Adjusting Insulin

If you take insulin and your blood glucose levels are consistently high (generally over 180 mg/dl three days in a row), you probably need a change in your insulin program or adjustments in your insulin doses. But before making any changes, be sure there are no other explanations for the high blood glucose results. Ask yourself the following questions:

- Did you eat too much without adjusting your insulin dose?
- Did you change your activity level?
- Did you make mistakes in measuring or timing your present insulin dose?
- Have you gained weight?
- Are you using new prescription or over-the-counter drugs that may be increasing your blood glucose?

If you answered yes to any of these questions, it will help you understand why you may or may not need to make changes in your insulin program. If you answered no to any of them, you probably need more insulin or a different insulin program.

Blood glucose that is high in the morning (fasting blood glucose) requires some detective work to determine the actual cause. The basal insulin—glargine, ultralente, overnight NPH, or the insulin pump basal dose—controls the morning glucose level. Although you might think an elevated morning glucose level was related to eating too much food the evening before, this is often not the primary cause. What you ate the evening before would have been used or stored within about four hours and would therefore have had most of its effect on your blood glucose in the middle of the night rather than the next morning. An exception would be if you ate a high-fat meal the night before, where the fat slowed the food absorption, prolonging the impact of the meal into the next morning Conversely, eating less food than usual at night can cause a different type of problem. Undereating at night and taking too much insulin can cause your blood glucose level to drop too low in the middle of the night. This could result in a rebound high blood glucose in the morning.

Thus, high blood glucose levels in the morning can have a number of quite different possible causes:

■   **TOO SMALL A DOSE OF THE OVERNIGHT INSULIN** — this can be either injected insulin or the overnight basal insulin dose in an insulin pump program. Sometimes the duration of the injected insulin may not be adequate, and sometimes, with insulin pumps, the timing of the basal dose increase may be incorrect.

■   **THE DAWN PHENOMENON** — an increase in the amount of insulin required during the latter part of the sleep cycle; this happens to everyone and is due to an increase in counterregulatory (anti-insulin) hormone levels that occurs naturally in the early-morning hours.

■   **NOCTURNAL HYPOGLYCEMIA** — this is low blood glucose that occurs in the middle of the night and causes a condition called *rebound hyperglycemia* (high blood glucose) or the *Somogyi phenomenon*. As a result of too low a level of glucose, the counterregulatory or stress hormones cause the liver to release too much glucose.

The actual adjustments for high blood glucose in the morning depend on which of the above was the most likely cause. One of the best ways to determine the cause is to check your blood glucose in the middle of the night. You will need several nights of checking to try to determine whether there is a pattern to the blood glucose levels. But regardless of the pattern seen, or whether any is seen at all, you and your doctor will need to make a best guess as to the reason, make an insulin adjustment, and then wait and see whether the problem is resolved. Adjustments can involve changing the type or dose of insulin you take at bedtime if there is not enough insulin or if its duration is not long enough, changing the insulin or insulin dose or changing the basal pump insulin dose to cover the dawn phenomenon, or decreasing the dose of insulin causing the low blood glucose in the middle of the night.

The guidelines for adjusting insulin for high blood glucose depend on many factors: the peak activity and the duration of the insulins you are taking, the times of day the injections are given, and the times your blood glucose is high. General guidelines for adjusting insulin when blood glucose is high are listed below. Always check with your healthcare providers before following the guidelines. Your doctor may recommend a different approach.

General Guidelines for Adjusting Insulin

- Look at your logbook. Check your glucose readings for the same time of day over three to five days. How many are within your target range? Are most too high? Too low? High and low, but few on target? Think about possible causes of the highs and lows. Could they have been prevented? If they are out of the target range, talk with your healthcare provider about making some changes.

- If two or more blood glucose checks done each day are high for three days in a row without any obvious temporary explanation, adjust for the high blood glucose that occurs earliest in the day. Do not adjust more than one dose or type of insulin at a time, unless directed by your healthcare providers.

- After adjusting your dose, wait three days for your blood glucose level to improve. If there is no improvement, make another adjustment to the same dose. Do not adjust your insulin a third time without consulting your healthcare provider.

- If your fasting or morning blood glucose is high, always check between 2 and 3 A.M. for "nocturnal" low blood glucose (during the night), a condition discussed above and in Chapter 17.

- Never increase an insulin dose until you are sure the high blood glucose is not caused by a "rebound," a condition also discussed above and in Chapter 17.

- Unless your healthcare provider advises you to do otherwise, do not reduce your insulin dose unless you are having insulin reactions (symptoms of low blood glucose).

- In general, if your fasting (morning) or pre-meal blood glucose checks are high, you need to adjust your basal insulin. The most common basal insulin is one of the long-acting insulins, such as glargine, although some individuals may use NPH or lente twice a day, or ultra-lente.

- If your post-meal blood glucose levels are high, you need to increase your rapid-acting insulin, such as lispro, aspart, and glulisine, or your regular insulin. To determine whether your post-meal blood glucose is high, check two hours after starting to eat. At this time, your blood glucose should be about 30 to 50 mg/dl higher than before the start of your meal. If it is higher, you need to change your bolus or pre-meal insulin dose. If you are counting carbohydrate, make sure that you are using the correct insulin-to-carb ratio and sensitivity factor. Your ratio and/or sensitivity factor may need to be adjusted.

- If your blood glucose levels are consistently above 200 mg/dl, call your healthcare providers. You probably need a change in your overall insulin program.

Special Circumstances

Follow these guidelines for the special circumstances described below:

- If your blood glucose is 250 mg/dl or higher and you are on insulin, check for ketones in your urine or blood. If ketones are present, follow your sick-day rules (see Chapter 19); call your healthcare provider if you are not sure what to do.

■ If your blood glucose is 400 mg/dl or higher and you have no obvious explanation, such as significant overeating, call your doctor or healthcare provider, especially if you are on insulin—and even if ketones are not present.

■ If your blood glucose is 250 mg/dl or higher, and you are sick, follow the sick-day guidelines in Chapter 19.

■ If your blood glucose is normal or low but you are spilling ketones, this is likely *starvation ketosis*. Starvation ketosis, commonly seen in pregnant women with diabetes, happens when there is adequate insulin but inadequate amounts of carbohydrate for glucose. Again, the body switches to burning fat for energy and ketones result. Do not increase your insulin, but instead try to consume additional carbohydrate. Remember, the dangerous situation is HIGH blood glucose AND ketones as a result of insufficient amounts of insulin.

■ Be sure to drink plenty of water. Try to drink a minimum of eight glasses each day.

■ If your blood glucose is over 180 mg/dl or over your target range for three days in a row, call your healthcare provider. He or she may want to change your diabetes medication dose, meal plan, or physical activity plan. Do this even if you are feeling well.

■ Ask yourself what may have caused the high blood glucose, and take action to correct it. If you are unsure, contact your healthcare provider.

Extreme High Blood Glucose Situations

Whenever you have extremely high levels of blood glucose, you and the people you live with must be prepared to act. Left untreated, this situation can result in coma and death.

Diabetic Ketoacidosis (DKA)

Serious problems may occur if your blood glucose gets so high that your body turns to its fat stores for energy. This happens because there is not enough insulin available for your body to use the glucose for energy, and it leads to the production of ketones, which build up in the blood and spill into the urine. Allowed to go untreated for a number of days, the combination of high blood glucose and ketones can lead to *ketoacidosis,* a serious and life-threatening condition. DKA is more likely to occur if you have type 1 diabetes, because your body makes little or no insulin. While it can occur in some people with type 2 diabetes, it is much less likely. Blood glucose levels of 250 mg/dl or above for several days or weeks may be an indication of an insufficient insulin supply, and increase the risk of DKA. However, DKA can occur quite rapidly if you become ill or are using an insulin pump that malfunctions.

Any illness, such as the flu, an injury, or surgery, or dental problems can lead to ketoacidosis if glucose levels are not monitored with subsequent increases in insulin doses if necessary. On days when you are sick, you are at a much greater risk for ketoacidosis. That's why it's vital that you follow the guidelines for sick-day care in Chapter 19 any time you are experiencing illness or other situations associated with severe stress. By following these instructions, you can prevent your blood glucose and ketones from rising to a point at which they result in ketoacidosis.

Ketoacidosis is a medical emergency. Symptoms include frequent urination, thirst or hunger, nausea, stomach pain, vomiting, chest pain, rapid shallow breathing, and difficulty staying awake. If you experience these symptoms, it is important to go to an emergency facility for treatment immediately.

Hyperosmolar Hyperglycemia State

Not all people who take insulin have ketones in their urine or blood when they are sick. In a condition called *hyperosmolar hyperglycemic state (HHS),* an individual with type 2 diabetes can become very ill without ketones. HHS, which is not very common, is characterized by very high blood glucose levels (usually greater than 600 mg/dl), without ketones, and with severe dehydration and confusion. It usually occurs in people who still make some insulin: older people or people with type 2 diabetes treated with insulin, diabetes pills, or lifestyle alone. HHS does not occur in people with type 1 diabetes—because they cannot make any insulin, they would develop ketoacidosis.

What to Do in Emergencies

If coma or unconsciousness occurs from high blood glucose, you need immediate emergency attention. You should be taken by ambulance to a hospital or emergency center.

Be sure that people at your home and/or work know what to do in the event of an emergency. Also, whenever you are sick, ask someone to check on you. And at all times, wear an identification tag that says you have diabetes.

Summary

Below is a summary of what to do when you experience the symptoms of high blood glucose:

1. Check your blood glucose to confirm that it is high. Compare it with the goal set by your healthcare providers.
2. Drink plenty of water or noncaloric caffeine-free fluids—at least eight glasses a day.
3. Follow your diabetes treatment plan. Eat your meals as advised by your healthcare providers. If you feel up to it, do the same amount of physical activity every day. Check your blood glucose level.
4. If you take diabetes pills, take the prescribed amount at the correct time.
5. If you take insulin, adjust it according to your directions.
6. Call your doctor if your blood glucose is over 180 mg/dl for three days in a row and you're not sure what to do.
7. If you are sick, have recently had surgery or undergone a medical

procedure, or are under a high degree of stress, follow your sick-day guidelines. If you are not sure what to do, call your healthcare provider.

8. If you use an insulin pump, follow the guidelines outlined in Chapter 16. Be aware that pump malfunction can lead to DKA rapidly. Do not delay taking action for a very high, or rapidly rising, glucose level with suspected pump malfunction.

CHAPTER 19

Managing Diabetes When You Are Ill

If you have diabetes, you need to take special care of yourself when you are sick. Being sick changes the way your body functions, including the way your cells use insulin. You must be prepared to make adjustments in your diabetes treatment program.

Any infectious disease, even the common cold, stomach upset, flu, or diarrhea, puts stress on your body. Stress can also result from an injury, surgery, or invasive dental work, such as having a tooth pulled. Moreover, severe emotional trauma such as a divorce or a death in the family also produces bodily stress. In response to such stress, the body makes chemical messengers called *hormones*. (Recall that insulin is a hormone as well.) Influenced by these hormones that are present at times of stress, the liver releases stored glucose into the bloodstream. This new supply of blood glucose provides your body with the additional energy you need to overcome an illness or a stressful event. But at the same time, it means more insulin is needed to keep your blood glucose level normal.

In large amounts, these same hormones work against the action of insulin, making the body's cells more resistant to it. For people who do not have diabetes, the pancreas makes up for this insulin resistance and the resulting increased insulin need by releasing more insulin. In people with diabetes, the situation can be vastly different. Even when you are well, your pancreas may not be able to make enough insulin to meet your needs. But when you get sick and the hormones described above make your body's cells more resistant to insulin, blood glucose will have more trouble getting into your body's cells and will build up in the bloodstream. Also, the hormones release glucose from glycogen (stored glucose), sending blood glucose even higher. Taken together, these responses have the potential to produce extremely high blood glucose and a need for more insulin.

Ketoacidosis

The situation can become even more complicated. If you have type 1 diabetes, the lack of enough insulin makes you unable to use the glucose in your bloodstream, and your body turns to its fat stores for energy. This causes the production of acids called ketones, which accumulate in the blood and spill into the urine. The excessive formation of ketones in the blood is called *ketosis,* and the presence of ketones in the urine is called *ketonuria.*

Allowed to go untreated, the combination of high blood glucose and ketones can lead to *ketoacidosis* (also called *diabetic ketoacidosis,* or *DKA*)— an extremely serious condition that can lead to diabetic coma and death. The symptoms of ketoacidosis are nausea, stomach pain, vomiting, chest pain, rapid shallow breathing, and difficulty staying awake.

While ketoacidosis is usually seen in people with type 1 diabetes, it can occur in those with type 2 diabetes, even those who are not normally treated with insulin. Recall that, over time, people with type 2 diabetes increasingly lose the ability to make insulin. Someone may be making just enough insulin to maintain adequate glucose control, but if he or she gets sick, insulin need is increased so much that it overwhelms the pancreas's ability to make it. In this setting, ketoacidosis can occur. There is also a rare variant of type 2 diabetes, seen in particular in African Americans, in which the possibility of ketoacidosis occurring is somewhat more likely. These people are often in diabetic ketoacidosis when they first seek treatment for diabetes. However, once the glucose is brought under control, they have type 2 diabetes, and may be treated with oral medications alone.

The important point is that even people with type 2 diabetes—at the time their diabetes is diagnosed, or in the setting of a significant illness—should check for the possibility of ketoacidosis.

Hyperosmolar Hyperglycemic State

If you have type 2 diabetes and become sick, you should be aware of a serious condition, also related to high blood glucose levels, called *hyperosmolar hyperglycemic state (HHS)*. It results when extremely high levels of blood glucose cause excessive urination and severe dehydration, but without ketones. It may also be caused by the stress of an illness, and it can occur in people who have had high blood glucose for a long time. In someone with type 2 diabetes, HHS is more likely to result from these stresses than diabetic ketoacidosis, the exceptions discussed in the previous section not withstanding.

HHS causes a severe imbalance in the body's chemistry. The body may still produce some insulin, which prevents the ketone formation found in ketoacidosis; nevertheless, the high blood glucose and dehydration can lead to coma or death. The symptoms that signal the onset of this state are excessive urination, excessive thirst, increased hunger, drowsiness, nausea, vomiting, abdominal pain, and rapid shallow breathing.

Guidelines for Sick-Day Care

Ketoacidosis and hyperosmolar hyperglycemic state are very serious conditions. That's why it is extremely important that you follow the guidelines described below during any period of illness or during other situations associated with severe stress. By following these guidelines, you will prevent your blood glucose and ketones from rising to dangerously high levels.

1. Always take your diabetes medication. NEVER SKIP YOUR INSULIN OR YOUR DIABETES PILLS, EVEN IF YOU ARE TOO SICK TO EAT. (See item 6 if you cannot eat.)
2. Check your blood glucose every three to four hours throughout the

day and night. If you are too sick to check, ask someone to do it for you. If you live alone, have a friend contact you if he or she does not hear from you in four hours. This may be necessary because your high blood glucose levels could make you sleepy and prevent you from following these guidelines. If you take insulin, also check for ketones if your blood glucose is 250 mg/dl or higher.

3. Call your doctor or healthcare provider if your blood glucose is 250 mg/dl or higher for two consecutive blood glucose checks. Do this whether you have ketones or not.

4. If you use insulin, you may need to take extra injections if your blood glucose is 250 mg/dl or higher. You can learn to do this yourself or you can call for help when you get sick. Either way, make sure you have the right information or know who to call under these circumstances.

5. It is important that you continue to eat and drink. If you can't follow your meal plan but can still eat some food, choose items from Table 19-1. Each item contributes about 15 grams of carbohydrate. You need to try to eat or drink about 50 grams of carbohydrate (or 3 carbohydrate servings) every three to four hours.

6. If you feel too sick to eat, drink six to eight ounces of fluids every hour. If you are unable to eat solid foods, you should switch back and forth between fluids that contain sugar, such as regular soft drinks and juices, for one hour, and drinks that do not contain sugar, such as diet soft drinks and tea or water, for the other hour. If you are unable to follow your meal plan, choose foods or beverages that contain salt. Clear soup, bouillon, and Gatorade are good choices. Call your healthcare provider at once if you throw up the beverages you drink.

7. Rest and keep warm. Do not participate in physical activities. Have someone take care of you.

8. Call your healthcare provider if you throw up, have persistent diarrhea, are in pain, or have questions.

Treat the Underlying Illness

It is very important to treat the illness that has made you sick. Be sure to follow the directions from the doctor caring for your underlying illness. For

TABLE 19-1 Foods for Sick Days

The following foods contain about 15 grams of carbohydrate, or are equal to one carbohydrate serving. Try to eat or drink 50 grams of carbohydrate (3 carbohydrate servings) every three to four hours.

½ cup applesauce

½ cup apple juice

⅓ cup grape juice

⅓ cup fruited yogurt

½ cup regular Jell-O

¼ cup milkshake

1 cup Gatorade

1 tablespoon honey

¼ cup regular pudding

½ of a twin-pop Popsicle

½ cup regular ice cream

½ cup eggnog

½ cup cooked cereal

Other foods you may try include salty foods such as broth, consommé, and tomato juice, and soft solids like toast, cooked cereals, and soups.

example, you may be advised to use an antibiotic for an infection, or to take acetaminophen or other nonaspirin medications for a fever. Always inform the doctor caring for your illness that you have diabetes.

Prevent Dehydration

When your blood glucose levels are markedly high, your kidneys cannot recycle all the glucose and the excess spills into the urine. The presence of excess glucose in the urine draws additional water from your body, causing you to pass large volumes of urine. This loss of water from your body may lead to dehydration. Thus it is very important to follow guideline number 6. It is also important to consume some salty foods. A good goal: *Drink one cup (8 ounces) of noncaffeinated fluid every ½ to 1 hour. Alternate salty fluids such as broth or bouillon with low-salt fluids.*

Prevent Ketoacidosis

As explained previously, diabetic ketoacidosis, or DKA, can lead to coma and death. To prevent ketoacidosis, it is very important to keep your blood glucose from rising too high. It is very important to follow guideline numbers 1 through 4. Remember: *Always take your usual insulin dose. Never omit it, even if you are unable to eat. Monitor your blood glucose and check for ketones. If your blood glucose is higher than 250 mg/dl and ketones are present, you always need extra insulin, called a sick-day dose. Extra insulin is also needed if your blood glucose is high but ketones are not present, in which case you won't need as much. Do not use extra insulin if your blood glucose is less than 250 mg/dl, even if ketones are present.*

Dosage and Timing of Extra Insulin

The extra amount of insulin you need is based on the total number of units of insulin you take each day when you are well. It is usually taken as rapid- or short-acting insulin. Below are guidelines for increasing your insulin doses. Check with your healthcare providers before following these guidelines—they may recommend a different approach for your situation.

- If blood glucose levels are high and *ketones are present,* the additional insulin used as a sick-day dose should be 20 percent, or one fifth, of your usual daily dose of insulin. To calculate the amount, divide the total number of units in your usual daily dose by 5. Take that amount in ADDITION to your usual insulin dose. For example, if your blood glucose first thing in the morning is over 250 mg/dl, you are spilling ketones, and you take 50 total units of insulin each day. 50 divided by 5 is 10. Therefore, you should add an additional 10 units of rapid-acting or short-acting insulin to your usual breakfast dose.

- If ketones are not present but your blood glucose is high, the additional insulin used as a sick-day dose of rapid-acting or short-acting insulin should be 10 percent, or one tenth, of your usual daily dose. To calculate the amount, divide the total number of units in your usual daily dose by 10. Take that amount in addition to your usual daily insulin dose. For example, in the case above, 50 units divided by 10 is 5. Therefore, you should add an additional 5 units of rapid-acting or short-acting insulin to your usual breakfast dose. Practice calculating a 10 percent or 20 percent increase in your present daily total.

Add up your daily rapid insulin amounts	Add up the daily long-acting insulin	Add the two totals	1) Divide daily total by 10 for your 10% increase 2) Divide daily total by 5 for your 20% increase
Total _____ units	Total _____ units	Daily Total _____	10% _____ 20% _____

- Check your blood glucose again in about three to four hours. If your blood glucose is still high and you are still spilling ketones, add another sick-day dose of 20 percent to your lunch insulin dose. If your blood glucose is high but you are *not* spilling ketones, add another sick-day dose of 10 percent to your lunch insulin dose. If you do not routinely take a lunch insulin dose, just take the sick-day dose. If your blood glucose is less than 250 mg/dl, do not take extra insulin, even if ketones are present. Just take your usual insulin dose.

- If you follow a sliding scale (see Chapter 15), your total daily dose will change each day. To calculate your usual daily amount of insulin, add up your morning and evening long-acting insulin. Go to the section of your sliding scale that lists your blood glucose from 100 to 150, which is the target pre-meal blood glucose range for most people with diabetes. Add all the rapid-acting insulin listed for breakfast, lunch, dinner, and bedtime in this column. Add that amount to your long-acting total to determine your typical insulin total for a day. Take 10 percent of that total if your ketones are negative or small, 20 percent if your ketones are moderate or large. Add that number to the dose listed on your sliding scale for your current blood glucose. Read the following:

EXAMPLE   In the morning Patty takes 10 units of NPH, and at bedtime 8 units of NPH. Her intermediate-acting insulin total is thus 18 units. Patty takes rapid insulin before each meal by the following sliding scale. Patty is ill before lunch and her glucose reading is 289 mg/dl, which by her scale would call for 4 units. Although her ketones are negative, she still needs to have 10 percent more of her daily total. Add the number of units before each meal from the 100 to 150 range on her scale which adds up to _____ units.

Blood Glucose	Before Breakfast	Before Lunch	Before Supper	Bed
100–150	2 units	2 units	3 units	0 units
151–200	3 units	3 units	4 units	0 units
201–250	3 units	3 units	4 units	1 units
251–300	4 units	4 units	5 units	2 units
301–400	5 units	5 units	6 units	2 units

Yes, seven units is correct. Now add this amount to the long-acting insulin total: 7 plus 18 = 25 units. A 10 percent increase would be 2.5 units, or 3 units. Now find the amount of rapid-acting insulin she was to take before lunch for her glucose level of 289 mg/dl and add the 3 units to that amount. Her before-lunch dose will now be _____ units.

Yes, seven units is correct. At supper Patty's glucose level is 260 mg/dl, and she has moderate ketones in her urine. Can you calculate a 20 percent increase for her suppertime dosage? Patty should take _____ units. Yes, she should take 10 units before supper (20 percent of 25 units per day = 5 units, added to the 5 units she would normally take for a glucose level of 260 mg/dl at suppertime = 10 units), and she should call her healthcare provider because she has moderate ketones.

- After taking two sick-day doses, if your blood glucose is still high, call your healthcare provider for further instructions. Do not take a third sick-day dose without consulting your healthcare provider.

- Sometimes people who are sick hesitate to use extra amounts of insulin. If you are not sure how much extra insulin to take, immediately contact your healthcare provider. High blood glucose with ketones is a medical emergency.

- If you are carbohydrate counting and using an insulin-to-carbohydrate ratio, use your sensitivity factor to correct blood glucose levels above your target glucose goal in the same way you normally would. If your blood glucose level is over 250 mg/dl, check your urine for ketones. If ketones are negative or small, calculate the additional insulin dose using the sensitivity factor. Then add up your typical total daily dose, which is all the insulin you take daily, and take 10 percent of that number. Use the **larger** of the two calculated doses—either the one calculated by the sensitivity factor, or the one that is 10 percent of the total daily dose.

  If your ketone results are moderate to large, calculate the additional insulin dose using your sensitivity factor. Add up your typical total daily dose, as above, and take 20 percent of that number. Once again, use the **larger** of the two calculated doses, either the amount determined by the sensitivity factor, or the amount that is 20 percent of the total daily dose.

  If your blood glucose level does not return to your target within 3½ to 4 hours, your sensitivity factor should be changed by 10 or 20 percent based on ketone results.

  EXAMPLE   10 percent change in sensitivity factor used for negative or small ketones:

  Blood glucose = 400 mg/dl
  Target blood glucose is 120
  Sensitivity factor = 50

Subtract 120 from 400 = 280 mg/dl, divide 280 by 50 = 5.6, or 6 units, multiplied by .1 (10 percent) = 0.6 plus 6 units = 6.6 (round up to 7 units).

EXAMPLE 20 percent change in sensitivity factor used for moderate or large ketones:

Blood glucose = 320 mg/dl
Target blood glucose is 120
Sensitivity factor = 50

Subtract 120 from 320 = 200, divide 200 by 50 = 4 units, multiplied by .2 (20 percent) = 0.8 plus 4 units = 4.8 (round up to 5 units).

- If you have type 2 diabetes and do not yet take insulin, you may be put on insulin temporarily to keep your blood glucose under control when you are sick, undergoing surgery, or have a serious injury. Once the surgery or illness has passed, you can be taken off insulin and return to your usual diabetes treatment program.

Nourish Your Body

The body needs extra energy to overcome an illness. That's why it's vital that you eat or drink some source of nourishment and calories when you are sick. Try to eat your usual amount of carbohydrate-containing foods. Follow guideline numbers 5 and 6 regarding the amount of carbohydrate to eat.

Prevent a Hyperosmolar Hyperglycemic State

Take the following steps to prevent this serious condition, which may occur in people with type 2 diabetes:

- If you take diabetes pills or insulin, always take your medication. Never omit it, even if you are unable to eat. Check with your doctor to see if you should increase your dose during your illness.

- Monitor your blood glucose every three to four hours. Set your alarm clock to wake you during the night. If you are too sick, ask someone to check your blood glucose for you.

- If blood glucose levels are 250 mg/dl or higher, check for ketones. If ketones are present, or if your blood glucose is consistently 250 mg/dl or higher, call your healthcare provider. It's very important to watch for the presence of ketones during an illness.

Watch for Danger Signs

Contact your healthcare provider if you have any of the symptoms listed below. Hospital care is necessary for these problems.

- Signs of dehydration, such as dry mouth, cracked lips, sunken eyes, weight loss, and skin that is flushed and dry
- Inability to drink the recommended amount of fluid, or persistent vomiting for more than one hour, or persistent diarrhea
- A fever of 101 degrees or higher
- Symptoms of ketoacidosis, such as nausea, stomach pain, vomiting, chest pain, rapid shallow breathing, or difficulty staying awake
- If after taking two doses of extra insulin in 24 hours, your blood glucose is still 250 mg/dl or higher

Over-the-Counter Medications

People with diabetes are often concerned that they use only sugar-free medications, such as cough syrups, when ill. This is good to do when you can. However, sugar-free preparations may not always be available. Keep in mind that "sugar" per se is not really the problem—it's how a person with diabetes is able to *handle* that sugar. In addition, the amount of sugar in these medications is usually relatively small. The ability of this small amount of sugar to cause elevated blood glucose levels is often less than the stress of coughing all night if you did not take the cough syrup. So try to use sugar-free medications when possible, but if the medication is necessary and a sugar-free version is not available, use what you have; if necessary, compensate with additional insulin or, with guidance from your healthcare team, diabetes pills if needed.

Examples of Sugar-Free Medications

Antacids	Antidiarrheals	Laxatives	Sugar-Free Cough medicine- Sore Throat	Analgesics
Amphojel	Kaopectate	Peri-colace	Chlor-Trimeton	Aspirin
Alternagel	Pepto Bismol	Milk of	Tabs	Acetaminophen
Gelusil	Imodium	Magnesia	Dimetapp	• Tylenol
Rolaids	Diasorb	Metamucil	Elixir	Ibuprofen
Maalox		(sugar-free)	Scot-Tussin	• Advil
Mylanta		Natural bran	DM Liquid	• Motrin
Riopan		foods	Cerose DM	• Nuprin
		Dulcolax	Liquid	
		Citrucel	Chloraseptic	
		(sugar-free)	Spray	
			Nice Throat	
			Lozenges	
			Cepastat	
			Lozenges	

Sick-Day Checklist

Keep the following items on hand in case you become sick:

- extra bottle of regular or rapid-acting insulin and syringes
- ketone strips
- sugar-free and regular gelatin (such as Jell-O)
- broth packets (salt-free if you are on a low-sodium diet)
- saltine crackers (salt-free if you are on a low-sodium diet)
- *caffeine-free* tea

- *caffeine-free* carbonated beverages (sugar-free and regular), such as ginger ale
- substitute foods: fruit juice boxes, applesauce, sherbet
- table sugar packets
- thermometer
- medications to relieve fever
- antidiarrheal agents, such as Imodium
- glucagon kit in case of hypoglycemia
- telephone number of the diabetes care team
- cold/cough/flu medicine recommended by healthcare provider (see sugar-free medication list)

CHAPTER 20

Long-Term Complications of Diabetes

If you have either type 1 or type 2 diabetes, you should be aware that your diabetes can cause a number of problems after you've had diabetes for years. These long-term complications can affect various parts of your body—your eyes, kidneys, nerves, blood vessels, heart, and other areas—and they are more likely to occur if your diabetes has not been well controlled. That's why it's so important to work closely with your healthcare providers to develop a program that keeps your blood glucose as close to normal as possible—to minimize or prevent these complications.

The landmark research study known as the Diabetes Control and Complications Trial (DCCT) revealed that people with type 1 diabetes can reduce their risk of developing complications by 50 percent or more by maintaining excellent blood glucose control. Physiologic insulin therapy, use of frequent blood glucose checking to adjust insulin doses, and carbohydrate counting facilitate the type of control that is needed. This approach is discussed in Chapter 15. Another landmark research study, the United Kingdom Prospective Diabetes Study (UKPDS), showed that people with type 2 diabetes can also reduce their risk of developing complications by controlling blood glucose and blood pressure. Type 2 diabetes changes naturally over time: beta cell function declines, resulting in decreased insulin production, and blood glucose levels gradually increase. This means that treatment must also change—progressing from nutrition therapy alone to nutrition therapy combined with diabetes pills or insulin therapy or both. To know whether your treatment program is continuing to be effective, checking your blood glucose is essential.

The message is clear. Whether you have type 1 or type 2 diabetes, you should work with your healthcare providers to achieve blood glucose levels as close to normal as possible to reduce the risks of long-term complications. Some people discover that despite their best efforts their diabetes is so difficult to manage that they can't achieve the type of control they want. And despite hard work, other people still develop complications. This can be very discouraging. But remember, by doing the best job you can with your diabetes day to day, you *are* lowering your risk of developing further complications later on, and you are slowing the progress of complications that may just be beginning.

Controlling blood glucose is the first step, but diabetes affects the whole body, including blood vessels and nerves. Controlling cholesterol and blood pressure can therefore decrease risks for complications even more! Your healthcare provider will perform the following tests, but you need to know the results and what they mean.

- A1C — A blood test that measures average blood glucose over the past two to three months and is the best way to measure overall glucose control. It should be measured two to four times a year, the goal being a value of less than 7 percent. (See Chapter 12 for more information.)

- BLOOD PRESSURE — Measures the pressure against the walls of your blood vessels. High blood pressure is more common in persons with diabetes and increases the risk of stroke, heart attack, and kidney and eye diseases. It should be measured at every visit, or at least once a year, with a goal of lower than 130/80 mmHg.

- CHOLESTEROL — A blood test that measures the amount of fat (lipids) circulating in your bloodstream. LDL cholesterol can clog the walls of the arteries but can be treated if caught early. Blood fats should be tested once a year, with an LDL cholesterol goal of at least less than 100 mg/dl; in people at high risk, such as those with diabetes and coronary heart disease, the recommended LDL goal is now 70 mg/dl. Further, the HDL cholesterol goal should be greater than 40 mg/dl for men and 50 mg/dl for women. The total cholesterol goal should be less than 200 mg/dl, and the triglyceride goal should be less than 150 mg/dl. Medications can be used to lower your cholesterol if needed, along with a meal plan low in saturated fat and trans fat.

- MICROALBUMIN — A urine test that measures how well your kidneys are working. If you catch problems early, they can be treated. Microalbumin measures small amounts of protein in the urine and should be measured at least once a year, with a goal of less than 30 micrograms per milligram creatinine. Medications referred to as ACE (angiotensin-converting enzyme) inhibitors or ARBs (angiotensin receptor blockers) can help control microalbumin and blood pressure.

- EYE EXAM — To protect your eyes, you should have a dilated-eye exam every year. Drops are put in your eyes to dilate your pupils, making it easier to see inside your whole eye. Medications or laser surgery can stop problems from getting worse, reduce the risk of vision loss, and in some cases restore useful vision.

- FOOT EXAM — Remove your shoes and socks for a foot check at each appointment with your healthcare provider. Check your feet daily to prevent problems. (See Chapter 21.)

In 2004 it was reported that only 37 percent of adults with diabetes had A1C levels less than 7 percent, only 36 percent achieved a blood pressure less than 130/80 mmHg, and 52 percent had cholesterol levels less than 200 mg/dl—and if goals for A1C, blood pressure, and total cholesterol were combined, only 7 percent achieved all three goals. The message is clear—there is a lot that can be done to prevent long-term complications in persons with diabetes, but unfortunately we are far from helping people meet goals that would aid in preventing or delaying these complications.

Heart and Blood Vessel (Cardiovascular) Disease

Both type 1 and type 2 diabetes increase the risk for cardiovascular (heart and blood vessel) disease. Compared with the general population, the risk is two or three times greater for people with type 1 diabetes, and the disease occurs at a younger age. In addition, before menopause, women with diabetes lose their natural protection against heart disease. Cardiovascular disease is very common in persons with type 2 diabetes and may be present even before the diagnosis of diabetes. The disease is common in older people as a result of aging, but it intensifies in people with diabetes. Furthermore, people with diabetes do not always have classical chest pain, so unusual shortness of breath or excessive fatigue should be reported to the healthcare provider so that they can be evaluated.

Many people have what is now termed *metabolic syndrome*, which is a cluster of conditions that increase the risk of developing vascular disease (heart disease, strokes, and peripheral vascular disease). The most recognizable components of this syndrome are abdominal obesity, elevated blood pressure (hypertension), elevated triglycerides (part of the lipid profile), low HDL (the "good" cholesterol), and glucose intolerance. Patients with diabetes and metabolic syndrome also have a much higher rate of cardiovascular disease. Much of the focus of complication prevention for people with type 2 diabetes is aimed at the vascular complications, and thus treatments target the abnormalities that are part of metabolic syndrome.

The heart and blood vessels are referred to as the *cardiovascular system*. This is the means by which blood is pumped from your heart and circulated throughout your body. As it circulates, the blood carries nourishment and oxygen to all of your body's tissues. It also removes waste products.

Problems occur when the walls of the blood vessels become thickened. It is now thought that this thickening is related to inflammation of the vessel wall, which then leads to the formation of plaques, which cause partial blockages. If these plaques rupture, clots form on that rupture site, causing a more acute, total blockage. If the blood vessel is providing blood to the heart, the result is a heart attack. This process is referred to as *atherosclerosis*.

The risk factors for vascular disease all help this process along. When blood vessels are inflamed, the plaques that contain fat are formed. High cholesterol levels allow this to happen more readily. Elevated cholesterol levels, especially LDL cholesterol; high blood pressure; cigarette smoking; diabetes; and diets high in saturated fat and cholesterol all damage blood vessels and/or help the plaques build up. Sticky blood platelets form blood clots when those plaques rupture, leading to the more complete blockage in blood vessels.

Thus the link between heart disease and the various components of metabolic syndrome, including diabetes, is quite convincing. Studies show that among people who have had a recent heart attack, one third to one half have had abnormal blood glucose levels, at least temporarily. Researchers have also learned that heart attack is a chief cause of death in people whose diabetes developed after age 30.

Why people with diabetes develop cardiovascular disease earlier than people who do not have the disease is not clearly understood, but studies suggest that the inflammatory process begins very early in the patient who is insulin resistant. This starts the process of damage to the lining of the blood vessels, called the endothelium, a single layer of cells found in all the blood vessels. When this process damages the endothelium, it is referred to as endothelial dysfunction, and it tends to occur in people with some or all of the components of metabolic syndrome.

As the atherosclerosis progresses, from a thickening of the blood vessels to a partial or complete blockage due to plaque rupture and clotting, a number of very serious consequences can follow. Partial blockage of the large coronary arteries that supply blood to the heart may cause chest pains (angina) as sections of the heart become damaged from lack of nutrients. If the blood supply is blocked altogether, a heart attack *(myocardial infarction)* may occur. A blockage in the circulation of blood to the brain may cause a stroke. Blockages in the blood vessels that supply blood to the legs and feet can cause pain in the thigh or calf muscles when standing, walking, or exercising. This condition is called *intermittent claudication* and is due to *peripheral vascular disease.*

Preventing Cardiovascular Disease

From the discussion above, it should be obvious that controlling your glucose is only one of the things you can do to reduce your risk of developing blood vessel disease. Being overweight, having high lipids (blood fats, cholesterol), having high blood pressure, and smoking are other other risk factors you can try to change. If you need to lose weight, read Chapter 8. And talk to your healthcare providers about adjusting your calorie intake and getting more physical activity.

Eating foods containing large amounts of saturated and trans fats and cholesterol increases the level of cholesterol in your blood, particularly LDL, or "bad" cholesterol. This can lead to clogging of the blood vessels, reduced circulation, and an increased risk of cardiovascular disease. A meal plan low in saturated fat and cholesterol is essential, so be sure to consult with your dietitian about these matters.

High blood pressure *(hypertension)* also speeds the development of atherosclerosis. If you develop high blood pressure, your doctor may suggest that you lose weight and reduce the amount of salt in your diet. If your blood pressure remains high, your doctor will treat it aggressively with medication.

Smoking increases the risk of blood vessel disease because *nicotine* narrows or constricts the blood vessels. This is bad news for people with diabetes, who are already at risk for blood vessel disease. Smoking adds additional risk and is particularly hazardous. Your healthcare team can discuss smoking cessation options with you.

People with schizophrenia and/or bipolar disorder are at increased risk for the metabolic syndrome. The cause may be genetic, but a lifestyle of decreased activity and poor dietary habits also contributes. Because certain antipsychotic medications may cause the metabolic syndrome to worsen, first consult a mental health provider if you have these metabolic conditions or are at risk for them.

What Action Can You Take?

In summary, the following are important steps you can take to reduce your risk of cardiovascular disease:

■   Be more physically active.
■   If you are overweight, losing even a few pounds can help improve
    blood fats and blood pressure levels.

- If you smoke—try to stop!
- Eat less saturated fat and less trans fat, and include more whole grains, fruits, and vegetables in your meal plan.
- Be sure your lipids are tested annually unless you have excellent lipid values, in which case they should be tested every two years.
- If your LDL cholesterol is greater than 100 mg/dl, it is recommended that you take a statin medication to lower it. Ask your healthcare provider about this.
- If your triglycerides are high and your HDL cholesterol low, ask your healthcare provider about fibrate or niacin medications. Combination therapy using statins and fibrates or niacin, along with nutrition therapy, is often necessary to achieve target lipid (fat) goals.
- Adults with diabetes should take aspirin. If you cannot tolerate aspirin, ask your healthcare provider about alternative therapies.
- If your A1C is not at target, ask whether your diabetes medications need changing.
- Some studies have suggested that use of ACE inhibitors or ARBs can reduce the risk of vascular disease.

High Blood Pressure (Hypertension)

Hypertension (high blood pressure) is defined as blood pressure equal to or greater than 140/90 mmHg and affects the majority of adults with diabetes. Blood pressure is the force of the blood on the walls of the arteries. Two levels are measured: the first number is the higher, or *systolic,* pressure, which occurs each time the heart pushes blood into the vessels; the second number is the lower, or *diastolic,* pressure, which occurs when the heart rests. As a result of the findings of research studies, it is recommended that a blood pressure of less than 130/80 mmHg be the goal for people with diabetes.

Hypertension requires aggressive treatment. It is a major risk factor for cardiovascular disease (discussed above) and also for retinopathy and nephropathy (discussed later in the chapter). Much of the hypertension among people with diabetes may be related to the insulin resistance syndrome, which is commonly present even before the diagnosis of type 2 diabetes. In persons with type 1 diabetes, it is often a result of early kidney problems.

Several large research studies have reported an increased risk of cardiovascular events and higher death rates from cardiovascular disease in persons with diabetes whose blood pressure is 120/70 mmHg or higher. The studies documented improved outcomes, especially a reduced risk of stroke, when blood pressure was controlled.

Preventing Hypertension

To achieve the goal of normalizing blood pressure, lifestyle modifications and medications may be prescribed for many people. In fact, multiple medications may be required to meet blood pressure goals. Your blood pressure should be checked every time you visit your healthcare provider. If your blood pressure is higher than 130/80 mmHg, it should be rechecked on another day to see if it differs. If hypertension is confirmed with another reading, treatment should begin immediately.

If your blood pressure is between 130 and 139 mmHg systolic, or between 80 and 89 mmHg diastolic, you may start treatment with lifestyle therapy. A diet low in sodium is recommended to help lower your blood pressure, so ask your dietitian to help you develop a low-sodium meal plan (see guidelines on page 86). Eating more fruits, vegetables, and low-fat dairy products, avoiding excessive alcohol (more than two drinks per day), and decreasing saturated fats have also been shown to be effective. Regular physical activity and losing even small amounts of weight (if needed) can also reduce blood pressure. You can see that these recommendations look similar to the lifestyle recommendations for lowering lipids.

If targeted goals are not met after three months, medications may be recommended in addition to the changes you have made in your lifestyle. (If your blood pressure is greater than 140/90 mmHg, medications may be recommended along with lifestyle changes from the beginning.)

Angiotensin-converting enzyme (ACE) inhibitors, angiotensin receptor blockers (ARBs), beta-blockers, diuretics, and calcium channel blockers are all classes of medications that have been shown to be effective in lowering blood pressure. However, either an ACE inhibitor or an ARB is usually the medication of choice in people with diabetes. If one is not tolerated, the other should be substituted. ACE inhibitors exert their action on angiotensin II, an enzyme in the kidney that can contribute to vascular damage within the kidney and increased pressure. The use of ACE inhibitors and ARBs reduces both blood pressure and microalbuminuria (see Kidneys, page 280). Some ACE inhibitors have been shown to have other effects as well, and may help reduce the inflammation that contributes to vascular damage, and perhaps also contributes to insulin resistance and other related risk factors. The most common side effect of ACE inhibitors is a dry cough. ARBs are less likely to cause a cough and therefore may be substituted for ACE inhibitors in treating hypertension. Because the two medications have different mechanisms of action, they may even be combined. Medications from the other classes are also often combined in treatment programs. Thus, if goals are not met with one medication, another is added. Many people with diabetes require three or more medications to reach target goals.

What Action Can You Take?

The following are some actions you can take to lower your blood pressure. You will notice that some of them are the same steps you can take to lower your blood lipids.

- Learn to check your own blood pressure, record the results, and report any changes to your healthcare providers.
- Be more physically active.
- If you weigh too much, losing even a few pounds can help lower blood pressure.
- Use less salt and eat fewer salty foods.
- If you smoke—try to stop!
- Ask about medications that can help lower blood pressure.

Eyes (Retinopathy)

Your eyes are very vulnerable to the effects of diabetes. For example, many people have *blurred vision* in the early stages of diabetes. This is caused by fluid that seeps into the lens of the eye, causing it to swell and altering its ability to focus properly. Once diabetes treatment begins, the lens resumes its normal shape and vision improves. Blurred vision can also result from fluctuating blood glucose. In such cases, the damage is not permanent. It lasts only a few weeks until you get your blood glucose in control. Therefore, unless you are really having functional difficulty due to poor vision, it is usually recommended that you wait until the glucose levels settle and your vision stabilizes before getting or changing an eyeglass prescription. You may also have other eye problems, many of which are not related to diabetes. For example, anyone can get *glaucoma,* which is caused by too much pressure in the eye. In fact, everyone past age 40 is at risk for glaucoma. Your ophthalmologist (eye doctor) can diagnose glaucoma with a simple test that measures your eyeball pressure. If detected, glaucoma should be treated promptly with, for example, eyedrops that allow proper fluid exchange.

Another problem that anyone can develop is *cataracts,* a condition in which the lens of the eye becomes cloudy. This problem usually comes with advancing age, and everyone is at risk. People with diabetes, however, are more likely to develop cataracts at a younger age, and poor diabetes control can speed the development of cataracts. Eye doctors can treat this problem with surgery.

All of the above conditions can occur in anyone, whether the person has diabetes or not. But there are some serious eye problems that are directly related to poorly controlled diabetes.

Preventing Retinopathy

The most serious eye problem that can occur with diabetes is damage to the *retina,* the thin, light-sensitive inner lining at the back of the eye. This damage, called *retinopathy,* involves small blood vessels in the retina that are easily harmed by high levels of glucose in the blood. About 90 percent of people who have diabetes more than 25 years will have some blood vessel changes in their eyes. Fortunately, complete blindness is rare if retinopathy is diagnosed early and treated promptly and correctly. As a matter of fact, many people who have blood vessel changes in their eyes don't realize it until their doctor tells them. So yearly eye exams by an eye doctor with expertise in diabetes eye care are a must for people with diabetes. Also, many advances have been made in treating and preventing eye disease associated with diabetes: we have truly entered a new era of hope that serious eye damage can be treated and prevented—diabetes is now considered the leading cause of *preventable* vision loss in working-age Americans.

How does retinopathy occur? To understand the problem, you first need to know how the eye works. The eye looks like a Ping-Pong ball and functions like a camera, with a lens in front and other structures in back. For you to see, light bounces off an object and then passes through your eye's lens, which focuses it on your retina. The retina translates the light signal into nerve impulses, which exit at the back of the eye along the optic nerve. The optic nerve then sends the message to your brain, which interprets the image. Wherever there is damage to the retina, the eye is unable to send these messages to the brain.

There are two stages in diabetic retinopathy—an initial stage, called *nonproliferative retinopathy*, and a more serious stage, called *proliferative retinopathy*, in which there is a greater loss of vision or even total blindness Another condition, called *diabetic macular edema*, can occur with either stage.

In the early, nonproliferative stage (formerly called *background retinopathy*) high levels of blood glucose cause damage to the blood vessels in the retina. They can actually leak fluid, which can collect and cause the retina to swell. Fluid collects in the central part of the retina *(macular edema)*, resulting in blurred vision. Macular edema can be treated with laser surgery when central vision is threatened.

A more dangerous stage of eye disease from diabetes is *proliferative retinopathy*. During this stage, abnormal blood vessels grow over the surface of the retina. These fragile blood vessels may rupture and bleed into the *vitreous humor*, the clear gel that fills the center of the eye. When this happens, the blood blocks the passage of light to the retina, and loss of vision or even blindness may occur. A further problem can occur when these blood vessels cause scar tissue, which may pull on the retina and cause it to become detached from the back of the eye. This type of retinopathy can also be treated with laser surgery to reduce the risk of vision loss. If hemorrhage does occur and vision is lost, or if the scar tissue threatens to detach the retina from the back of the eye, a *vitrectomy* (a surgical procedure to remove the blood and scar tissue from within the eye) can frequently successfully restore vision.

Treating Eye Disease

If you experience any changes in your vision, notify your doctor immediately. An eye examination can determine the cause of your vision change, and you can begin timely treatment. Today treatment can dramatically reduce your risk of severe vision loss. Techniques include *laser surgery,* in which a bright, powerful beam of light is focused on the retina. The light scars the area of the retina affected by retinopathy, stopping the formation of new blood vessels. Laser surgery is usually done on an outpatient basis in the eye doctor's office. It may cause some minor discomfort, but that disappears quickly. After treatment, you may experience a slight decrease in vision. But the overall benefits far outweigh any minor drawbacks. The technique is a virtual eyesight saver. Other treatments include vitrectomy surgery, as discussed above. Some new treatments for eyes that do not respond well to laser surgery include the injection of steroids directly into the eye.

Remember, your eyes can become damaged without your knowing it, because the damage can occur in areas that do not affect vision. And you often feel no pain. Only careful eye examinations at regular intervals will detect the damage. If you have type 1 diabetes, it's a good idea to have your eyes examined by an eye doctor expert in diabetes care at least once a year. If you have type 2 diabetes, your eyes should be examined when your diabetes is diagnosed and at least once a year thereafter. Under certain circumstances, you may need immediate attention. Call your eye doctor's office if you experience any of the following symptoms:

- sudden loss of vision
- severe eye pain
- the sensation that a curtain is coming down over your eyes

Your eye doctor will want to see you right away.

Presently, there is no known cure for diabetic retinopathy, and no known means to prevent it from occurring. However, it is clear from major nationwide clinical studies that the risk of severe vision loss (being able to see only the largest letter on the eye chart five feet in front of you) from proliferative retinopathy can be reduced to less than 5 percent, and the risk of moderate vision loss (your vision decreasing by 50 percent) from diabetic macular edema can be substantially reduced, by proper eye care and laser treatment when necessary.

What Action Can You Take?

What can you do to preserve your vision? While there is no foolproof system to prevent retinopathy, whether you have type 1 or type 2 diabetes, the important things to do are:

- Keep your A1C level below 7 percent.

- Keep your blood pressure below 130/80 mmHg.

- If you smoke—try to stop.

- Have at least annual, complete eye examinations through dilated pupils by an eye doctor experienced in diagnosing and managing diabetic eye disease.

- If there is a problem, seek early treatment. Remember that appropriate laser treatment and surgery can significantly reduce the risk of vision loss and blindness from diabetes.

- Control associated risk factors for the onset or progression of retinopathy, including kidney disease, anemia, high cholesterol, and abdominal obesity.

Kidneys (Nephropathy)

Your kidneys are also at risk of damage from high blood glucose. The most serious kidney disease is called *nephropathy*, which can occur in people who have had diabetes for a long time, particularly if their diabetes has been poorly controlled.

Kidney damage is a serious problem because your kidneys are very important organs. Each person is born with two kidneys, which lie toward the back of the body, one on either side of the spine and slightly above the waist. As blood flows through the kidneys, tiny filtering units called *nephrons* filter out waste products and other substances, passing them out as urine. Over time, high blood glucose can damage these filtering units, making it impossible for them to carry out their job. Once the damage begins to occur, it can't be repaired. Certain urine tests can help your doctor pick up very early problems. If these are detected, your doctor can recommend a course of treatment, which may slow or even prevent the development of end-stage renal (kidney) disease, which requires a kidney transplant or dialysis.

If the kidneys lose their ability to function, you may experience the following symptoms, found in end-stage renal disease:

- Swelling of the ankles, hands, face, or other parts of your body
- Loss of appetite, accompanied by a metallic taste in your mouth
- Skin irritations, caused by the buildup of waste products
- Difficulty thinking clearly
- Difficulty managing your blood glucose
- Fatigue, caused by your body's inability to cope with the buildup of fluid and waste materials

You may not notice all of the above-mentioned symptoms. And they usually don't occur suddenly. In fact, the onset of symptoms is generally gradual. Nonetheless, they do signal loss of kidney function. People in the early stages of kidney damage may experience no symptoms. So to detect kidney problems at an early stage, your healthcare provider will test your urine and blood for the presence of minute amounts of protein and other substances, which are the earliest signs of decreasing kidney function. By identifying and treating the problem early on, the process may be slowed or even stopped, so be sure to ask your healthcare provider if he or she is performing these tests, and what the results show.

Once damaged, the kidneys usually continue to deteriorate as years go by. Eventually, they may fail completely. When the kidneys are operating at 10 percent capacity or less, you must find other ways to carry out their tasks.

This may involve a blood-cleansing method called *dialysis*. There are two types of dialysis. With the first type, *hemodialysis,* blood is cleansed by a machine at a hospital or clinic or sometimes at home. The blood is circulated through the machine, which removes all impurities and returns it to the patient. The procedure must be performed three or four times a week, with each procedure lasting three to five hours. With the second type, *peritoneal dialysis,* a fluid flows into the body through a tube that has been permanently inserted in the abdomen. This fluid absorbs the wastes and is then drained and replaced by new fluid. This procedure, which can be done at home, takes about 40 minutes each time and must be repeated three or four times a day.

An alternative to dialysis is *kidney transplantation.* This is a surgical procedure in which the person receives a healthy kidney from a donor. People can live with just one kidney, so this causes little threat to the donor, who is often a close relative of the person receiving the transplant.

Preventing Kidney Damage

Living with with kidney damage can take a great deal of energy and effort, and it's in your best interests to do everything you can to keep your kidneys as healthy as possible. If kidney damage does occur, it cannot be repaired. But there are steps you can take to slow the progression of the damage.

Reduce High Blood Pressure. Keeping your blood pressure at proper levels is very important. High blood pressure puts further strain on the kidneys, and it should be treated promptly with appropriate medication and changes in your food intake.

Keep Your Blood Glucose in Control. Certain types of kidney damage are linked to poor diabetes control. Therefore, one of the best ways to take care of your kidneys is to keep your blood glucose in the normal range. Monitor your blood glucose regularly. Stick to the meal plan and physical activity programs devised by your healthcare providers. Take your diabetes medicines as prescribed.

Treat Urinary Tract Infections. Urinary tract infections can damage your kidneys, and they should be treated immediately by your doctor. Get regular checkups and know the signs of such an infection—cloudy or bloody urine, a burning sensation, frequent urination, or the feeling that you constantly have to urinate. The earlier these infections are detected and treated with antibiotics, the better for the life of your kidneys.

Test for Microalbuminuria. Your urine should be tested regularly for *microalbumin*. This test, usually done on the urine sample you leave during a routine medical exam, measures very small amounts of protein in the urine. When the kidneys are working normally, they return the protein to the blood rather than letting it pass out of the body in the urine. If protein is present in the urine, it means the kidneys are not filtering substances properly. While the presence of microalbumin does not signal the level of problems indicated by the presence of larger amounts of protein, it does suggest that some early kidney damage is occurring. If your doctor diagnoses microalbuminuria, he or she may want to start treating you with medication that might help protect your kidneys from further damage. This medication is also used to treat high blood pressure, but your healthcare provider may prescribe it (even if you don't have high blood pressure) because research shows it may slow kidney damage. Eating a low-protein diet can ease the kidneys' workload, possibly slowing the loss of kidney function. Your dietitian can show you ways to reduce protein in your diet.

Test for Creatinine. Be sure your healthcare provider tests your blood for *creatinine*, a waste product derived from the activity of the muscles. Normally, your kidneys can remove this substance from your blood. A buildup of creatinine in your blood signals that your kidneys are losing their ability to function normally.

Will these preventive measures really help? Yes! According to recent research studies, whatever you do today to keep your kidneys functioning as normally as possible will increase your chances of healthier kidneys in the long run. Good control of diabetes is the key to preventing kidney damage.

What Action Can You Take?

In summary, you can do the following:

- Keep your A1C in the target range of less than 7 percent.
- Ask your healthcare provider to have your urine microalbumin and your serum creatinine checked at least yearly.

- Keep blood pressure below 130/80 mmHg. High blood pressure can damage kidneys.
- Ask about ACE inhibitors and ARBs, medicines that help control microalbumin and blood pressure.

Nerves (Neuropathy)

Chronic high blood glucose can also damage your nerves, producing *neuropathy*, a condition that can be very debilitating and painful. Neuropathy strikes in many forms. Some people say it feels like walking on pins and needles or walking on steel wool. If your hands are affected by neuropathy, you may feel like you are constantly wearing a pair of gloves.

Why does diabetes affect the nerves? The precise cause of the neuropathy that leads to pain in the feet and hands still remains uncertain. It is likely that it is caused by effects of the diabetes on both the arteries that provide blood to the nerves and the impact of the metabolic changes that diabetes can cause. The metabolic effects of elevated glucose hyperglycemia can lead to the production of substances that can be toxic to nerves or interrupt their function.

There are two main types of neuropathy, depending on which nerve cells are damaged: *sensory neuropathy* affects feelings in your legs or hands, and is also referred to as peripheral neuropathy; *autonomic neuropathy* affects nerves that control various organs, such as your stomach and urinary tract.

Sensory Neuropathy

If you have diabetes, you may be painfully familiar with sensory nerve damage. It usually affects the extremities—legs, arms, or hands. It can also affect nerves that send signals to your body's skeletal muscles. Symptoms may include numbness, coldness, tingling, or the feeling that you are walking on steel wool. Occasionally there is pain that feels like tightening bands across the chest or abdomen. Sometimes cold or wet weather makes the condition worse. The pain is often worse at night, making the weight of bedclothes unbearable.

Sensory neuropathy can occur in nearly any nerve. The feeling ranges from minor discomfort to severe pain. Eventually, the pain may disappear—not necessarily because the condition is better but because the nerves have died. Once dead, the nerves can never grow back, and all sensation at that site is lost. The loss of feeling results in numbness. By maintaining better control of your blood glucose, you can help prevent extensive nerve damage.

If you lose sensation in a certain part of your body, you may face another problem. You may have trouble recognizing minor injuries. For example, you may not feel the development of a blister on your foot, which may then become infected. Or you may unknowingly place your feet in scalding water. The foot bones, too, may suffer because of the lack of feeling. The final result may present significant difficulties, including the possibility of the loss of a limb.

Sensory neuropathy may also affect muscles triggered by sensory nerves. Throughout the body, constant tiny electrical impulses travel from your nerves to your muscles. This process normally helps preserve muscle tone. When neuropathy destroys the nerve cells, they cannot stimulate the nearby muscle, resulting in muscle wasting *(amyotrophy)*. If this occurs in your thighs, you may experience a painful condition that causes the thigh muscles to decrease in bulk and strength. You may have difficulty rising from a chair or climbing stairs. Your doctor can try to treat this condition with pain relievers and nerve-quieting medications. You may also be advised to increase your physical activity to help restore muscle strength. Recovery is usually slow, so don't expect overnight changes.

If the muscles responsible for raising the foot are weakened, your foot slaps with each step *(foot drop)*. You may be advised to wear a brace, and recovery usually takes place in time. *Charcot foot* is another problem that can evolve as a result of nerve damage. In this rare condition, the small bones of the foot become misaligned and the foot becomes deformed. If you develop this problem, you may require bed rest or other treatment to keep weight off the affected foot. Individuals are often advised to exercise the large muscles of their legs to prevent further muscle wasting. See Chapter 21 for more information on this condition.

Occasionally neuropathy affects a single nerve that operates a muscle or group of muscles. If the muscles of the eye are involved, you might experience double vision. The condition may continue for three to six weeks or more. But in time, most people completely recover. A less common type of sensory neuropathy involves the muscles in the chest or abdomen. The person feels sharp, burning pain that seems to encircle the body. People often mistake this for chest pain. This condition, called *truncal neuropathy*, usually disappears gradually. Of course, any type of chest pain should be evaluated by a healthcare provider since it can be caused by a variety of problems.

Autonomic Neuropathy

Autonomic neuropathy affects involuntary nerves in the body. These include the nerves that control the actions of the stomach, intestines, esophagus, bladder, penis, and even the circulatory system.

If neuropathy strikes the nerves controlling your digestive tract, you may have trouble processing or disposing of food, a condition called *gastroparesis*. Symptoms of gastroparesis that affect the upper gastrointestinal tract can include bouts of nausea and vomiting, and a feeling of early satiety (the feeling of being full, even though only a small amount of food has been eaten). Symptoms of neuropathy can also affect the lower gastrointestinal tract, typically causing alternating diarrhea and constipation. Your healthcare provider can prescribe medications to help with both of these problems. For nausea and vomiting due to gastroparesis, you may be given medications to increase the motility of your digestive tract and help food move along. Also, if your stomach is emptying slowly, it can affect the timing of your food absorption in relation to the time that your diabetes medications are working. You may achieve a better match between your food and diabetes medications if you delay taking your insulin or diabetes pills until after you eat. Eating four to six small meals daily can minimize feeling overfull after a meal. Solid foods will pass through your stomach more quickly if they are well chewed. Hard-to-chew foods can be ground or pureed. Low-fat, low-fiber foods will also pass through your stomach more quickly than high-fat, high-fiber foods. Some high-fiber foods move through the stomach with great difficulty and may leave behind a residue known as *bezoar*.

For diarrhea, your healthcare provider may prescribe diphenoxylate and atropine (often sold under the brand name Lomotil) or loperamide

(Imodium). Keep in mind that gastrointestinal conditions unrelated to diabetes are much more common than those listed above, which *are* caused by diabetes. Therefore, if you have any of the symptoms described above, be sure to check with your healthcare provider and let him or her determine the cause of your difficulty.

Sometimes diabetes damages the nerves that control the contraction of blood vessels. If you have this condition, your blood pressure may fall when you stand or when you sit up from a lying position. When you have been lying down and get up quickly, you may feel weak and dizzy. If severe, this condition, called *orthostatic hypotension,* can be helped by a certain medication that will raise your blood pressure. Of course, this poses a problem if you already have high blood pressure. Your doctor will have to carefully balance your prescriptions of pressure-raising and pressure-lowering drugs.

Autonomic neuropathy may also affect your bladder, making it difficult to tell when it is full. To handle this problem, you may find it helpful to establish a routine of going to the bathroom regularly, perhaps every two hours.

Diabetes may affect your sexual function, a complication particularly common to men. Nearly one half of all men with diabetes develop *erectile dysfunction (ED, or impotence),* the inability to have or maintain an erection. It is thought that erectile dysfunction caused by diabetes results, in some cases, from damage to the nerves that control the small valves located in the blood vessels leading to and from the penis. These valves regulate the flow of blood into the penis to make it rigid. When the nerves are damaged, the man has trouble having or maintaining an erection. For information on ways to treat this problem, see Chapter 24.

Much less is known about how diabetes may cause specific nerve problems that affect sexual function in women, although it has been suggested that vaginal dryness may occur. Also, high levels of blood glucose may make women more susceptible to vaginal yeast infections, which in turn can make intercourse more painful.

Treating Neuropathy

To treat sensory neuropathy, your healthcare provider may recommend pain relievers such as aspirin or acetaminophen (Tylenol). To help reduce nerve inflammation, you may be given nonsteroidal anti-inflammatory drugs such as naproxen (sold under several brand names, including Naprosyn) or ibuprofen (Motrin, Advil, and Nuprin). The extent to which nerve irritation may be relieved by drugs varies. In the past, medications such as promazine (Sparine) or amitriptyline (Elavil) were used. If these medications, often known as antidepressants or mood elevators, are recommended to you, your doctor is not suggesting the problem is in your head—it's just that these drugs in modest doses seem to help people with neuropathy.

More recently, people have used gabapentin (Neurontin) with some success. Keep in mind, though, that the Food and Drug Administration has not approved this medication to treat painful neuropathy, because of a lack of scientific data demonstrating its effectiveness. However, many physicians and patients report success, and thus this medication has been used for this purpose. Recently, two medications have been introduced with indications for treatment of diabetic neuropathy pain. Duloxetine (Cymbalta), a medication also used to treat depression, has been demonstrated to be effective against neuropathy pain. Another medication similar to gabapentin called pregabalin (Lyrica) has specific indications for treatment of pain, including that caused by diabetic neuropathy. Other medications are also being tested and may be approved for this purpose.

Some people find relief by wearing a body stocking or panty hose to minimize the rubbing effect of clothes. Others are helped by analgesic ointments such as Ben Gay. Relaxation techniques—biofeedback, self-distraction, imagery, and meditation—also benefit some people. Ultimately, the best treatment for painful neuropathy is to control your glucose levels as best you can. With time, this often provides relief. If you are suffering from neuropathy, talk to your healthcare providers about possible treatment options.

What Action Can You Take?

- Maintain blood glucose within normal or near-normal levels.
- Inform your doctor about any tingling or pain, as well as numbness or loss of feeling, especially in the extremities.

■   If you have a loss of sensation in any part of your body, be careful to avoid injuries to that area and check it daily for signs of injury or infection.

The Skin

The skin is the body's largest organ. It serves as your protective "armor," the first line of defense against invading organisms. People with diabetes have the same skin problems as other people, but they also have problems specific to poorly controlled diabetes. One is excessively dry skin, caused by dehydration. This essentially means you don't have enough fluids in your body's tissues, often the outcome of poorly controlled diabetes. Dry skin can be treated with a skin lotion containing lanolin and, of course, by achieving better control of high blood glucose.

Sometimes "shin spots" appear on the front of the legs. These are quite harmless and are nothing to worry about. However, you also have the possibility of getting fungal infections, which are discussed in Chapter 21.

Fatty plaques *(xanthomas)*, which are orange-yellow in color, may appear around the knees or on the shins or elbows. They are sometimes related to high blood levels of cholesterol or triglycerides. You can help this condition disappear with proper diabetes control and by reducing dietary saturated fat and cholesterol (see Chapter 6). Your doctor may also prescribe medications that can lower blood fats.

The most specific skin problem in people with diabetes has a jaw-breaking name—*necrobiosis lipoidica diabeticorum*, usually just referred to as NLD. A relatively harmless condition, it can nevertheless be quite disfiguring. It is believed that NLD results from inflammation of the skin in which the skin thins out, becoming discolored and dimpled. What actually is happening is the destruction of the layer of fat in the skin.

For unknown reasons, NLD occurs more often in women than in men, generally in the teen years. It is most often found on the front of the legs between the knees and ankles and first appears as a pink or red discoloration, which later becomes shiny and tight, much like the skin of an apple. Although generally harmless, this condition can be alarming. You can be assured that the discolored areas often improve, although it may take years. The main danger of this condition is that the area may break open, form a sore, and become infected.

There is no satisfactory treatment for NLD. Ointments are generally ineffective, although some cases have improved with cortisone treatment. Skin grafts are sometimes necessary for severe cases, which fortunately are rare. Researchers are experimenting with new treatments. For example, some scientists propose that NLD may be caused by the clumping of platelets, tiny cells that are part of the blood-clotting mechanism, which leads to blockage and inflammation of blood vessels and the beginning of NLD; they suggest using "anticlumping" medications to slow the progression of the condition. To date, this treatment is still experimental, but it may offer hope in the future.

Another condition that is associated with insulin resistance in diabetes is *acanthosis nigricans*. It is characterized by a thickening and darkening of the skin in patchy areas in the skin folds of the armpits, neck, or groin, ranging in color from tan to dark brown. It is usually a sign of insulin resistance, and any overweight person with this symptom should be tested for prediabetes.

Sorting It Out

You should be aware of the wide range of long-term complications that can arise from your diabetes. But don't make the mistake of thinking that all of your medical problems are related to your diabetes. You may ignore a completely different problem that needs prompt attention. How can you sort it out? Many people see one doctor for their primary care and a diabetes specialist for their diabetes. This is strongly recommended by organizations like Joslin Diabetes Center and the American Diabetes Association. As a general rule, if you are unsure about a particular problem or wondering whether it is related to your diabetes, ask a member of your healthcare team.

If you have a new health problem, bring it up when you see your primary-care doctor. Don't wait until you see your diabetes specialist. And be sure to see your diabetes specialist at *least* every six months, and an ophthalmologist at *least* once a year to check your eyes. Also, plan to work with other members of your healthcare team—the nurse, dietitian, and others—to solve any specific problems you may have.

The emotional strain of dealing with diabetes and the threat of long-term complications can take a toll. The members of your healthcare team can help you sort out your feelings. They can also direct you to a specialist who is trained to help you cope emotionally with a lifelong disease. This topic is covered more fully in Chapter 26. Many diabetes centers have support groups in which people with diabetes share their problems and help one another find solutions. You can also check with the American Diabetes Association, the Juvenile Diabetes Foundation, or local diabetes societies for listings of groups in your area.

During the past decades, major advances have been made in diagnosing, treating, and preventing the long-term complications of diabetes. Researchers have produced remarkable treatments for problems with the eyes, kidneys, and nerves; blood vessel disease; and other problems associated with diabetes. As research continues, you can expect even more improvements in treatments. But success in the immediate future rests with you and your healthcare providers. By learning about long-term complications and watching for signs, you are pivotal in arresting their progress. And by learning how to prevent them—particularly with good diabetes management—you have the promise of a healthier you.

CHAPTER 21

Foot Care

People with diabetes have a greater chance of developing foot problems. In fact, they spend more days in the hospital with foot complications than with any other problem. However, many of these complications are preventable. For that reason, your healthcare providers will ask you to pay special attention to your feet.

Why are you at higher risk for these problems? A combination of the following factors sets the stage for foot trouble:

- People with diabetes often have less sensation in their feet due to nerve damage *(neuropathy)*, as discussed in Chapter 20.
- People with diabetes tend to have more narrowing or blockage in their blood vessels, also discussed in Chapter 20.
- Many people with type 2 diabetes who are older or are overweight often can't reach down to properly inspect or care for their feet.
- People who have had diabetes for a long time frequently have eye complications that affect their ability to see where they are placing their feet and to examine their feet adequately.
- People with diabetes that is not well controlled have a higher risk for infection because their ability to fight it is reduced.

Symptoms of Foot Problems

One of the most common problems for people with diabetes is nerve damage that results in a decrease or loss of feeling in the feet. For example, you may step on a tack without noticing any pain. Or you may be totally unaware of a severe burn on your feet after walking barefoot on hot pavement. The loss of feeling also makes you unaware of a sore or injury, which can then more easily become infected because you don't take care of the injury.

Another common condition in diabetes is impaired circulation. Blood vessels narrow with age, but this process is accelerated in people with diabetes. The legs and feet are among the first to be affected. Signs of poor circulation include:

- Cramps that occur in the legs while walking but go away after resting.
- Slow-healing cuts and scratches.
- Redness of your feet when you are sitting, or whiteness when they are propped up on a stool or chair.
- Lack of normal hair growth on the legs and feet.
- Pain in your feet and legs, especially at night, which can be relieved by hanging them over the side of the bed. This is a sign of more advanced disease.

The feet may prove vulnerable to infection because of the nerve and circulation problems that frequently complicate diabetes, particularly if it is not well controlled. Infections begin with damage to the skin, which serves as a protective barrier. Once damaged, the barrier is no longer intact and provides an entryway for invading organisms, leading to infection. Damage to your skin can result from an injury, irritation, or foot deformities. Common foot problems include corns and calluses, ingrown toenails, fungal infections (athlete's foot), and sores caused by pressure on the foot, perhaps from poorly fitting shoes.

Unless treated promptly, a foot infection can lead to a chain of events that worsen with time. In the presence of infection, the body responds with inflammation and swelling. Diminished circulation decreases the body's ability to move disease-fighting cells to the infection site. Moreover, elevated blood glucose levels make these cells less effective in battling the infection. And if you have neuropathy, you cannot feel the pain of infection. In fact, your nerve function may be so reduced that you continue to walk on the injured part. The situation is particularly dangerous when there is pus or drainage from a sore and the foot is red, hot, and swollen. If you ever have this problem, *go to the emergency room at once.* You need the immediate care of a medical doctor to stop the infection and avoid permanent, severe damage that, in the worst cases, can lead to losing a foot or toe.

Another problem that can develop is *Charcot foot.* This is a condition that affects approximately 1 of every 700 people who have diabetes, and it is usually limited to those who have moderate to severe loss of feeling in their feet. Charcot foot is more common among people who are overweight, but it can also occur in thin people. No one is quite sure how Charcot foot begins. However, it is thought to be caused by an incidental trauma or a twist of the foot that injures some of the ligaments that support the arch of the foot. Once the ligaments have been damaged, the bones begin grinding against one another and the arch may collapse. The damage often goes unnoticed because the person has already lost feeling in the foot. With the collapse of the bones in the arch, the person's weight is distributed differently along the sole of the foot, introducing pressure points and irritation that may lead to sores and infection.

If your foot swells without explanation and is warm to the touch with no apparent break in the skin, you may have Charcot foot. When these symptoms occur, be sure your healthcare provider or foot doctor (podiatrist) examines your foot. Charcot foot must be differentiated from the red, hot, swollen foot caused by infection. With infection, you should go to the emergency room immediately.

Rest is the primary treatment for Charcot foot. Depending on the severity of the damage, no weight should be placed on it for several weeks. Permanent foot deformities can be avoided if the condition is diagnosed and treated early.

Guidelines for Daily Foot Care

To minimize the risk of foot problems from diabetes, it's important to follow a daily routine of foot care and inspection.

- **EXAMINE YOUR FEET.** Each day, look at your feet in good light. Be sure you examine the bottoms of your feet. If you cannot bend over to see them, place a hand mirror on the floor and hold each foot over it. If your eyesight is poor, have someone examine your feet for you. Look for areas of redness, as well as dryness or breaks in the skin, especially around the toenails and between the toes. Notify your healthcare provider immediately about sores or infections that do not seem to be healing properly. Redness, swelling, and increased warmth are signs of infection.

- **WASH YOUR FEET.** Wash, but do not soak, your feet in warm, soapy water each day. Soaking softens the skin and makes it more susceptible to infection. Never use hot water. Always test the temperature of the water with your elbow—this will prevent burning your feet if you have nerve damage and cannot feel the water temperature. Use a mild hand soap. Rinse your feet well after washing, and dry them carefully, especially between the toes.

- **CARE FOR YOUR SKIN.** After washing and examining your feet, lubricate them to prevent dryness. Creams are a better choice than lotions because they hold moisture in the skin longer. Begin applying the cream at your heels and work toward your toes. Apply the cream at bedtime and put on clean, dry socks to promote absorption. Do not use perfumed lotions, because they contain alcohol, which dries rather than lubricates. Do not put any lotions or creams between your toes. If your feet perspire, use talcum, baby powder, or mild foot powder to absorb the moisture. Do not allow the powder to cake between the toes.

- **FILE YOUR TOENAILS.** File your nails with an emery board. Never use scissors or clippers, because you might cut yourself and risk infection.

Don't file your nails shorter than the ends of your toes. Shape them according to the contours of your toes and the toes next to them. If you have impaired vision, have a friend or podiatrist trim your nails when needed. Consult a foot doctor for ingrown toenails or fungal nail infections that lead to discoloration and thickening. These conditions need expert care.

■ **CARE FOR CORNS, CALLUSES, BLISTERS, AND WARTS.** Corns and calluses can increase pressure on the feet and are signs of potential ulcers. If neglected, they can lead to irritation and possible infection. Properly fitting shoes can relieve and prevent these thickened areas of skin. Use a moisture-restoring cream to soften them. Do not tear off loose skin, and never use corn- or callus-removal products. Don't cut corns or calluses—do not perform bathroom surgery! Watch for discoloration on or around corns and calluses, which could indicate a more serious problem, such as an ulcer beneath the skin. Because of the potential for foot ulcers, corns and calluses should be examined regularly by a foot doctor who may decide they should be reduced in size or even removed altogether.

Blisters should be treated with antiseptic. Warts are difficult to treat and may disappear if left alone. Like calluses, plantar warts (on the soles) lead to point pressure and may ulcerate. If a wart begins to spread or causes you pain when you're walking, consult your health-care providers or podiatrist.

■ **WEAR GOOD SHOES.** In addition to daily foot care, you should be concerned about your footwear. Buy shoes that protect and cover your feet and have been properly fitted—when you're buying footwear, try the shoes on in the afternoon when your feet are slightly swollen, and wear the socks or stockings that you plan to use with them. Wear swimming shoes when you go into a pool, lake, or the ocean. Make sure your shoes allow room for your toes to rest in their natural positions; avoid pointed shoes that squeeze your toes together. When you wear slippers around the house, be sure they are sturdy enough to prevent stubbing your toes. Always check inside your shoes for foreign objects before putting them on. Break new shoes in gradually to prevent blisters from forming.

- **ALWAYS WEAR SHOES.** Don't go barefoot (especially on the beach) or wear sandals, clogs, or flip-flops—your feet need more protection.

- **WEAR PROPER SOCKS AND STOCKINGS.** Wear socks made of materials that wick moisture away from the skin. Wear a clean pair every day; if your feet sweat, change your socks several times a day. Make sure socks are the correct size and free of seams and darns. Never wear socks or stockings with constricting tops; they can decrease the circulation in your legs. Constricting garters or girdles should also be avoided. Check your socks for drainage, which may be your first sign of a new ulcer or blister.

- **EXERCISE YOUR FEET.** Walking is the best physical activity for your feet, provided your shoes fit properly. Walking helps the circulation in the feet. After exercising, be sure to check your feet for signs of irritation or blister formation.

- **AVOID INJURY FROM HEAT AND COLD.** Don't let your feet get too hot. Avoid sunburn, walking barefoot on hot pavements, electric heating pads, hot-water bottles, and bathwater that is too hot (test it first with a bath thermometer). Beware of exposed radiators and steam rooms or saunas as sources of potential burns. Cold and frostbite can also harm foot tissue, so be extra protective of your feet in cold weather.

Have Your Feet Examined Regularly

Regular examination of the feet is very important.

- Everyone with diabetes should have a foot exam at least once a year. Examinations should occur more often if you have neuropathy, poor circulation, and/or any foot deformities.

- A foot examination should include visual examination of your feet, including the skin integrity, checking of your foot pulses, and checking of sensation using items such as a monofilament, pin, and/or tuning fork.

- Assist your provider in checking your feet by wearing shoes and socks that are easily removed, and do take them off during your appointment.

- Referral to a podiatrist (foot doctor) is often recommended if you have foot deformities, pressure points, or nail deformities, or just for good preventive maintenance.

- Special shoes may be recommended if you have foot deformities, ulceration on your feet, prior amputation, or nerve damage. Medicare and some insurance companies will cover part or all of the cost for prescription footwear.

First-Aid Treatment

Once in a while, something will happen to your feet, so it's important to know the basic guidelines for first-aid care.

Cuts and Scratches

Treat cuts and scratches promptly. Wash the affected area with warm water and soap. *Do not soak.* You may apply antibiotic ointments such as Bacitracin, Neosporin, Polysporin, or ST37. Never use strong antiseptics such as iodine, Betadine, mercurochrome, boric acid, Epsom salts, creosol, or carbolic acid. Cover the affected area with a dry sterile dressing and paper tape or a Telfa bandage. Do not use adhesive tape or Band-Aids, as they may cause allergic reactions or irritations. Change the dressing every day. Do not apply heat treatments, such as a hot-water bottle or a heating pad, to the cut or scratch. Stay off your feet as much as possible and call your healthcare provider if affected areas do not improve within 24 hours. If red, swollen areas develop or a yellowish drainage occurs, contact your doctor immediately. Do not assume the condition has improved just because there is no pain.

Athlete's Foot

Athlete's foot is caused by a fungus that grows in a warm, moist setting. Symptoms are itching, tiny blisters, and the scaling of skin between the toes or on the soles of the feet. If these symptoms appear, consult your healthcare provider to make sure it is athlete's foot rather than some other skin problem. Since the fungus of athlete's foot grows in a warm, moist setting, you should wash and carefully dry your feet and change your socks or stockings more than once a day. Feet that perspire heavily are more likely to get athlete's foot, so keep your feet as dry as possible. If your skin is too moist, apply talcum, baby powder, or a mild foot powder to absorb the moisture. Changing your socks will also wick moisture away from the skin. Treat athlete's foot with an over-the-counter antifungal ointment such as Lotrimin, Lamisil, or Tinactin. Avoid sneakers and boots. Do not use any other remedies without the consent of your healthcare providers or podiatrist. If these measures don't work within seven to ten days, stronger prescription drugs may be needed, so consult your provider.

Prevention Is the Best Strategy

Today you have every reason to be hopeful about preventing and treating foot problems. Again, good management of your blood glucose is essential to the health of your circulatory and nervous systems. The longer these systems stay healthy, the less chance you have of developing serious foot infections.

It's also comforting to know that damaged feet that once would have been lost are now being saved. This success is due to a number of factors—better care of diabetes, the use of antibiotics, and improved surgical techniques. For example, narrowed or closed blood vessels that cannot transport blood down to the legs and feet can often be replaced by grafting blood vessels from other parts of the body or using synthetic vessels. Drugs are also available that increase the flexibility of the membranes of red blood cells, allowing them to pass through partially clogged arteries. Of course, the best strategy is prevention. Exercise can improve circulation, and with daily inspection and care of your feet—and by keeping your diabetes in control—you can help prevent foot problems, and keep those that develop from becoming limb-threatening.

What Action Can You Take?

The following are ten rules for foot care:

- Never soak your feet!
- Never apply heat of any kind to your feet.
- Never cut your toenails—file them.
- Never wear shoes that do not fit.
- Never go barefoot.
- Never use strong medicines on your feet.
- Never allow corns or calluses to go untreated.
- Never perform bathroom surgery on your feet.
- Never keep your feet too moist or too dry.
- Never assume that the sensation and circulation in your feet are normal. Instead treat your feet as though they are a potential for trouble—which they are!

PART FIVE

Special Challenges of Diabetes

CHAPTER 22

Diabetes in Children and Adolescents

If your child has diabetes, you probably have many questions: *What should I do when my child's blood glucose is too high or too low? What can my child eat? How do I take care of my child on a day-to-day basis? How can I help my child eat better? What should I do if my child has the flu? How can I get my child to be physically active?* The list can go on and on.

Before answering these and other questions, it's important to emphasize that clinicians have more treatment options than ever before to help treat your child's diabetes. There are new types of insulin that can help keep your child's blood glucose under good control. There are new glucose monitors to help you, your child, and your child's other caregivers monitor blood glucose. Counting carbohydrates provides more flexibility in food choices. And your healthcare team is available to provide the education and support that your child, you, and your family need.

Technology has revolutionized the management of type 1 diabetes. Delivery systems for insulin, blood glucose monitors, new insulins, and insulin pumps have greatly improved treatment programs. Unfortunately, our advances in technology also have a a downside: labor-saving devices, transportation, computers, and video games, together with calorie-dense foods that are readily available and inexpensive, have contributed to a dramatic increase in type 2 diabetes in youth.

The increasing number of children diagnosed with type 2 diabetes is of concern today. In some medical centers, more than 40 percent of new cases of diabetes in children are type 2 diabetes. The increase in the number of cases of type 2 diabetes in youth has been most dramatic among ethnic and racial minorities.

Both type 1 and type 2 diabetes in youth require parents or other caregivers to be knowledgeable and involved in the care of their child's diabetes and in lifestyle changes that facilitate improved glucose control. If your child has type 1 or type 2 diabetes, the key is to approach the illness in an organized and positive manner. Children have an amazing capacity to adapt. In fact, they are often more able than adults to accept changes in lifestyle, perhaps because they have not yet developed habits that are hard to break. With your help—and the expert advice from a healthcare team—your child can continue to lead a happy, healthy, and active life.

Basic Skills for Caregivers

When your child is diagnosed with diabetes, your first step as a parent or caregiver is to focus on the immediate treatment program your child needs. In time, you can learn more about the intricacies of diabetes—knowledge that will make you even more aware of the various treatment options. But you should learn about diabetes gradually. It's unrealistic to try to learn everything at once. This is not the time to worry about the possible problems that may occur in people who have had poorly controlled diabetes for a long time. There will be plenty of time to develop strategies that will help prevent long-term complications. What you need to do is accept the fact that your child has a condition that needs to be managed on a daily basis, learn the basics, and move forward with a positive outlook.

If Your Child Has Type 1 Diabetes— What Parents and Caregivers Need to Know

As your child's caregiver, your first goal is to learn the following "basic skills":

- *insulin injections*—how to give insulin injections with a syringe, an insulin pen, or an insulin pump
- *low blood glucose*—how to recognize, treat, and prevent low blood glucose
- *high blood glucose*—how to recognize, treat, and prevent high blood glucose
- *monitoring*—how to monitor your child's blood glucose and ketone levels
- *nutrition*—what kinds of food to prepare, how much to offer, when to offer these foods, and how to adjust insulin doses based on what your child eats
- *physical activity*—how to adjust insulin and carbohydrate intake for times when your child is more physically active than usual
- *rules for sick days*—how to handle your child's diabetes during sick days (sick-day rules will be discussed later in the chapter)

In this chapter, you will become acquainted with these skills. For detailed information, be sure to read other chapters on these topics. And of course, continue to rely on your child's healthcare providers as your primary source of information—they will tell you what you need to know for your child's diabetes. In this chapter, you will also learn the ways in which diabetes can affect normal behavior at various stages of your child's development. Understanding these changes is a very important part of your child's care.

If Your Child Has Type 1 Diabetes— What Your Child Needs to Know

How much do children need to know about their diabetes? First of all, they need to know that it is not their fault that they have diabetes—

nothing they could have done would have prevented it. They need to know that with your help and their healthcare providers' help they will be able to manage their diabetes and live healthy, active lives. Treatment depends on your child's age and maturity. Some children can learn to measure and inject their own insulin by early adolescence. However, it is recommended that parents and caregivers share responsibility with their children for insulin injections until puberty is completed, usually by midadolescence. Every child is different in his or her capacity to cope with the demands of diabetes, but all children need and deserve their parents' help and support well into the teenage years. Before you give your child the responsibility for measuring and injecting insulin, remember that this is a serious and complex matter. Your child needs to be mature enough to handle the job, and in general, children are not capable of having sole responsibility for insulin injections until they are older adolescents.

How about checking their blood glucose? Children need to understand the rationale for regular checking, whether or not they can do these checks themselves. Most important, they need to learn the symptoms of a "low blood glucose reaction" (also called an insulin reaction) and how to take appropriate action. Later, as they begin to appreciate the overall goals of diabetes treatment, they will want to accept a greater role in their care. In fact, children quickly learn that maintaining good health is the ticket to joining their friends in many of the normal activities of youth.

If Your Child Has Type 2 Diabetes— What Parents and Caregivers Need to Know

As your child's caregiver, your first goal is to learn the following "basic skills":

- **LIFESTYLE CHANGES**—when we speak of "lifestyle changes," we are speaking of
  - healthy eating
  - increasing physical activity—encouraging your child to be more physically active
  - decreasing sedentary behavior—sometimes the most effective way to do this is just by turning off the television

■ FOOD AND MEAL PLANNING—what kinds of food to prepare and how to help your child lose even a small amount of weight (or to stop weight gain); losing even a small amount of weight can often return blood glucose to normal and decrease insulin resistance

■ MONITORING—how and when to monitor your child's blood glucose levels

■ COMMUNICATION AND BEHAVIORAL MODIFICATION—to help adolescents change and maintain lifestyle programs requires family and friends to be involved and supportive

■ MEDICATION(S)—a basic understanding of what oral diabetes pills might be used in children and when and why insulin injections may be necessary

In this chapter, you will become acquainted with some of these skills. But achieving treatment goals requires a team approach. Whereas type 1 diabetes usually occurs throughout childhood during the time when parents perhaps have more influence, type 2 diabetes usually occurs in adolescence, when peer influences are stronger. In addition to a physician, other healthcare team members can help you provide your child with guidance and support. The team should include a psychologist or social worker, a dietitian, a nurse, and an exercise specialist.

If Your Child Has Type 2 Diabetes— What Your Child Needs to Know

It is easy to understand why your child may have problems with the necessary treatment program for type 2 diabetes. Adolescence is a time when teens struggle for independence and desire to be like their friends, and because they feel they are invulnerable, they may engage in risk-taking behaviors for excitement. Developing type 2 diabetes could not come at a worse time. Your child therefore needs to understand that it is important to work as a family to manage his or her diabetes, and that while lifestyle changes may be difficult, they are essential. Adolescents are not generally motivated by reference to rewards in the future—rather, motivation for learning to manage their diabetes may more likely come from immediate gratification, such as improving acne, regulating menstrual cycles, improving their physical appearance, and gaining increased energy.

A Message to Parents: Handle Your Emotions

As you learn the basic skills of caring for your child or teenager, it's important to focus on your feelings as well. First, think about how you initially reacted to the news that your child has diabetes. Perhaps you felt overwhelmed, confused, or angry that this happened to your child or teenager and your family. You may even have felt guilty because you may feel you are at fault for your child's diabetes. You may have mistakenly blamed your child for being lazy or cranky, when, in fact, diabetes was causing most of the problems. These feelings are all part of the normal "coping" process that begins at diagnosis.

If you can eliminate such negative feelings, you'll be less likely to fall into an emotional trap that can stand in the way of helping your child manage his or her diabetes. Below are some positive attitudes to develop in caring for your child or teen.

Learn to Share Responsibility. If you are the parent of a younger child, you will be carrying most of the burden of caring for your child's diabetes. In essence, you are the one who will help plan, carry out, and assess your child's treatment. In raising any child, a parent's goal is to gradually transfer responsibility to that child. But when a child has diabetes, it's not quite the same. You will have to achieve a more delicate balance between encouraging your child's independence and still requiring a level of interdependence and shared responsibility. It is important to talk with your healthcare team about this very significant issue.

Sometimes, you may believe that you alone can meet your child's special needs. But you should realize that it's necessary to transfer some responsibility to other people—family members, relatives, school staff, coaches, and friends. This is particularly important as your child becomes a teen or if your child is a teen when he or she develops diabetes. Your healthcare providers can be an important resource in helping you educate family, friends, school personnel, and your child's or teen's friends about diabetes.

Set a Good Example. Perhaps one of the most difficult aspects of having a child or teen with diabetes is that it may require you as a parent to also make lifestyle changes. You can't expect your child or teen to follow a meal plan if you do not eat healthfully as well. For example, children and teens often drink regular soft drinks and juices in large quantities. It's important that water, diet soft drinks, and flavored drinks sweetened with sugar substitutes are readily available for them to drink. If you continue to drink regular soft drinks and eat inappropriate snacks, it will be very hard for your child or teen to make changes. It may also be important for you to start a physical activity program and encourage the whole family to be active.

Be Positive, Honest, and Hopeful. If your child or teen has diabetes, the whole family needs to be involved. At times, this may strain the family's ability to understand and support your child or teenager. Sometimes you will feel very alone. If you feel alone in the struggle, you may become despondent and fail to do some of the things you should be doing to help your child. As a parent, you may be going through other struggles, such as financial pressures or stress at work, which may also get in the way of your child's treatment, perhaps causing you to give up and essentially leave your child "on his own."

How can you cope? Be honest about all your feelings. First of all, talk to your child's healthcare team about your feelings. They can help you face the situation realistically—and with a great deal of hope. They can help you keep your child's welfare in the forefront. Second, connect with other parents of youngsters with diabetes. Ask your healthcare providers to help you meet people in similar situations, or contact Joslin Diabetes Center or the American Diabetes Association for information about family support groups in your area.

Remember, kids often take their cues from their parents. If you maintain a "can do" spirit, it will rub off on your child or teen. You will also be able to teach your child or teen more about diabetes. For example, he or she may think that diabetes will just disappear someday. Diabetes, however, will never go away. It will be with your child or teen *always,* and you need to help your son or daughter accept this fact.

Goals of Treatment

The goals of treatment are to lower blood glucose levels and keep them as near normal as possible. However, very young children are at more risk than older children from severely low blood glucose levels that will affect brain development. Therefore, for them blood glucose goals are slightly higher than for school-age children. Tight glycemic control is not recommended for children under the age of 2 and should be applied cautiously in children less than 8. Most children younger than 6 or 7 are unable to recognize symptoms of low blood glucose and as a result cannot respond appropriately. As with adults, goals and treatment programs for children need to be individualized. Be sure to discuss this issue with your child's healthcare providers and learn what their recommendations are. Table 22-1 gives the Joslin Diabetes Center's glucose goals for younger children with diabetes.

Why Do Children Develop Type 1 Diabetes?

Children develop diabetes for the same reasons that older people do. In the case of type 1 diabetes, hereditary factors may set the stage for autoimmu-

TABLE 22-1	Glycemic Control Goals for Younger Children with Diabetes		
Age	Plasma Glucose Goal Ranges (mg/dl)		A1C
	Before meals	Bedtime/Overnight	
Toddlers and preschoolers (0–5)	100 to 180	110 to 200	less than or equal to 8.5 (but greater than or equal to 7.5)
School age (6–11)	90 to 180	100 to 180	less than 8%
Adolescents and young adults (12–20s)	90 to 130	90 to 150	less than 7%

nity. In other words, a child may be born with certain genes, the basic blue-prints of life, that increase the chances he or she will develop diabetes. Then something triggers the immune system to mistakenly destroy the body's own beta cells—the cells in the pancreas that produce insulin. Once this happens, the child has diabetes. Environmental factors unknown at this time are perhaps what causes the immune system to destroy the beta cells. There is still much to learn about the causes of type 1 diabetes in children, including both genetic and environmental factors.

Type 1 diabetes affects boys and girls in equal numbers. Although it can develop at all ages, from the early months of childhood through the teenage years and even into adulthood, the most common time is during the early teenage years, though we are seeing an increase in the number of very young children with type 1 diabetes. In children, the symptoms of type 1 diabetes often seem to appear very rapidly, in contrast to adults, who may develop type 1 diabetes more slowly. The symptoms in children may include tremendous thirst and frequent urination. The child may eat large amounts of food yet experience an unexplained but very rapid weight loss. If the condition is not recognized early, dehydration may occur because of the loss of fluids from excessive urination. Vision can be blurred from temporary changes in the lenses of the eyes. Overall, your active and robust child may become weak, irritable, and have little energy. Schoolwork often takes a plunge. Your child may also complain of pains in the legs and abdomen or have difficulty breathing. If these symptoms are present in a child, he or she should be checked by a healthcare provider immediately.

Although the symptoms often are abrupt—that is, they seem to happen suddenly—in reality the destruction of the pancreas's beta cells has been gradual over a period of years. When the level of destruction reaches the point at which the beta cells are no longer able to produce adequate insulin, symptoms appear, and then the need for treatment is urgent. Today, though there is yet no way to stop the destruction of the beta cells, a great deal of research is being done and we have high hopes for the future.

Treatment of Type 1 Diabetes in Children

One goal of the treatment plan developed by your healthcare providers to manage type 1 diabetes in your child will be to relieve the symptoms caused by his or her high blood glucose levels. Also of concern is the prevention of acute complications such as ketoacidosis and hypoglycemia (too low a blood glucose level). Moreover, the treatment plan will reduce your child's chances of developing long-term complications from diabetes. As your child follows this plan, he or she will feel better and have more energy.

Blood glucose levels have an impact on how your child grows and develops. For this reason, your child's blood glucose levels should be as well controlled as possible. While this may seem difficult at times, it should be your overall goal. But always approach the treatment plan with a bit of realism. It is important that children feel included in family, school, and holiday celebrations, and there may be times that to maintain the social and emotional health of your child, you have to compromise. It is unrealistic, for example, to try to "fine tune" blood glucose levels at a child's birthday party.

Your Healthcare Team Is Vital

If your child has diabetes, it's vital that you seek the guidance of a healthcare team. The team should consist of people with a special knowledge and interest in how children develop—both physically and emotionally. They should have up-to-date training and experience in the management of type 1 diabetes.

The team should include a pediatrician who is specially trained in diabetes, a pediatric diabetes nurse specialist, a dietitian who works mostly with children and teenagers, and a mental-health professional (a social worker or clinical psychologist who understands emotional and social problems in the family). The team should work with the child's own pediatrician and others involved with the child, such as teachers, the school nurse, the school guidance counselor, and sports coaches.

Your healthcare providers are there for you now and in the future. At first they will help you and your child understand and follow the initial treatment plan. The team will also help you continue the treatment into the years ahead, making the proper adjustments as your child grows and develops. This support is an important part of the overall treatment.

If you don't live near a medical center that is staffed with a diabetes treatment team, your child will probably receive routine care and emergency treatment from your local doctor. But you may find it very beneficial to travel to a specialized diabetes center. If you choose this course, it's essential for everyone involved—you, your family doctor, and the members of the child's diabetes team—to maintain constant communication.

Treatment Stages of Type 1 Diabetes in Children

Children often go through the following treatment stages in type 1 diabetes:

- **ACUTE ONSET, OR NEWLY DIAGNOSED.** This is the first sign that your child has diabetes. Symptoms include fatigue, frequent urination, thirst, and, of course, high blood glucose. During this stage, your child's blood glucose levels may be controlled with small doses of insulin.

- **REMISSION, OR "HONEYMOON."** During this stage, your child's diabetes seems to improve or even go away. This "remission" usually lasts only a short time. The diabetes has not been cured—soon it will come back and become an even greater challenge to control. During this stage, it is important to continue your child's insulin doses. By giving small amounts of insulin, you protect the remaining beta cells and help prolong the honeymoon stage. The remission often ends with an infection or another acute illness, or with the onset of puberty and increased growth.

- **INTENSIFICATION.** During this stage, managing your child's diabetes becomes more intense. Diabetes is not getting worse, but it is more difficult to control. You must carefully check your child's blood glucose levels, and the amounts of insulin must be increased or adjusted. You and your child may get discouraged because the blood glucose levels tend to fluctuate without any obvious cause and despite your careful efforts.

- **TOTAL DIABETES.** At this stage, the pancreas's beta cells have been almost or totally destroyed. The body depends solely on an outside supply of insulin to convert food into energy or store it for future use. Diabetes becomes somewhat harder to control because the body is no longer producing any insulin to supplement the injected insulin. If insulin is omitted, your child is at immediate risk of developing ketoacidosis, a dangerous condition caused by the buildup of ketones in the blood (see Chapter 18).

Insulin

Insulin is the primary treatment for children and adolescents with type 1 diabetes. Before your child developed diabetes, insulin was present at all times in the bloodstream. The pancreas automatically secreted insulin in response to eating, and the level of insulin increased with the amount of carbohydrate eaten. Now that your child has diabetes and is being treated with insulin, the goal is to try to copy that pattern as closely as possible. In general, one daily injection or premixed insulin injection won't be enough. Most children with type 1 diabetes need a program that replaces insulin in a pattern resembling what they would have had if they did not have diabetes—referred to as a physiologic insulin program (see Chapter 15). They usually need a basal, or background insulin supply, provided by insulins such as glargine or another long-acting insulin (or two or more injections of intermediate-acting insulin such as NPH or lente) or basal insulin provided by an insulin pump. They also need bolus doses of rapid-acting insulin (lispro, aspart, or glulisine) at mealtimes to keep blood glucose at the desired level.

The insulin programs outlined in Chapter 15 for type 1 diabetes are also used in the treatment of children and teenagers; study this chapter to gain an understanding of the various insulin-dosing schedules. Insulin doses are changed daily based on the results of frequent checking of blood glucose and the amount of carbohydrate eaten. Some children and adolescents also use insulin pumps, which require intensive education, careful monitoring, and ongoing evaluation by medical professionals familiar with pump use. See Chapter 16 for information on how pumps can be used effectively.

Your child's insulin doses will need to be adjusted continuously. Insulin needs change as a child grows and develops, so it is important that your child be reevaluated at least every three months, or at time intervals recommended by your healthcare team.

Physical activity can reduce the body's insulin needs, although it will never completely replace injected insulin (see Chapter 9). If your child's activity level varies, it may be necessary to adjust his or her insulin dose or to increase carbohydrate intake. For example, if your child is going away to summer camp, starting an active summer job, or beginning a new sports season after an inactive school year, he or she may need less insulin, more carbohydrate, or both.

Both parents and all your child's caregivers should learn to prepare and give insulin. Detailed guidelines are provided in Chapter 14. In early adolescence, some children may begin to participate in their own care and give their own injections, but only with parental supervision. Don't rush your child to accept this responsibility until he or she is mature enough to understand the dangers of using an inaccurate dose of insulin.

Nutrition

The nutritional needs of children with diabetes are the same as those of children who don't have diabetes. Your child needs no special foods, vitamins, or minerals. The eating program that your dietitian will develop provides everything needed for energy and growth. However, the key to meal planning is to coordinate insulin with the times your child eats, the amount of food eaten, and his or her physical activities. This topic is discussed in detail in Chapter 4.

By learning carbohydrate counting and insulin-to-carbohydrate ratios, flexibility is possible. Children's appetites and schedules vary so much that an insulin program that covers the child's usual lifestyle is essential. For example, children often prefer snacks—if a rapid-acting insulin is used at meals, it may not cover snacks. Some children can eat 15 grams of carbohydrate for a snack without needing to take additional rapid-acting insulin. If the snack is larger than that amount, an additional injection of rapid-acting insulin may be needed to cover the snack. One of the advantages of insulin pump therapy is the ease of giving bolus insulin when the child chooses to eat.

Many youngsters are influenced by peer pressure about food—pressure to eat or drink or not to eat or drink something. The fear or embarrassment that they will have a low blood glucose reaction in front of their friends may cause teenagers to overeat. Children sometimes test the limits of their diabetes by experimenting with overeating and undereating. In dealing with these issues, the approach should be similar to the one the family uses to effectively solve other types of parent-child conflicts. Try to get to the bottom of the issues causing the conflicts. Set firm but realistic guidelines in consultation with the dietitian on your healthcare team.

Physical Activity

Physical activity is an important part of a healthy lifestyle. Children and teenagers should be encouraged to participate in regular sports activities and various exercise activities. To do this safely may require changes in insulin doses or carbohydrate intake. For additional guidelines, see Chapters 9 and 10.

- **LOWERING OF BLOOD GLUCOSE.** The benefits of physical activities and exercise are many. An added benefit and risk for children and teens with diabetes is that physical activity will lower blood glucose at the time of the activity and afterward. Low blood glucose occurs after exercise due to a "lag" effect caused by the body's cells becoming sensitive to insulin. This effect persists even when the person has stopped exercising. In addition, once exercise is completed, the body replenishes the storage form of glucose (glycogen) by drawing upon glucose in the blood. As a result, the blood glucose levels may continue to drop. Additional carbohydrate is usually needed to prevent these drops in blood glucose.

    There are times when your child's overall activity will increase, such as during summer vacations. At these times, your child may need less insulin. Teenagers are usually taught to reduce their insulin dose when they participate in sports—the amount of the reduction depends on the results of blood glucose checks done before and after physical activity. Parents and teenagers should discuss with their healthcare providers how to handle changes in insulin doses to accommodate exercise. If your child is an active athlete, you should consult an exercise physiologist.

■ **BEWARE OF HIGH BLOOD GLUCOSE.** There are times, however, when exercise will cause blood glucose levels to rise. This usually happens after exercise events of high intensity, such as activities with a lot of start-and-stop action—singles tennis, track events, football, and so on—activities that cause participants to become breathless. If blood glucose is elevated because of high-intensity activities, extra insulin should NOT be given. Over time, the blood glucose will correct itself, as long as an adequate amount of insulin was given in the first place. If extra insulin is given, hypoglycemia will occur. Work with your healthcare provider (an exercise physiologist, if available) to help determine the appropriate insulin doses for this type of exercise.

Occasionally, if individuals are insulin deficient for a period of time and then try to participate in exercise, high blood glucose levels and ketones can result. Some insulin is needed for exercise to effectively lower glucose levels. If your child has high FASTING blood glucose—of 250 mg/dl or more with ketones, or 400 mg/dl or higher without ketones—it is likely that there is insufficient insulin present. He or she should not do any strenuous activity until blood glucose levels are under better control. Extra insulin is usually needed.

Why Do Children Develop Type 2 Diabetes?

Risk factors for type 2 diabetes in children are similar to risk factors for adults—ethnic background, family history of type 2 diabetes, being overweight, being physically inactive. A major risk factor for children is being overweight or obese, especially for children who have a family history of type 2 diabetes. Only about 5 percent of families with a child with type 1 diabetes have a family history of type 1 diabetes, whereas more than 90 percent of families with a child with type 2 diabetes have a family history of type 2 diabetes.

It may be difficult to determine whether a child has type 1 or type 2 diabetes. One third or more of children with type 2 diabetes have ketones in their blood or urine or ketoacidosis at diagnosis, problems usually associated with type 1 diabetes. Type 2 diabetes in children usually develops during the teenage years. They may have signs of insulin resistance such as high blood pressure or blood fat problems, but may or may not have the other usual symptoms of diabetes, such as thirst, frequent urination, and so on. Type 2 diabetes is often diagnosed incidentally at a routine school or sports physical examination. But other youths with type 2 diabetes may experience weight loss and other symptoms common for type 1 diabetes. In addition, acanthosis nigricans, patches of thickened, velvety skin, brownish gray in color, can frequently be found in the neck area and in other parts of the body that bend or rub against each other. They are present in 60 percent to 70 percent of children who develop type 2 diabetes, and are a sign of insulin resistance.

Insulin resistance appears to be central to the development of type 2 diabetes in youth, probably a result of obesity and genetics. Insulin resistance requires the beta cells to release more insulin than normal in order to maintain normal blood glucose levels. Eventually, the ability of the beta cells to produce this additional insulin begins to wane. When these cells are unable to keep up with the insulin requirements brought on by the presence of insulin resistance, blood glucose levels become elevated. Puberty, a known time of insulin resistance, may be another reason type 2 diabetes is usually diagnosed at this time.

Treatment of Type 2 Diabetes in Children

As with type 1 diabetes, the goal of treatment of type 2 diabetes is to normalize blood glucose. However, unlike youths with type 1 diabetes, youths with type 2 may also have high blood pressure and blood fat problems that require treatment.

Initial treatment depends on the level of blood glucose. For some, insulin therapy is needed. Others can be treated with lifestyle changes involving eating and exercise. Unless there is some success with weight loss, most youths will require some form of medication. Some children do well with metformin. (See Chapter 13 for more information on metformin.)

If glucose goals are not met within three to six months with the use of metformin, other treatment is needed. Sometimes other diabetes pills are tried, but insulin may be required. Insulin may be started at bedtime alone. Frequent blood glucose checking is necessary to be sure morning blood glucose levels are around 120 mg/dl.

Making lifestyle changes in eating and physical activity takes time. Remember, changing one's lifestyle involves changing eating behaviors, increasing physical activity, and decreasing sedentary activities. Families and youths are likely to do better if eating and activity habits are changed gradually. Start with a few easy changes such as adding a daily serving of fruit or vegetables. Or start by adding a few minutes of activity each day. Remember, too, that parents should set a good example for their child with diabetes, by serving and eating healthful foods, and by being active regularly.

Nutrition

The following are general guidelines for changing eating behaviors:

- Decrease or eliminate excessive amounts of high-carbohydrate foods, such as extra-large desserts, and drinks, such as regular soda and large glasses of juice.

- Substitute water, low-fat milk, or diet soft drinks for regular soft drinks.

- Help your child learn carbohydrate counting—how many carbohydrate servings to eat for meals and snacks.

- Have meals at regular times without distractions such as television, homework, or video games.

- Control portions; it's not just a matter of what foods kids eat but how much is eaten. Help kids recognize proper portion sizes for various kinds of food, especially snack foods.

- Be sure time is allowed for breakfast, and be sure breakfast is eaten.

- Do not stock the pantry and refrigerator with high-fat, calorie-dense foods and beverages. Read labels and control purchasing.

- Do not use food as a reward.

- Introduce one new fruit or vegetable each week, with the goal of eating five servings of fruits and vegetables a day.

- Set a goal of three servings a day of low-fat dairy products, such as low-fat milk, yogurt, and cheeses.

- Help kids choose healthy foods for school lunches.

- Limit eating out to three times per week.

- Serve as a role model for avoiding temptation and enjoying healthy eating.

Physical Activity

The following are general guidelines for helping children change activity behaviors:

- Encourage and praise physical activity such as yard work, taking stairs instead of elevators, walking, biking, and so on.

- Set a goal of 40 to 60 minutes of physical activity each day.

- Set a goal of less than two hours of sedentary activity each day.

- Use pedometers (to measure the number of steps taken) or other gadgets to increase interest in exercise.

- Take a 5-to-10-minute activity break for every 30 minutes of watching TV, playing video games, or sitting at the computer.

- Establish rewards that are not food related for meeting physical activity goals.

Monitoring Diabetes in Children

Checking Blood Glucose

Checking blood glucose is the best way for you or your child to determine daily blood glucose patterns. It helps you and your child and your child's healthcare providers make decisions about how to manage variations in your child's lifestyle. The concepts and techniques behind monitoring are covered in detail in Chapter 12 and Chapters 17, 18, and 19.

At times, you may think of checking as a bothersome chore, something forced upon you and your child by your healthcare team. Instead, see it for its many benefits. It is a very effective tool to evaluate how well your child's diabetes is being managed. Blood checks will help you determine whether your child's blood glucose is too low or too high. The results will also give you an idea of how to make adjustments in insulin or carbohydrate to match your child's activity level.

Most children tolerate blood checking well. Many school-age children are able to use glucose meters and perform the check by themselves. There is no right age to learn—only the right time for your child. The best approach is to know how and when to monitor and what to do with the results. Use the results to help adjust insulin, carbohydrate, or physical activity to improve control of your child's diabetes.

Ask your healthcare team for times when you should check your child's blood glucose. They will tailor a monitoring program specifically to your child's needs. Whenever you check, write down the results and show this record to your healthcare team. Be sure to note any significant variations in activity or food consumption. Using this record, you and your healthcare team can spot patterns in your child's blood glucose levels and make appropriate adjustments. Diabetes experts recommend that morning (fasting) blood glucose values be between 70 and 150 mg/dl. Any bedtime blood glucose that is less than 120 mg/dl may require an increased amount of carbohydrate for the bedtime snack.

When checking blood glucose, try to avoid using the word *test*, and avoid *good* or *bad* to describe the results. Children or teens may think you are being judgmental, which can cause resentment and anger, feelings that may lead them to lose interest in controlling their diabetes. Children have been known to give false results in order to please their parents. The words *high* and *low* are more appropriate to describe blood glucose.

Glycosylated Hemoglobin (A1C)

The A1C test, described in Chapter 12, provides a good idea of how well your child's blood glucose has been managed over the previous two to three months. This test is particularly useful with children because their blood glucose levels fluctuate, making it hard to assess the results of regular blood checks. But remember, the results of the A1C test represent only an average of what the blood glucose levels have been. Therefore, the test should never be used as a substitute for blood glucose checking. It should be used in addition to daily checking of blood glucose.

Your healthcare team may set a goal for your child's A1C level. For adults with diabetes, the goal is usually an A1C less than 7 percent. However, the activity level and eating habits of children vary, so reaching a level under 8 percent can be difficult. Keep in mind that goals depend on age and must be tailored to each child.

Diabetes and Child Development

The treatment of children with diabetes will vary according to their stage of growth and development. As a parent, you should be aware of the changes in treatment at different ages.

Infants and Very Young Children

Increasingly, type 1 diabetes is being found in children age 5 and younger. Infants need relatively small amounts of insulin, so you or your pharmacist will probably be advised to dilute the clear (rapid-acting or short-acting) insulin from the usual U-100 strength to U-50 (half strength), U-25 (quarter strength), or U-10 (one-tenth strength) to allow dosing at one-tenth unit increments. This can be done with the diluting solution provided by insulin manufacturers. Be aware that the amounts of insulin needed will increase as your child grows. This is very important to discuss with a diabetes specialist.

Through Age 12

Many youngsters with type 1 diabetes can master some parts of their diabetes care. Early on, they can be actively involved in food selection, preparation, and meal planning, learn to spot symptoms of low blood glucose and how to treat it, and help with blood checking. But your child probably won't be ready to take responsibility for injecting insulin until after early adolescence, so you shouldn't hurry him or her into taking on this responsibility. It's critical that the right dose of insulin be given at the right time. If not, serious problems can occur.

Once children reach a maturity level that allows them to take on more of their diabetes care, parents should continue to oversee all aspects of care. Some parents are overly concerned that unless their child takes full responsibility early on, the child will end up being too dependent as a young adult. This is not true. Your child will eventually learn to accept his or her role in self-care. Older children are often eager to take over the injections when there are personal payoffs, such as an overnight visit to a friend's house or a camping trip or class outing.

Before the effects of chronic high blood glucose on growth were understood, some children with diabetes did not grow to normal height. That picture has completely changed. Today, with new insulins and monitoring methods, children whose blood glucose is controlled will grow at a normal rate. If your child's growth and development are not proceeding as expected, check with your doctor. Your child may need changes in his or her treatment program. Of course, there are reasons for poor growth and development that are unrelated to diabetes, such as thyroid or gastrointestinal problems. Both of these can be more common with diabetes, but your doctor can help find and treat them.

Teenagers

All children—whether they have diabetes or not—gradually learn to accept responsibility and strive for independence. When a child has diabetes, the quest for independence is more complicated. In their teen years all children undergo rapid growth and sexual changes. For a child with diabetes, these bodily changes make it harder to control blood glucose. The upshot is that teenagers with diabetes need closer medical supervision—just when they want to be more independent and "do their own thing." They may also be at a stage when they temporarily reject the values of their parents or other authority figures. Diabetes often becomes the battleground for this struggle. Some teens test the limits of their condition, wanting to find out whether they really have diabetes and what happens if they don't follow their treatment programs. This may mean overeating, omitting insulin injections, or refusing to check their blood glucose.

The teen with diabetes is quite sensitive to "being different." He or she may omit insulin injections, eat spontaneously with his or her peer group, and omit checking in order to prove "nothing is wrong." As a parent, you should expect such lapses once in a while, tolerating them up to a point. However, if your teen shows severe self-destructive behavior—actions that result in repeated episodes of ketoacidosis and visits to the emergency room, or even just deteriorating diabetes control—it is a signal that the family needs the help and support of a professional counselor. In such cases, a behavioral specialist can be a very important member of your teen's diabetes treatment team.

Puberty and Menstruation. In general, the onset of puberty usually proceeds on schedule in children with diabetes. Poor diabetes control, however, can delay puberty. For example, in girls it may mean a delay in menstruation, which can cause anxiety and distress for the child and her parents. But be assured that if thyroid function and other hormones are normal, this delay will correct itself as your daughter's diabetes control improves. During menstruation, many women notice a rise in blood glucose levels for a few days before the beginning of the monthly flow. At these times, your daughter may need to temporarily increase her insulin dose. Boys don't experience such dramatic changes during puberty.

Everyday Activities

School

Children with diabetes should participate fully in all school activities. But they should understand the need to keep their diabetes well regulated during the school day. This will not only help them in their normal growth and development, it will help minimize high or low blood glucose reactions that may be distressing and call attention to them as "different."

Teachers should be told about your child's diabetes, and made aware of medication needs, but encouraged to consider the child just like everyone else in the classroom. Parents should meet with the child's teacher at the beginning of every school year to explain the nature of diabetes, the need for blood glucose checking and insulin injections (for example, at lunch), and the need for following the child's meal schedule. Most important, your child's teacher should be informed about the symptoms of low blood glucose—how to recognize and treat them. School nurses and other staff may also be part of your child's care away from home. It is useful to prepare written instructions for your child's teachers.

Organized Sports

Youngsters with diabetes are encouraged to participate in athletic activities of all types. Just be sure that your child's coaches and teammates know about the possibility of a low blood glucose reaction—what the symptoms are and how to treat the problem. On days of strenuous activity, your child may need to check blood glucose more often and eat additional foods or beverages containing carbohydrate. He or she should always keep some carbohydrate on hand to deal with low blood glucose. Diabetes is not an obstacle to success in sports. Many professional athletes—in baseball, hockey, football, basketball, tennis, and other sports—have effectively managed type 1 diabetes.

Camps and Other Special Programs

Just because your child has diabetes doesn't mean he or she must be excluded from summer camp. Since the 1920s, camps have been available for young people with diabetes, including camps devoted just to children with diabetes. The Joslin Diabetes Center runs the Elliott J. Joslin Camp for Boys in Charlton, Massachusetts, and works closely with the Clara Barton Camp for Girls, in nearby Oxford. For lists of camps in the United States, contact the American Diabetes Association. There are also camps in other countries.

The primary purpose of these camps is to provide fun and recreation while ensuring good diabetes treatment and helping children learn more about caring for their diabetes. A successful camp experience often leaves children feeling less isolated and more comfortable with themselves. They can gain confidence in caring for their diabetes and also see how their peers cope with similar situations. Camp also relieves the anxiety and depression that some children feel regarding being "different." An added bonus is that such camps provide parents with confidence that their child is safe and medically supervised by experts while having fun away from home.

CHAPTER 23

Diabetes and Pregnancy

Thanks to improvements in diabetes management over the past 50 years, women with diabetes now give birth to very healthy babies. In fact, infant survival rates among women with diabetes are now nearly identical to those among women who do not have diabetes.

Today women can control their diabetes by monitoring their blood glucose and making adjustments to their insulin doses. In addition, numerous medical tests have been developed to monitor the well-being of the mother and child throughout the months of pregnancy. Such medical advances have significantly reduced the risks of pregnancy to the mother and improved the chances of survival for the unborn baby. However, it's still important to realize that diabetes does make pregnancy more difficult. And babies born to women with diabetes do have an increased risk of birth defects. But if good diabetes control is achieved before conception and during pregnancy, the risks of miscarriage and birth defects are greatly reduced and a healthy baby is the expected outcome.

But before discussing pregnancy and diabetes in women with pre-existing diabetes, it will be helpful to review changes that occur in all women who become pregnant, including a special group of women who develop *gestational diabetes*—diabetes that is first diagnosed during pregnancy.

Metabolic Changes During Pregnancy

During pregnancy all women, whether they have diabetes or not, require more insulin than they did before they got pregnant. This is because the placenta, which provides nutrition and fuel to the growing baby, produces hormones that increase insulin resistance. As the placenta grows, more insulin is needed to overcome this resistance and to keep blood glucose normal. By the end of pregnancy, women normally need up to twice the amount of insulin they did before becoming pregnant.

A lack of insulin can create problems with the type of fuel the body burns during pregnancy. In general, the body gets its energy from blood glucose. If there isn't enough insulin in the bloodstream to help convert the available glucose into usable energy, the body turns to fat and protein for energy. In *any* woman who is pregnant, the body is more likely to turn to fat than protein, saving the protein for the growth of the baby.

The majority of women who don't have diabetes can keep up with the increased need for insulin during pregnancy. They continue to use blood glucose efficiently. But pregnant women with diabetes—who don't have enough insulin to meet their needs—are more likely to burn fat instead of glucose. When this happens, blood glucose and ketones can build up in the bloodstream, leading to the dangerous condition called *ketoacidosis* (see Chapter 18). Preventing this condition is one of the main reasons that you must take special care of yourself during pregnancy if you have diabetes. You must regularly check your blood glucose and test your blood or urine for ketones.

However, some women who don't have diabetes, just like someone with type 2 diabetes, cannot produce enough insulin during pregnancy to overcome the insulin resistance. Their pancreases, which under normal circumstances are able to supply enough insulin to keep blood glucose normal, can't keep up with the increasing demand for insulin during pregnancy. This leads to the development of glucose intolerance, which is referred to as *gestational diabetes* (*gestation* refers to the time the baby is developing in the womb). Some of these women will have only a minimal insulin deficiency and will be able to adequately control their blood glucose with a meal plan. Others may have a more severe deficiency and require insulin along with nutrition therapy to control their blood glucose.

For women with gestational diabetes, when labor begins, the increasing insulin resistance that was present during pregnancy is dramatically reversed and the need for extra insulin disappears. For women with preexisting diabetes, insulin requirements also drop dramatically, and after giving birth these women may require only half of their prepregnancy insulin dose. However, their insulin requirements eventually return to their prepregnancy levels.

Gestational Diabetes

Gestational diabetes is more likely to occur in women who are overweight, over age 30, and have a family history of diabetes, but it may also occur in women who have no known risk factors for this condition. You are at high risk for gestational diabetes if you had it in a previous pregnancy, are overweight, have a family history of diabetes, or are spilling glucose in your urine. If you are African American, Hispanic American, Asian American, Native American, or a Pacific Islander, you are also at higher risk of developing gestational diabetes. If you are at high risk, you should be tested as soon as possible. If the test is normal, you should be tested again between the twenty-fourth and twenty-eighth weeks of your pregnancy. This is the time when most women are routinely tested for gestational diabetes. First a *glucose challenge test* is done, in which blood glucose is checked an hour after you consume a sugary drink. If your blood glucose is 140 mg/dl or higher at this time, a *glucose tolerance test* is recommended. This test measures blood glucose three hours after a sugary drink. However, if you have a fasting glucose greater than 126 mg/dl or a random glucose greater than 200 mg/dl, you have diabetes and there is no need for a glucose challenge or glucose tolerance test. You should be treated for gestational diabetes.

Treatment of Gestational Diabetes

The American Diabetes Association is currently reviewing its goal of treatment for gestational diabetes, and at this writing it appears as if the new recommendations will be to target the fasting glucose at 60–99 mg/dl, and the peak post-meal glucose (approximately 1 hour after the start of the meal) at 100–129 mg/dl. To do this, nutrition therapy is the most important form of treatment. Food choices are based on appropriate weight gain, normalization of glucose, and whether or not ketones are present. Some women, in an effort to avoid insulin, stop eating adequate carbohydrate and calories. Without enough glucose to burn, the body switches to burning fats, which produces ketones. Ketones may affect the baby and should be avoided. If blood glucose is normal or low and ketones are present either in the blood or urine, the solution is to increase carbohydrate intake. Therefore, if you try to go for a period of time without eating, and as a result your blood glucose drops too low, you are both depriving your growing baby of the glucose it needs and potentially causing ketones to be produced, neither of which is ideal for your baby.

Distribution of meals and snacks is also important. Your baby is feeding continuously, using glucose and other fuels from your body. Therefore, smaller meals and snacks, particularly a bedtime snack, are frequently recommended. Rarely, some women may need to drink a glass of milk or eat some other form of carbohydrate during the night to avoid spilling ketones in the morning.

Your dietitian will work with you to design a meal plan that ensures you are eating enough food for a gradual weight gain. This will allow your baby to continue to grow normally. You will also learn about carbohydrate counting (see Chapter 4). Your meal plan will probably involve a moderate restriction of carbohydrate and calories. In particular, foods containing carbohydrate are often not well tolerated at breakfast, and careful attention to the amount of carbohydrate in food at breakfast is important. However, carbohydrate is needed and can be handled better as the day progresses.

Regular physical activity lowers fasting and post-meal blood glucose. It is an important adjunct to watching your food intake. You are encouraged to do some type of physical activity, such as a brisk walk, for 15 minutes or longer for a minimum of three days a week, or according to your healthcare provider's recommendation.

Checking your blood glucose is also important. Initially it is recommended that you check your fasting blood glucose (before breakfast) and again one hour after the start of each meal. Your diabetes educator can teach you how to do blood glucose checking correctly.

Some women will also require insulin by injection to adequately control blood glucose. However, even if a woman requires insulin during pregnancy, she usually does not need to continue taking it after delivery. If she does, it is likely that she was in early stages of diabetes before pregnancy, and the pregnancy just made it obvious.

If you can achieve good glucose control with lifestyle changes alone (that is, with a meal plan and physical activity), recommendations for monitoring of the baby and delivery will be similar to those for all women who are pregnant. However, if you require insulin therapy or develop high blood pressure, more careful monitoring will be needed. The most common risk is that your baby may become too large (macrosomic), which can lead to birth injury. Your doctor will try to estimate your baby's size to determine when and what is the best time and means of delivery.

Your doctors will also be checking your baby's blood glucose after birth. Your baby may have become used to receiving extra amounts of glucose from you, and its pancreas may have compensated by making extra insulin. At birth this supply of glucose is no longer available, but your baby may not be able to immediately turn off the release of insulin. As a result, your baby's blood glucose may drop too low. This can be easily treated by giving the baby glucose, but your doctors must keep checking to see whether this is a problem.

If you have ever had gestational diabetes, be sure to tell any future doctors you may consult during a subsequent pregnancy—or for any reason—so they can keep a lookout for changes in your metabolism. To decrease the risk of developing diabetes in the future, you should engage in regular physical activities (see Chapters 9 and 10) and try to maintain your weight as close to normal as possible.

How Is Pregnancy Different if You Already Have Diabetes?

If you have diabetes and needed to take diabetes pills or insulin *before* you became pregnant, then you will need to take insulin and you will need more insulin as the pregnancy progresses. In fact, by the time you are close to delivery, you need much more—often twice as much. During your pregnancy you will have to pay special attention to the balance of insulin, carbohydrate, and physical activity. You will also need to eat additional calories and protein—for your own needs and those of your developing baby. With the advice of your healthcare team, you will need to make gradual and continuing adjustments to your treatment program. Note also that diabetes pills have not been proven safe and effective for use in women with preexisting diabetes who are pregnant, which is the reason insulin is recommended for everyone who is pregnant. Both aspart and lispro more effectively control postprandial glucose levels than regular insulin, which is important in a pregnant woman. Glargine, detemir, and glulisine are not recommended for use during pregnancy.

Planning Pregnancy

For women who already have diabetes, special prenatal care should begin before the baby is conceived. That's because critical organ growth occurs during the first several weeks of pregnancy, generally before a woman even realizes that she is pregnant. If the mother's blood glucose levels are elevated during this time, the risk of birth defects and other health problems developing in the unborn child increases significantly. Poorly controlled diabetes before conception and during the early weeks of pregnancy can result in birth defects in 5 to 10 percent of pregnancies, (and as high as 30 percent with very poorly controlled diabetes) and miscarriages in 15 to 20 percent of pregnancies. The miscarriage rate may even be higher, as many may not even be recognized when they occur early in pregnancy.

If you have diabetes and are considering having a baby, the best way to ensure your baby's healthy development is to be sure that you have excellent control of your diabetes *before* you become pregnant. It cannot be emphasized enough how important good control is prior to pregnancy. It is recommended that the A1C be 7 percent or below prior to pregnancy to reduce the risk of birth defects to close to the rate in women who do not have diabetes. Very high A1C levels can be associated with a 30 percent risk of birth defects. Of course, this "excellent control" must continue throughout the pregnancy. Women with diabetes who are planning a pregnancy should see their healthcare providers for an A1C test, which monitors blood glucose levels over the previous two to three months and helps determine when it may be best to conceive. Your healthcare providers will also review your blood glucose checks with you and help you adjust your insulin dose until your blood glucose goals are achieved. Diabetes educators and dietitians should teach or review with you the skills necessary for intensive glucose management. You may also be advised to start prenatal vitamins before you become pregnant. Studies have shown that folic acid, for one, reduces the risk of certain birth defects. For these reasons, family planning before conception is advised so that these measures can be carried out in a timely manner.

Pregnancy requires a strong commitment from you to check your blood glucose frequently and to participate in an aggressive approach to diabetes management. In addition, women with diabetes usually need to be in the care of an obstetrician who deals with "high risk" cases. And after delivery, the baby needs the care of a doctor who specializes in newborns.

Many women wonder whether pregnancy will worsen any complications from diabetes. To answer that question, your doctor will do a full evaluation. It is advisable to have such an evaluation *before* getting pregnant. That way, your healthcare team can inform you of any additional risks you may face during your pregnancy. While some complications of diabetes may temporarily worsen during pregnancy, after the baby is born, a woman usually returns to the level she might have expected if she hadn't been pregnant. However, you and your healthcare providers should pay special attention to the following conditions that can be serious, even if they worsen just for a short time.

- **Retinopathy.** One of these serious conditions is a change in the blood vessels on the *retina*, the delicate, light-sensitive membrane lining the back of the eye. (This condition is discussed in detail in Chapter 20.) If you have this problem and it has reached the stage at which new, undesired blood vessels are forming on the retina *(neovascularization)*, you may lose your vision. Getting pregnant can make matters worse, because pregnancy can speed the changes in the eyes associated with diabetes. If new blood vessels are detected, you should postpone your pregnancy.

Another eye problem, called *background retinopathy*, often occurs in people with diabetes. With this condition, the risk of losing sight is much lower than with the condition described above. Background retinopathy may progress somewhat during pregnancy, but it usually doesn't reach a threatening stage.

If you have diabetes, it is very important to know the condition of your eyes, especially if you are considering pregnancy. Your eyes should be examined by a physician called an *ophthalmologist*, particularly one who is an expert in diagnosing and treating diseases of the retina. If retinopathy is detected and it is in a risky stage, your doctor may advise you to postpone pregnancy to avoid more severe damage. Retinopathy can be successfully treated with laser therapy, and once stabilized, it is much less likely to worsen during pregnancy.

All pregnant women with diabetes should have their eyes checked by an ophthalmologist two or three times during pregnancy. If the condition of the eyes worsens, the doctor will be able to detect the problem early on and begin treatment without delay. As with other complications from diabetes, any eye changes you have during pregnancy may improve gradually after delivery.

■ **Hypertension and kidneys.** Before you become pregnant, it is also a good idea to check how well your kidneys are functioning. Your doctor can determine this by performing simple tests on your urine. If your kidneys are functioning well, they will very likely continue to do so during pregnancy. If, however, protein is being lost in the urine, pregnancy can make the problem worse. It can lead to high blood pressure *(hypertension)*, and your body may begin to retain fluids *(edema)*. If this occurs, you must take great caution and care. You may even need prolonged bed rest. Sometimes premature delivery of the baby is necessary to protect the health of the mother.

■ **Neuropathy.** Even with good diabetes control, damage to your nerves *(neuropathy)* can get worse during pregnancy. The symptoms include tingling, numbness, or discomfort in the legs or feet. See Chapter 20 for more information on relieving symptoms of nerve problems.

Managing Diabetes During Pregnancy

If you have diabetes and are pregnant, it's best if you are cared for by a team of experts in this area of medicine. Such a team is made up of a diabetes specialist *(endocrinologist)*, an obstetrician who specializes in high-risk pregnancies *(perinatologist)*, an eye specialist *(ophthalmologist)*, a nurse educator, a dietitian, and a mental health professional. Another member, who should be present at the baby's delivery, is a specialist in the care of newborns *(neonatologist)*.

If you don't live near a diabetes center where such a team is available, consult your primary-care doctor as well as your obstetrician and pediatrician. Overall, you will need two kinds of care—for your diabetes and for your pregnancy—and this care should be closely coordinated by all members of your healthcare team.

The Course of Pregnancy

First trimester. As soon as pregnancy is confirmed, you should begin visiting your healthcare team regularly. Visits every two to four weeks are often recommended, the frequency dictated by the degree of glucose control. Communications between visits occur by phone or fax/e-mail to review glucose patterns. However, even more frequent visits would be recommended if glucose control were poor, as the first trimester (the first three months) is critical to the developing child (fetus). During this time the basic body structures begin to form, and if diabetes is uncontrolled, major structural damage to the baby can occur, resulting in birth defects.

At your first visit, you should see your diabetes specialist and your obstetrician. In addition, it is important to see a nurse educator, who will review the goals of diabetes care during pregnancy, and a dietitian, who will prescribe a revised meal plan that includes additional calories and protein to cover the increased needs of your pregnancy. Iron and vitamin supplements are often prescribed. Close and frequent monitoring of your blood pressure, weight, and eyes is important. If your pregnancy causes nausea and vomiting—called *morning sickness,* even though it can occur at any time—your insulin doses may need to be decreased slightly at first.

Throughout your care, urine cultures are frequently done to make sure you don't have a urinary tract infection. If you develop a fever, cloudy or bloody urine, urinary burning or urgency (constantly feeling that you have to urinate), contact your doctor at once. In the later stages of pregnancy, it is sometimes difficult to distinguish the symptoms of a urinary infection from the pressure of the baby on the bladder, so let your doctor decide what is actually happening.

Second trimester. During the second trimester (months 4 to 6), weekly checkups should continue. Also, you will continue to closely monitor and care for your diabetes. Many women find that their diabetes becomes more stable now than in the first trimester, although insulin doses must still be increased. During this period, your healthcare providers will watch closely for increases in blood pressure and fluid retention, and decreases in kidney function. In addition, various tests may be done to determine the health of the developing baby. Anemia is a common problem during this period, and treatment with iron supplements may be necessary.

Third trimester. Weekly checkups continue through the third trimester (months 7 to 9). Many women find that their diabetes remains relatively stable, although their insulin dose may have to be increased—many now need twice as much insulin. Also, the regimen may need to be intensified (made more physiologic to match normal insulin patterns, like those of someone who does not have diabetes). As with all diabetes, insulin adjustments vary from person to person. Your goal is good control, regardless of the insulin dose needed. Often, toward the last few weeks of pregnancy, the amount of insulin needed will begin to decline.

During the third trimester, any signs of high blood pressure, fluid buildup, or kidney problems are of concern. An ultrasound test (described later in this chapter) is performed periodically to check the baby's growth and development, and the baby's heart is closely monitored. Additional tests may be performed, some of which are routinely done for all pregnancies—for example, testing the hemoglobin level in your blood to make sure you are not anemic. Other tests may be done based on your specific situation. For example, your doctor may want to measure your thyroid function because women with diabetes are more likely to have thyroid disturbances.

Glucose Goals During Pregnancy

Throughout your pregnancy, the goal of your diabetes treatment program is to achieve blood glucose levels as close to normal as possible. As noted, the treatment goal recommendations are currently under review by the American Diabetes Association, and it appears that the new recommendations will be to target the fasting glucose at 60–99 mg/dl, and the peak glucose approximately 1 hour after the start of the meal at 100–129 mg/dl.

To achieve this control, you should ideally check your blood a minimum of six times a day—before breakfast, lunch, and dinner, and two hours after each of these meals. You may also have to check overnight as well. Before adjusting your insulin doses, consider all other possible reasons for any change in your blood glucose—what you ate, the timing of the insulin dose in relation to meals, or any changes in your physical activity.

Nutrition, Weight Gain, and Physical Activity

The expression "You're eating for two" takes on added meaning for pregnant women who have diabetes. As with your regular diabetes care, your meal plan is a very significant part of your treatment during pregnancy.

For this reason, during the early stages of your pregnancy you should meet with a dietitian skilled in nutrition for pregnant women with diabetes. Together, you will develop a plan for the first trimester of pregnancy. At the beginning of the second trimester, this plan may change to meet the increasing needs of the growing baby. During pregnancy you will need extra calories and protein and may be advised to take supplements of vitamins and minerals, such as iron, folic acid, and calcium. In addition, you may need between-meal and bedtime snacks to prevent hypoglycemia.

Nutrition. Proper nutrition is very important to your health and the health of your baby. If you have any of the problems found in the list in Table 23-1, call your dietitian or doctor.

Nonnutritive sweeteners such as aspartame, sucralose, and acesulfame-K are safe for use during pregnancy; however, moderation is often recommended. Because saccharin crosses the placenta and is cleared slowly

---

TABLE 23-1   When to Contact Your Dietitian During Pregnancy

You should contact your dietitian (or physician) for a review of your meal plan if you notice any of the following.

1. **KETONES** are present in your blood or urine when your blood glucose is within or near the normal range. This may indicate that you are not eating enough, and in particular not enough carbohydrate-containing foods.

2. **WEIGHT LOSS** may indicate that you are not eating enough.

3. **INADEQUATE WEIGHT GAIN** (less than 2 pounds per month during the second and third trimesters) may indicate that you are not eating enough.

4. **EXCESSIVE WEIGHT GAIN** (more than 1 pound per month in the first trimester, and thereafter 7 pounds or more per month, or more than 2 pounds per week) may indicate that you are eating too much or that your body is retaining fluid.

5. **WIDELY FLUCTUATING BLOOD GLUCOSE LEVELS** may indicate that you are eating too much at certain times of the day.

---

by the fetus, Joslin does not recommend its use during pregnancy. Alcohol use during pregnancy is not recommended. And of course, tobacco, whether you have diabetes or not, or are pregnant or not, is hazardous to health.

Weight gain. Your meal plan is designed to help you gain the proper amount of weight during your pregnancy while maintaining good blood glucose control. This weight gain is important to ensure the growth of your baby. In addition, you need to have enough carbohydrate in your diet so that your body doesn't burn fat for energy, leading to the production of ketones. How much weight should you gain? First, check the body mass index (BMI) chart in Chapter 8 and determine what your BMI was before you became pregnant. If it was between 20 and 25, you should plan to gain 25 to 35 pounds during pregnancy. If your BMI was 26 to 29, you should gain only 15 to 25 pounds, and if it was over 30, you should gain only 15 pounds or less. If your BMI was less than 20, you should gain 28 to 40 pounds.

About half the weight gained during pregnancy is due to the growth of tissues in the mother that support the growth of the baby (extra blood, breast enlargement, and fat stores). The other half is for the baby itself, the placenta (the tissue in the womb that supplies nourishment to the baby), and the amniotic fluid (fluid that surrounds the baby).

Your healthcare providers will closely monitor your weight during pregnancy. How fast weight is gained will vary from woman to woman. But on average, expect to gain only about 3 pounds in the first trimester. During the second and third trimesters, expect to gain about ½ to 1 pound per week. Weight gain should be steady and progressive. If you are losing weight, your healthcare team will want to evaluate and treat the problem.

Physical activity. If you have diabetes and are pregnant, you may continue to do forms of physical activity that are moderate and safe. In fact, most women with diabetes can continue the activity plan they had before pregnancy. But this is not the time to start a new and involved exercise program. As with all pregnant women, you must be careful as your pregnancy progresses. The extra weight you are carrying in your abdomen causes a change in your center of gravity. Rather than engaging in activities that can easily throw you off balance, choose forms of activity that are safer, such as walking on a well-paved sidewalk or in a shopping mall.

Adjusting Insulin

Guidelines for adjusting insulin doses are found in Chapters 14 and 15. A physiologic insulin regimen or an insulin pump may be needed to achieve near-normal blood glucose levels—research has shown that precise control during pregnancy is important to the health of the baby.

During pregnancy the body's cells become more resistant to insulin. As a result, blood glucose rises more rapidly and drops to lower levels before the next meal. You may need to eat snacks between meals to avoid low glucose before the next meal.

Insulin pump therapy may help women who are unable to achieve good control with multiple injections. As with all other methods of insulin treatment, good blood glucose control using an insulin pump should be established before pregnancy.

The benefit to the baby of near-normal blood glucose should be balanced with the risk to the mother of having a severe low blood glucose reaction. People who can no longer tell when their blood glucose is low are particularly at risk (see Chapter 17). If you have a low blood glucose reaction, you can lose control of your car while driving, lose consciousness, or have a seizure. You may be unable to take anything by mouth to raise your blood glucose into the normal range; in these infrequent situations, an injection of glucagon can be given (again, see Chapter 17). Family members should be taught how to give such an injection. Blood glucose should be tested before driving.

Testing for Ketones

Your doctor will also ask you to test your urine or blood for ketones because of the increased risk of ketoacidosis during pregnancy (the test for ketones is described in Chapter 12). Ketoacidosis can be dangerous both for you and for your baby. You should check for ketones each morning before eating or taking insulin. If ketones are present two days in a row, even though your blood glucose is normal or close to normal, you should call a member of your healthcare team. The causes vary, but you may need a change in your insulin program or a larger nighttime snack.

On days when you are feeling well and your blood glucose is above 250 mg/dl, always check for ketones. Call your doctor immediately if ketones are more than a "trace." On days when you are sick, it's even more important to monitor for ketones—even if the illness is minor, such as a common cold, an upset stomach, the flu, or diarrhea. (To learn how to take care of your diabetes on sick days, see the guidelines in Chapter 19.) Why is monitoring so important? Because you need to do everything you can to prevent ketoacidosis, which can harm you and your baby, and can ultimately lead to the death of the baby. Fortunately, since the advent of home blood glucose checking and physiologic insulin programs, ketoacidosis is quite rare.

Preeclampsia is a condition that is defined by a combination of findings—high blood pressure (hypertension), and protein in the urine, and fluid retention. It is more likely to occur in young women and those with preexisting high blood pressure and a previous pregnancy complicated by preeclampsia. Preeclampsia is more common in women with diabetes, particularly if they have renal disease or preexisting hypertension. The presence of renal disease itself may lead to worse outcomes of a pregnancy. Preeclampsia, which can also occur in pregnant women who do not have diabetes, can progress to a serious condition called *eclampsia,* which involves seizures. (This problem is different from the impairment of kidney function described earlier in the chapter.) By closely monitoring your health, your doctor will be able to diagnose preeclampsia early and begin treatment, which often includes bed rest. If preeclampsia is severe, the baby may have to be delivered early to protect the health of the mother. This could have ill effects on the baby, since its lungs may not be able to support life on their own. A respirator may be necessary to help the baby breathe.

Monitoring the Baby's Health

Depending on your specific needs, your healthcare team may decide to perform a variety of tests to make sure that your baby is developing properly. These tests will also help predict the time of delivery.

- ALPHA-FETOPROTEIN (TRIPLE SCREEN): This is a blood test that is performed at 16 to 18 weeks to detect possible defects in the baby's brain or spinal cord. Since the test is not very precise, an ultrasound is performed if it is abnormal, to further evaluate the baby.

- ULTRASOUND: This test uses sound waves that pass through the mother and baby and are translated into images of the baby's internal organs and bony structures. The test does not use X rays, which could be harmful to the developing baby. Ultrasound is usually first performed at week 16 or 18 and is used to estimate the expected delivery date. It is usually repeated between weeks 26 and 28, and again near the time of delivery to be sure that the baby is growing properly and to measure weight and size. The size is important in determining whether the baby can be delivered normally or if a cesarean delivery (surgery) will be necessary. Additional ultrasound testing can and may be done to assist in performing the amniocentesis.

- **NONSTRESS TEST:** This test uses a sound-pickup device, but it is different from the one used for ultrasound. Often done in the last few weeks of pregnancy, it measures the heart rate of the baby as it changes with movement.

- **OXYTOCIN CHALLENGE TEST, OR STRESS TEST:** In this test, also done in the final weeks, a small amount of medication is given to the mother to cause a small uterine contraction. The response of the baby's heart is then observed.

- **AMNIOCENTESIS:** This test on the amniotic fluid surrounding the baby is used to check the baby's lungs. A needle is passed through the skin (after it is numbed) and uterus into the fluid. Higher "test scores" mean the baby's lungs are more mature and less likely to have trouble breathing at birth. Amniocentesis can also detect birth defects, including genetic abnormalities.

Delivery

Women with uncomplicated pregnancies whose diabetes has been in excellent control may be safely delivered at 39 to 40 weeks (full term). Other women may be scheduled for delivery at 38 weeks. Based on the estimated size of the baby, your doctor will recommend a delivery through the birth canal (vaginal delivery) or a cesarean delivery (surgery). Once the baby is born, it is usually cared for in the newborn intensive care unit of the hospital, where it can be closely observed.

As soon as the baby is born, the mother's need for insulin drops significantly. For a few days, in fact, you may need less than what you used before pregnancy. However, as the body returns to normal, your insulin needs will probably be about the same as before you were pregnant.

Breastfeeding

Breastfeeding is encouraged in women with diabetes. However, you may prefer to bottle-feed your baby. The decision will depend on personal choice and the advice of your healthcare providers.

Women who breastfeed often need an increase in calories, similar to what they ate while pregnant, but this varies from person to person. You may be advised to eat a snack before nursing to prevent low blood glucose. Also, be sure to get enough calcium in your diet.

Your Decision

The decision to become pregnant requires more thought and planning if you have diabetes. But it is comforting to know that medical science has reduced your risks significantly and that with the help of your healthcare providers, and by taking good care of yourself and keeping your blood glucose in good control, you can have a healthy baby.

CHAPTER 24

Sexual Issues

A person diagnosed with diabetes often asks, "Will diabetes or its treatment affect my sex life?" The good news is that, in general, people with diabetes are able to perform sexual activities normally and lead satisfying sex lives. However, diabetes can have an impact on sexual and reproductive issues affecting both men and women, and some problems and possible solutions are discussed below.

Sexual Functioning in Men

The effects of diabetes on vessels and nerves involved in normal functioning of the penis can lead to various forms of sexual problems. In the past the term *impotence* was used interchangeably with *sexual dysfunction*. Today, however, the term *erectile dysfunction* (ED) is used. ED is defined as the consistent or repeated inability to achieve or maintain a penile erection long enough to permit satisfactory sexual intercourse. ED is now recognized as a common and significant problem for many men—whether or not they have diabetes. Men previously just lived with the condition. Today drugs and other forms of therapy allow most men with ED to have satisfactory sex lives.

Erectile Dysfunction

During an erection the penis gets harder and longer, and it rises. Although this sounds simple, many events inside the body must take place in a precise sequence for an erection to happen. Sexual stimulation is the first step. This causes nerves and cells in the corpora cavernosa (two long chambers inside the penis) to release nitric oxide. This chemical relaxes muscles in the penis to allow more blood to flow in. The extra blood causes the chambers to expand and stiffen. At the same time, other muscles do just the opposite—they close, trapping the blood within the penis and keeping the penis erect. The increase in blood entering the penis and the slowing of blood leaving causes the erection. An erection ends when muscles relax, the blood drains out, and the penis becomes flaccid.

Men with diabetes develop ED more often than other men. Older age, having diabetes for a number of years, poorly controlled blood glucose levels, and having other complications of diabetes increase the likelihood of developing ED. *Neuropathy*—that is, damage to the nerves—can result from chronically high blood glucose levels, which explains why men with poorly controlled blood glucose are at higher risk for ED. The nerves involved in an erection work by controlling small valves that are located in the blood vessels leading to and from the penis. When ED occurs in men with diabetes, it may be due to damage of the nerve fibers controlling these valves. As a result, the valves don't function properly. But keep in mind that nerve damage from diabetes can occur in other parts of the body as well, a topic discussed in Chapter 20.

In some men (with or without diabetes), the cause of ED may be the hardening of the blood vessels that supply the flow of blood to the penis. These vessels can become narrowed or blocked, like blood vessels in other parts of the body, causing blood circulation to be decreased. The chemical messengers inside the penis are affected as well: the activity of nitric oxide, which relaxes the corpora cavernosa, is decreased, so less blood flows into the penis.

For men with diabetes, just as for other men, psychological factors such as performance anxiety and relationship problems can also cause a dampening of sexual stimulation. Whatever the cause, ED in men with diabetes tends to develop gradually; it doesn't suddenly occur one day. Over time, a man will notice that his penis is less rigid or that he can't maintain an erection as long as he used to. Nighttime and morning erections are affected. With this decline, the man doesn't necessarily feel a loss of sexual desire, nor does it mean that he is infertile. That's why ED can be so frustrating—he simply is unable to perform sexually.

One of the problems in discussing ED is that it is difficult to know what is normal. Modern life tends to emphasize sex—in the news media, advertising, movies, magazines, and books—which raises people's expectations to unrealistic levels. We do know that ED can occur at any age, and the result is sometimes the opposite of what might be expected. For example, some men who have diabetes can perform sexually into their seventies, while some men who do not have diabetes experience ED in their forties or fifties.

Men with diabetes who are experiencing ED should first discuss the problem with their healthcare provider. Sometimes it can be caused by medications used for other medical conditions. Tests can also be done to determine whether the production of sex hormones is normal. In addition, you may be advised to be evaluated by a *urologist*, a doctor who specializes in the urinary tract, and a psychologist, who can help you sort out any stresses in your life.

Treatment of ED

The first step in treating ED is to achieve optimal control of blood glucose. If controlling glucose, changing any medications that are known to affect erectile function, or sessions with a qualified psychologist do not reestablish normal sexual function, other treatment methods should be considered.

Three oral medications are commonly used today to treat ED—sildenafil (Viagra), vardenafil (Levitra), and tadalafil (Cialis). All three drugs have been shown to be effective in men regardless of the severity or the cause of ED. In addition, they have been shown to be effective in men with ED due to diabetes. They work by enhancing the effects of nitric oxide—the chemical that relaxes muscles in the penis to allow more blood to flow in. These drugs do not cause an erection by themselves. Sexual stimulation (foreplay) is also required.

Sildenafil was the first medication on the market. Released in 1998, it revolutionized the treatment of ED. Vardenafil was approved for use in 2003. Each of these should be taken about an hour before intercourse and is effective for about four hours. Tadalafil was also approved for use in 2003. This drug is not designed to be taken on demand. It becomes effective in approximately two hours, but once effective the benefit of the drug continues for the next 24 hours.

In general, these drugs should not be taken by men who take nitrates. Interactions are also possible with other drugs, so be sure that whoever is prescribing the medication knows your complete medical history. Because the drugs may cause some change to vision, it is recommended that you consult with your ophthalmologist.

There are other options if the ED pills cannot be used or don't work. Some drugs can be self-injected into the penis to increase blood flow. The only approved injected ED drug is alprostadil (Caverject, Caverject Impulse, Edex). It causes an erection within 5 to 20 minutes and lasts an hour or less.

Alprostadil is also available as a suppository pellet (MUSE, Vivus), which is inserted into the urethra with an applicator. It initiates an erection within 8 to 10 minutes with its effects waning after 30 to 60 minutes.

A vacuum device is another option. In this method a cylinder is placed over the penis. A tube at the end of the cylinder leads to a pump that draws air out of the cylinder, which creates a vacuum that pulls blood into the penis to cause an erection. A snug elastic ring on the tube is slid onto the penis to hold in the blood during sexual activity (maximum time is about a half hour). Removing the elastic ring allows the blood to flow out and the penis to become smaller again.

Counseling may help even when ED has a physical cause. If you are experiencing ED, a member of your healthcare team can discuss the various treatments available and help determine what is best for you.

Retrograde Ejaculation

Another problem that a small number of men with diabetes encounter is known as *retrograde ejaculation,* which refers to a backward flow of semen, the fluid that contains sperm. Normally, during sexual activity, the semen is ejaculated outward. But some men with diabetes have a type of nerve damage that allows the semen to flow backward into the bladder, where it is destroyed. If this occurs, fertility can be reduced or prevented altogether, a serious problem for young men wishing to start a family.

The nerve damage that causes retrograde ejaculation is different from the damage that results in ED. And fortunately the condition is quite rare. Tell your healthcare provider if you have any early signs of this problem. Such signs may be an incentive for you and your partner to begin having children sooner rather than later. But remember, there are many other causes of infertility. If a couple is experiencing any difficulty in conceiving a child, both partners should be checked by a fertility expert.

Women's Health Issues

Women with diabetes should be aware of changes related to diabetes that can affect female function and sexuality. From puberty through childbearing to menopause, reproductive hormones influence glucose and insulin levels. Furthermore, a major decision in the life of a woman is whether to become pregnant. For women with diabetes, it is especially important that their diabetes be under excellent control *just before* and *during* pregnancy. For more information on this topic, see the discussion in Chapter 23.

Menstruation

An area related to female function is *menstruation,* the regular monthly flow of blood from the uterus. Poor control of diabetes (with chronically high blood glucose) may cause a delay in the onset of puberty or may create menstrual irregularities. Some women with diabetes notice a rise in blood glucose for a few days before the monthly flow begins. If you notice this pattern and take insulin, your healthcare provider may advise you to increase your insulin at this time. However, there is often a drop in insulin needs at the start of menses. With experience, you should learn to reduce your insulin dose in anticipation of the start of menses rather than waiting to see the actual drop in glucose levels. Failure to reduce insulin doses in time may result in low blood glucose reactions. Women who control their blood glucose with an oral medication or by nutrition therapy alone may also need an adjustment in medication, food, or physical activity if they notice a rise in blood glucose before menstruation.

Birth Control Options

Because it is vital that women with diabetes have their blood glucose under control *before* becoming pregnant, birth control measures become vitally important in preventing pregnancy until all conditions are optimal for both mother and developing baby. Regardless of the degree of glucose control, sexual activity with no protection leads to a high chance of pregnancy.

In general, women and men with diabetes use the same birth control measures as people who don't have diabetes. The choice, which depends on your preference, is often between an oral contraceptive and a barrier method. *Birth control pills* (oral contraceptives) have been used by millions of women for the past few decades. The birth control pills of the 1970s had much higher doses of hormones (estrogen and progestin) than those used today. Women with diabetes who choose birth control pills should choose a low-dose combination pill of estrogen and progestin, or a minipill containing only progestin. In most cases, insulin needs do not change on low-dose pills, but women with diabetes should have their blood pressure, A1C, cholesterol, and eyes checked regularly—before and during the use of oral contraceptives. If used properly, birth control pills are highly effective in preventing pregnancy. But because they do not protect against sexually transmitted disease, condoms are recommended for additional protection.

Other options are contraceptive patches that provide predetermined levels of estrogen and progesterone to suppress ovulation and control the cycle. There are also two injectable forms of hormone contraception—Depo-Provera and Lunelle. Both have been shown to be safe and effective.

Barrier methods have a higher failure rate than oral contraceptives. *Condoms* are thin latex sheaths that cover the penis and are used in combination with spermicide creams in preventing pregnancy. They also reduce the risk of contracting the AIDS virus and other sexually transmitted diseases from partners. The use of a *diaphragm*, a flexible device placed in the woman's vagina to block the passage of semen, is another way to prevent pregnancy. *Intrauterine devices* (IUDs) do not have any disadvantage specific to women with diabetes, nor are they associated with an increased incidence of infection in women with diabetes.

At some time in your life, you or your partner may want to consider more permanent ways to prevent pregnancy. In men, this can be done through *vasectomy*, in which part of the sperm-carrying duct is removed. Women may wish to consider *tubal ligation*, in which the fallopian tubes, which conduct eggs from the ovaries to the uterus, are tied off. Although these procedures are usually permanent, they will not impair sexual function or enjoyment.

Clearly, there is no single form of contraception that is perfect for everyone. Your healthcare provider will help you and your partner decide what's best for your situation.

Vaginal Dryness and Infections

Some women with diabetes notice that their vagina doesn't naturally become lubricated upon sexual activity. This can make sexual relations uncomfortable, and while the problem can occur in all women, it may be more likely in women with poorly controlled diabetes. High levels of blood glucose also make women more susceptible to vaginal yeast infections, which in turn can make intercourse more painful. Several water-based lubricants are available without a prescription and may increase your comfort during sex. And of course, you should renew your efforts to get your diabetes in control.

Hormone Replacement Therapy

Menopause is defined as the cessation of menstrual periods and is accompanied by loss of the hormones estrogen and progesterone. Their loss can result in hot flashes and vaginal dryness. *Hormone replacement therapy* (HRT) is the addition of low-dose estrogen and progesterone in postmenopausal women with the intent of reversing the uncomfortable effects of menopause. Use of HRT is controversial, with research suggesting both benefits and risks. Taking estrogen after menopause has been linked to a higher risk of heart attack, stroke, breast cancer, and gallbladder problems. Because of this, doctors now exercise great caution in prescribing estrogen after menopause. A major problem is lack of data as to the hormone's effects in women with diabetes, as most studies do not include many women with diabetes. If you have problems with menopause, discuss how best to alleviate them with your healthcare provider.

Heart Disease and Osteoporosis

Diabetes is reported to double a woman's risk of developing heart disease. Women with diabetes lose their natural protection against heart and blood vessel disease, especially premenopausal women. As a result, risk reduction for heart disease for women with diabetes should be as aggressive as for men. See Chapter 20 for additional information on risk factors and treatment of heart disease.

Women with type 1 diabetes are at increased risk for *osteoporosis*—loss of bone mass that leads to an increase in bone fractures. The risk for women with type 2 diabetes is similar to that of women who do not have diabetes. If you have type 1 diabetes, you should be evaluated for osteoporosis. Steps you can take to lessen your risk of developing osteoporosis include getting appropriate amounts of exercise, taking calcium and vitamin D supplements, and avoiding smoking and excessive alcohol use. You can prevent falls that cause bone fractures by using night-lights and muscle strengthening exercises, and removing hazards in the house that can contribute to falls.

Issues Affecting both Men and Women

Urinary Tract Infections

People with diabetes, particularly those with poor control, are more prone to urinary tract infections and bladder problems. This is because, in the presence of high blood glucose, the cells of the immune system are less effective in destroying bacteria that enter the body. Urinary tract infections can make sexual activity very uncomfortable, especially in women. If you have cloudy or bloody urine, burning in the urinary tract, or constantly feel as if you have to urinate, contact your healthcare provider immediately. The infection should be treated at once with antibiotics before it has a chance to spread to your kidneys. Do not have sexual relations until it is cleared up.

Genital Infections

Compared with the general population, people with poorly controlled diabetes tend to have more problems with genital infections caused by types of fungus commonly called yeast infections. These infections, which can be very annoying, affect the vagina and the top of the penis. They are usually related to poor diabetes control, which reduces the body's ability to resist infection and also leads to high glucose content in the urine, encouraging the growth of these organisms. Yeast infections can be treated with medicated creams and ointments or oral medications. Check with your healthcare provider about which product is best for your particular infection. However, keep in mind that these organisms are often resistant to any treatment until your diabetes control is improved. So get back on track as soon as possible.

Like the general population, people with diabetes can contract sexually transmitted infections. Those who are sexually active should have regular medical examinations to screen for such problems.

Sexual Dysfunction

Physical exams, blood tests, and honest dialogue are key to diagnosis and treatment when either party experiences a lack of sexual arousal or desire. People with poorly controlled diabetes, high blood fats, or high blood pressure are more prone to sexual dysfunction. Medications for blood pressure, blood fats, depression, and many other conditions sometimes affect sexual function and may require adjustment. Smoking, drinking, taking drugs, or consuming nutrition supplements containing stimulants—even too much caffeine—can impede sexual function when other physical problems are present. Many new treatments are being developed for these problems, so it is important to work with your healthcare provider to find the cause of the dysfunction and then treat it.

Sexual Activity and Low Blood Glucose

Some people with diabetes are concerned that the exertion of sexual activity may cause them to have a low blood glucose reaction, as can happen with other forms of physical activity. As with physical activity, however, the situation varies from person to person. If you experience low blood glucose after sexual activity, correct for it the same way you do with other types of activity—by adjusting your insulin or eating a snack (see Chapters 9 and 10). For example, you might try drinking a sugar-containing beverage just before sexual relations or possibly eating a snack afterward. Checking your blood glucose before and after sex can help determine the timing and the amount of the snack. Keep in mind, also, the "lag effect," whereby the glucose level drops sometime after the activity. Sexual activity at bedtime may result in hypoglycemia during sleep that may not be readily recognized.

Premarital Counseling

If you have diabetes, the prospect of marriage often raises several questions. For example, you may wonder, "Will my children have diabetes?" The answer to that question is very complicated and, as noted earlier, the degree of risk depends on which type of diabetes you have, whether one partner has diabetes or you both do, or whether anyone else among your extended family has the condition. Your healthcare provider can help you sort out answers to this important question.

You may also wish to consider a few other issues. A lifelong condition such as diabetes, as everyone who has it is aware, presents some challenges. If you have diabetes and are thinking of getting married, you should talk it out honestly with your prospective spouse. Once you both understand all the issues that may arise, you will be better able to handle them. Below are a few topics you might address:

- At present there is no cure for diabetes. People with diabetes can and do lead active and productive lives. But it requires a lifelong commitment to medical care. That's why it's so important for prospective partners of people with diabetes to understand the basics about diabetes and its care. They should also be prepared to support their spouse's self-care program.

- Pregnancy in a woman with diabetes may be more difficult and require more attention than in women who don't have diabetes (see Chapter 23). However, in recent years medicine has made great strides in this area, and risks of complications have been greatly reduced.

- Special problems with insurance may arise that must be handled with understanding, planning, and sensitivity.

Of course, all couples must deal with the ups and downs that life together can bring. In the marriage of a person with diabetes, knowledge and understanding by both partners, aided and abetted by generous doses of love, can go a long way toward creating and sustaining a stable and happy relationship.

PART SIX

Living Well with Diabetes

CHAPTER 25

Living Well with Diabetes As an Older Adult

If you are an older adult with diabetes, the treatment of your diabetes is not much different from that of a younger person with diabetes. The goal is to improve the quality and length of your life by preventing or slowing the onset or progression of the complications associated with diabetes. Poorly controlled glucose interacts with other issues related to aging to accelerate complications, so one goal is to help you maintain as near normal glucose levels as is possible. Some people may assume that diabetes is just something that happens as you get older, and they may not be very concerned about it. They may remember family members who developed diabetes and complications as they aged and assume either that developing diabetes is not serious or that there is nothing that can be done to prevent the problems they observed. However, diabetes *is* a serious disease, even when it is diagnosed in older adults. It does cause complications and can interfere with daily living. But something can be done and you need to see that it gets done! You need to take responsibility, with the help of your healthcare provider, for getting good medical care for your diabetes.

When diabetes occurs in older adults, it is usually type 2, but it can also be type 1, which can occur at any age. Older adults may have type 2 diabetes for a number of years before it is diagnosed, and when it is diagnosed, it may be viewed as "mild" diabetes. This approach puts the older adult at increased risk over time for developing complications of diabetes. Some older adults may have had type 1 diabetes for 30 to 40 years, and because of better treatment are living long and productive lives. Other older adults may be diagnosed for the first time with type 1 diabetes. While it can be hard for your doctor to determine exactly what type of diabetes you have, the goals of treatment are the same regardless of the type—helping you control your glucose, lipids (blood fats), and blood pressure to prevent (or for some, treat) the complications of diabetes.

Treatment Goals

For *healthy* older adults, Joslin Diabetes Center recommends a pre-meal blood glucose level of 90 to 130 mg/dl. Adjustments should be made in your treatment program if your glucose is regularly less than 90 mg/dl or greater than 140 mg/dl. The general goal for A1C levels is less than 7 percent. These targets may be adjusted if you have a history of low or unrecognized blood glucose, or if you have a medical condition that would increase the likelihood of harm should you have a hypoglycemic reaction. Ultimately, treatment goals should be individualized, so you should check with your healthcare providers as to what yours should be. Nutrition, physical activity, and monitoring programs are the foundation for helping you achieve your treatment goals.

Nutrition

The goals of your nutrition program are to help prevent unpredictable highs and lows in glucose levels, improve LDL cholesterol if elevated, achieve and maintain a healthy weight, and promote healthy food choices for optimal nutrition. A dietitian can help you design a meal plan that is convenient for your lifestyle. If finances are a concern, a dietitian can also help you get the most for your "nutrition dollar." Many people have a set pattern of meals and foods that they like. It is important that you share this information with your healthcare providers. In this way, a treatment program can usually be designed for you that will not be disruptive to your schedule and lifestyle.

From the standpoint of food choices, there are several things you can do to help control your blood glucose levels. The first is to space your meals and snacks throughout the day. It's also important that you don't skip meals (even if your blood glucose is high), especially if you are on diabetes medications. But even if you are not on medication, spacing of meals provides a more gradual amount of glucose to your body throughout the day. It is also helpful to learn about carbohydrate and fat portions. And rather than eliminating certain foods that you enjoy, work with your dietitian to determine the right portions for you. Chapters 4 and 5 discuss carbohydrate and fat choices.

Physical Activity

Physical activity is very important for everyone, but it is especially beneficial for older adults and for older adults with diabetes. Physical activity can help lower blood glucose levels, strengthen your heart and blood vessels, help with weight control, and keep your joints and bones healthy. It is important to find some activity you enjoy doing and then do it on a regular basis. Check first with your physician to see which activities may be best for you. You may need medical evaluation of your heart and your feet before starting a program of increased activity. If you haven't been doing any regular physical activities, such as routine walking, start with 5 minutes a day; as you feel comfortable, gradually increase the length of time you engage in the activity. To promote fitness, moderate physical activity for at least 30 minutes per day should be a part of your daily routine. Walking at a brisk pace (3 to 4 miles per hour) is an example of moderate physical activity. Chair exercises or brief daily walks are good activities to start with. If you are not familiar with chair exercises, ask your healthcare provider for information. See Chapters 9 and 10 for more information on physical activity. And ask your healthcare provider about exercise programs for older adults.

As an older adult participating in physical activities, foot care is especially important for you. Be sure you wear shoes that are supportive and fit properly. Checking your feet daily for signs of irritation or pressure can help decrease your risk of foot injury or infection.

Monitoring

If you have been newly diagnosed with diabetes, you will also learn how to check your blood glucose each day. The results help you and your healthcare providers determine how well your treatment program is working. How often you should check your blood glucose should be discussed with your healthcare providers. Some adults do fine checking first thing in the morning and before supper or bedtime two to four days a week. Others may check first thing in the morning, as well as before and two hours after the start of their largest meal. Chapter 12 has more information on monitoring.

Medications

To improve your glucose control, you may need to add a medication to your treatment program. Your doctor or other healthcare provider may start with a low dose of one of the diabetes pills (Chapter 13 discusses the different types of pills). Many adults will benefit from a combination of diabetes pills. They can be combined because they act at different sites in your body. Some of these pills should not be used if you have other medical conditions, such as heart failure, liver problems, or kidney failure. Be sure to discuss the status of these conditions with your physician when he or she is prescribing diabetes pills, particularly if you have different physicians caring for these other medical problems.

There may come a time when diabetes pills no longer keep your blood glucose at the level of control needed and insulin therapy will be needed. You should not view this as your fault or think that if you had just done something differently, insulin would not have been needed. Rather, this change reflects the natural progressive nature of diabetes and the fact that the longer you have diabetes, the less insulin the beta cells of the pancreas can produce. Many people eventually need to take insulin injections to control their blood glucose levels. Chapter 14 reviews the different types of insulin. But even when medications are added to your treatment program, it is important to continue being careful of your food choices and participating in regular physical activity.

Testing for and Treating Complications of Diabetes

Your healthcare providers will continue to screen you for complications. The sooner a problem is discovered, the easier it is to treat. Your blood pressure should be checked at every visit to your healthcare provider. As with glucose control, you may need a combination of blood pressure medications to keep your blood pressure under control. Your eyes and kidneys should be tested every year. If you have heart problems along with your diabetes, it is important that you achieve optimal glucose and blood pressure control, not smoke, engage in regular physical activities, and reduce your lipid (fat) levels. Your LDL cholesterol level should be less than 100 mg/dl. A daily dose of aspirin is also recommended.

Summary—Tips for Staying Healthy with Diabetes

- Try to keep your blood glucose in your target range.

- Eat healthy foods and work with a dietitian to create a realistic meal plan that you can follow.

- Be as physically active as possible.

- Have regular dilated eye exams by an eye doctor who specializes in diabetes.

- Don't forget to bring your blood glucose monitoring logbook to every visit with your healthcare provider.

- When your blood glucose is in good control, you'll feel better—so work with your healthcare team to get your blood glucose levels under control.

- Check your feet daily for any redness, or cracks in the skin. Devices are available to make it easier for you to see your feet (or ask a family member or friend to help you).

- Have your healthcare provider check your feet at each appointment. Ask whether you should see a podiatrist.

- If you have trouble seeing well, ask your pharmacist about monitors designed for the visually impaired. Some of these monitors have very large numbers or can actually talk. Also, use magnifying devices to help you see the numbers on insulin syringes and to help you recognize different pills (ask your pharmacist about these).

- Ask your doctor about diabetes education classes or refresher programs. Diabetes education is paid for by Medicare.

- Don't be too proud to let others help you. You may have family members or friends who would be happy to help you if they knew you could use some assistance—helping with your medicines, perhaps driving you to medical appointments, taking walks with you, or even just talking. (Perhaps you can offer them something in exchange—flowers from your garden, a home-cooked meal, some good advice . . .)

- Your doctor can recommend a social worker or a diabetes educator who will have good ideas for making things easier for you.

The important message for you is that you need to control your glucose, blood lipids, and blood pressure just as aggressively as do younger adults. You have a lifetime of learning experiences that you can draw on and that will help you successfully manage your diabetes and live a rewarding and satisfying life despite having diabetes. By learning everything you can about diabetes and working with your healthcare providers as an active team member, you will live well with diabetes.

CHAPTER 26

Coping with Diabetes

If you have diabetes, you face a wide range of special challenges. The first of these challenges is physical. You have to learn how your body works—how it uses the food you eat for energy—and how diabetes affects it. You need to conscientiously practice a variety of treatment and monitoring procedures to help you avoid high and low blood glucose levels and the threats they pose to your health.

Other challenges you face are emotional. You need to cope with how diabetes makes you feel—and how you feel about having diabetes. You and your family will inevitably have concerns, anxieties, and fears as you live with this condition over the weeks, months, and years. But most people find that, over time, they are remarkably resilient and able to deal effectively with their diabetes. It's always important, however, to remember that there are a number of ways diabetes can affect your emotions—and a number of ways that your emotions can affect your diabetes.

When you have diabetes, it's easy to believe you are the only person who feels a certain way. It's easy to become reluctant about sharing your feelings with others. However, it's important to realize you are not alone. Many other people are struggling with the same feelings and emotions you are.

Blood Glucose and Emotions

Both high and low blood glucose can cause obvious changes in your mood. For example, low blood glucose can make you nervous or irritable. By contrast, high blood glucose can make you feel tired, which can cause you to feel listless or depressed. The effect on your emotions of the varying glucose levels may be the result of feeling poorly because of the high and low glucose values rather than because of any direct effect of glucose on the mood control center of the brain itself. But don't fall into the trap of attributing all of your feelings—particularly negative ones—to your blood glucose levels. Remember, you may actually be responding to other circumstances in your life.

Try to distinguish between feelings related to blood glucose levels and those caused by other factors. Blaming all your feelings on your diabetes may prevent you from uncovering the true source of your distress, and that can keep you from solving a problem and feeling happier. It can also be frustrating to family members and friends, because it prevents them from interacting and sharing honest feelings with you. If you are upset or depressed about something, try to identify the source of the problem. This strategy can help you find the right road to a solution.

Stress and Diabetes Control

The stresses of everyday life can negatively affect your diabetes. For some, stress may directly influence their blood glucose levels. For others, the influence may be more indirect—for example, it may make it difficult for them to give their diabetes management the necessary time and effort. You may find that emotional stress from tense circumstances at home or work can raise or lower blood glucose levels. There are two basic ways this can happen: on the one hand, stress hormones can be released in your body, causing blood glucose levels to fluctuate; on the other hand, stressful situations can cause you to change key behaviors, upsetting your daily routine and making it harder to care for your diabetes. You might try to avoid stress to offset its effects, but it's not always possible to do this, so you might try to anticipate and prepare yourself to handle the stressful situations. If stress becomes overwhelming, you may wish to try counseling. Many diabetes centers have professional counselors who are trained to help people with diabetes handle stresses that can impinge on good diabetes management. It will be helpful if the counselor that you see has some understanding of diabetes. It will also be helpful for your counselor to speak with the members of your treatment team. In addition, exercise and relaxation techniques can help some people handle stress more effectively.

As you manage the care of your body and your emotions, it's important to avoid isolating yourself from other people. At times, you may be tempted to withdraw because you feel that people unfamiliar with diabetes cannot possibly understand your experience. While it may be true that some people will not understand, many others will. Seeking the support of your family and friends and making connections with other people who have diabetes can be helpful. It's particularly important to share your concerns with your healthcare providers. Be sure to include members of your family in visits to your healthcare providers in order to increase communication among all involved.

You may also find it helpful to participate in a diabetes support group, in which people share how they have addressed the unique challenges of their diabetes. Your healthcare providers and the local affiliate of the American Diabetes Association can tell you where these groups meet in your area.

Unique Stresses of Diabetes

People with diabetes have unique day-to-day stresses. Below are a few of the more common difficulties people with diabetes have discussed with clinicians at Joslin Diabetes Center. You may find that you can identify with many or all of them, which is only normal, because diabetes affects people's bodies and feelings in very similar ways. What differs is how people cope with these issues. Diabetes is a full-time job that requires persistent effort and commitment. That's why we recommend that you don't fly solo. Ask for support and help from family members and friends as well as from your healthcare providers.

Chronic Condition

Diabetes is a *chronic* disorder, something that never goes away. It requires daily care and attention, and for many people that can be emotionally draining, particularly if there are other stresses in their lives. One person describes it this way: "It's not the rolling of a boulder up a hill but the stone in your shoe that wears you down."

Diabetes is all about learning what to do, then doing it day after day despite changing circumstances. How do you deal with this irksome "stone"? First of all, there's nothing wrong with admitting that you hate diabetes. That's right, *hate* it. No one could expect you to feel otherwise. At the same time, you must *tolerate* it enough to convert your emotional energy into taking good care of yourself. Such honesty about your feelings will help you strike a healthy emotional balance. You will be able to better handle your everyday care.

Practically everyone who is diagnosed with diabetes goes through various emotional stages. For the first few weeks, you were probably *shocked* by the news, perhaps overwhelmed and confused by it all. You may then have gone through a stage of *denial*, thinking that you didn't really *have* diabetes, or if you did, it wasn't really a big deal. In fact, some people continue to deny the seriousness of having diabetes for a long time, facing the reality of the situation only when complications set in after many years of poorly controlling their blood glucose.

Another common reaction is *fear* or *anxiety* over the possibility that diabetes will lead to long-term problems with your eyes, kidneys, nerves, or other body systems. Because these complications are more likely to occur when diabetes is not in good control, it's vitally important that you reach the stage of *accepting* your condition. A growing understanding that good blood glucose control can prevent or minimize complications will give you some feeling of control over your future health. Of course, there will still be days when you feel distressed and overwhelmed by your diabetes, even after you've accepted the realities of having it.

"Invisible" Nature

Diabetes is an invisible condition, a disease that generally remains hidden. If you walk into a room, you can easily spot someone with a runny nose from a cold, but you can't tell who has diabetes. This invisibility factor can bring internal and interpersonal conflict. On one hand, you feel the "same" as other people, with many of the same desires and needs. On the other hand, you feel "different." Unlike people who don't have diabetes, you have to watch what you eat and sacrifice some of your independence to take care of your health. Coping with this tension—simultaneously feeling the same and different—can take some work. To put these feelings in practical perspective, talk them out with your family members and healthcare providers.

The hidden nature of diabetes makes it "a disease in the absence of illness." In other words, you may not experience any immediate symptoms or feel ill, even though subtle changes may be occurring throughout your body that, without good diabetes management, can lead to long-term complications. This lack of physical consequences can lead to lapses in your treatment program. After all, it's easy to remember to take a decongestant when you have a stuffy nose. It's not so easy to follow a meal plan, participate in regular physical activity, check your blood glucose, and take medication when there are no apparent warning signs. You may find it hard to keep your diabetes program on track as a result. Others may find it difficult to remember your need to keep a schedule or watch what you eat.

Staying with your treatment program requires concentration. You'll often need to think about when you ate or exercised; you'll need to remember to check your blood glucose and take your diabetes pills or insulin. You will need to develop a routine, something that's easier for some people to do than others. Adapting to a new lifestyle can take discipline and a lot of patience, qualities that do not come easily to many people. Be patient. Set realistic goals that are achievable. Over time, you can improve your care, step by step.

Frustration

Diabetes can cause frustration and anger. At times, you may be upset that you have diabetes in the first place. You may feel overwhelmed as you struggle to learn the basic things you need to know to care for your condition. There may be days when caring for your diabetes seems to get in the way of your job, your personal relationships, and just plain having fun. Feeling angry or frustrated, you may slack off on your eating plan, physical activity, medication, or monitoring. In fact, experts have identified more than 250 factors that can interfere with following a treatment program—everything from blaming the weather to living alone.

How can you deal with frustration? One way is by realizing that everyone with diabetes has good days and bad days. There will be times when you follow your treatment plan closely but don't see the results you hoped for. There will be times, and temptations, that make it hard to stick with your treatment plan. At a workshop for people with diabetes, the question was asked, "What's the biggest thing that gets in the way of sticking to your treatment program?" Without hesitation, everyone in the group shouted, "Food!"

So if you're having trouble with a meal plan, you're certainly not alone. The group pointed out additional hurdles: accommodating other people's schedules, taking care of family members, and traveling with diabetes. You have probably faced these hurdles too. To manage your care, you may have to change how you feel about your diabetes and how you cope when things don't go right. You may get frustrated when you're seemingly doing everything possible to control your blood glucose but not getting good results. That may cause you to ask, "What's the use?" And you may get despondent or angry, taking it out on yourself or other people. You may be tempted to abandon your program. At times like these it is very important to logically follow what you know about how to take care of yourself rather than react to how overwhelmed you feel.

Your relationships with family members can also be impacted by diabetes. Perhaps your loved ones care too much or care too little. Indeed, it is not uncommon to have arguments over what you eat and how you manage the other aspects of your diabetes.

You (and your family members) need to realize that you will have days of unexplained high or low blood glucose levels. And you need to realize that it's hard to stay motivated over a long period of time. Be honest about how you feel about this lifelong commitment. In fact, many of the ways you choose to cope with these feelings will require this type of honesty—a clear assessment of the task before you and how you will face occasional disappointments and failures. At those times, rather than throwing in the towel, try to see your diabetes treatment as a long stretch of highway. Once in a while you may veer off the road onto the shoulder, or run out of gas, or get a flat tire. But with the help of your healthcare providers, family, and other people with diabetes, you can get back on the road.

Unpredictability

Diabetes can be very unpredictable. It varies from person to person. Its impact on your body often changes over time, requiring adjustments as you get older. It can change with physical stresses, such as being sick. There even are moments when a sudden change in your blood glucose will occur for no apparent reason. As one person with diabetes put it, "It's just one crazy thing after another." Such unpredictability can be very unsettling, and people can become so anxious about experiencing something like a low blood glucose reaction that they may stay home as much as possible. Or they may keep blood glucose levels on the "high side" most of the time in order to avoid having a low blood glucose reaction.

To cope with the unpredictable nature of diabetes, it's important to learn as much as possible about your condition. That way, you'll be prepared for high or low blood glucose, what to do on sick days, how to order in restaurants, and how to travel with diabetes. By being prepared to deal with a variety of situations, you will feel more at ease. Indeed, you'll discover that much of life can go on as before.

A Paradox

Diabetes is a medical problem that must come first in your life. Yet you don't want it to take over your life, and that can create some challenges for how you think about yourself. Are you well or sick? Master or victim? In control or helpless? Optimistic or pessimistic? Independent or dependent? The way you respond to these questions will depend, in many ways, on your personal characteristics and how you approach life in general. Coping with the paradox of diabetes—it has to come first, yet you can't let it define you—takes emotional honesty, maturity, and support. But by sorting it out, you will be better able to manage it. Yes, your treatment program will be of utmost importance. But your diabetes has never been and never will be *you*. You are a person with many qualities, feelings, thoughts, and skills that you can use to find personal fulfillment as well as to make contributions to your family, job, and community. By defining yourself in this positive way, your diabetes care becomes a means to an end. Your care is a way to maintain your health so that you're able to be who you really are!

Hope for the Future

It is only natural that once your diabetes was diagnosed, you became concerned about your future. After all, you probably have heard that serious complications can develop in people who have had diabetes for many years. You may know someone with eye disease or even blindness due to diabetes. You may have heard about people who have had a foot or leg amputated or whose kidneys failed from the effects of poorly controlled diabetes. Naturally, this can make you concerned and anxious and cause you to question what the future will be like.

Various complications do occur in some people with long-standing, poorly controlled diabetes. However, it must be emphasized again that there is every reason for hope. Research shows that intensive treatment and monitoring procedures—which help you maintain good control of your blood glucose levels—can help prevent, delay, or reduce the severity of complications.

While there is no guarantee that every person will bypass the complications of diabetes, such problems are much less likely to occur if you maintain good blood glucose control. In both the Diabetes Control and Complications Trial and the United Kingdom Prospective Diabetes Study those who followed intensive therapy had a dramatic reduction in the development of complications. The primary finding in both studies was that any improvement in blood glucose control is linked to a clear reduction in risk of complications.

Success stories of people with diabetes abound, and they can help motivate you to stay on track with your program. You may wish to consider ways to improve your diabetes control. You might also like to meet people who are successfully managing diabetes. Successful management usually also requires the help of specialists skilled in diabetes management.

Be Open About Your Diabetes

Some people try to keep their diabetes a secret, believing that if it is found out, they will be considered "different" and will become the object of some type of special attention. They worry about being denied promotions by employers or becoming distanced from friends and acquaintances. Some of these concerns are legitimate. There are people who do not understand diabetes and need to learn more about it. Furthermore, there are employers who are unfamiliar with diabetes and may refuse to employ or promote a person who has it. It is unrealistic, therefore, to say that this is a groundless concern.

On the other hand, not letting others know you have diabetes also has its difficulties. You may feel tense and isolated as you try to care for your diabetes while hiding it from the people around you. Letting others know about your condition can bring about the positive support that is so important in dealing with your diabetes. Particularly for people on insulin, someone who works with you may need to know how to help you in case your blood glucose drops too low and you have a low blood glucose reaction.

Family members, friends, and fellow employees can offer encouragement as you strive to follow a meal plan, participate in physical activity, take medications, and monitor your condition. Some people with diabetes ask a friend or family member to learn along with them as they work at mastering the art of managing diabetes. They then have a partner who can share their disappointments and victories—and also help in time of need.

Keys to Success

The following checklist highlights ways that may help you deal with your diabetes. Review this list on a regular basis, refocusing your feelings and thoughts as other circumstances in your life change.

- **BE AWARE OF THE STUMBLING BLOCKS.** Identify factors that can interfere with your management of your diabetes. Are you tempted to eat second portions of food? Is it inconvenient to check your blood glucose at work or school? Do you frequently eat out at restaurants? Does your working style cause you to lose track of time? By concentrating on major stumbling blocks to your diabetes care, you will be able to find ways around them.

- **LEARN ABOUT DIABETES.** Learn the importance of meal planning, physical activity, medications, and checking your blood glucose. It's very important that you have correct and up-to-date knowledge about how to take care of yourself.

- **MANAGE STRESS.** Identify factors in your life that cause tension, wear you down, or make you anxious. Work with your healthcare team to reduce these stresses.

- **BE PREPARED.** Unlike people who don't have diabetes, you may have to plan aspects of your day. Also, you need to be ready to handle high and low blood glucose levels. Being prepared can help you feel more at ease and in control.

- **SET ACHIEVABLE GOALS.** With the help of your healthcare team, set practical and achievable goals. Approach your diabetes care in a step-by-step manner.

- **BE REALISTIC.** You're not always going to be in perfect control of your diabetes. You will have good days and bad days. When you occasionally have a bad day, don't dwell on it. Simply try to continue without guilt or blame. The goal is to do the best that you can, and accept that you won't be perfect.

- **ASK FOR SUPPORT.** Tell your family and friends that you appreciate their support. Define the boundaries of what is personally helpful (something that is supportive to one person may not be supportive to another). Tell family and friends specific ways they can help you follow your treatment program. Bringing family members along to meet with your healthcare team can be a constructive way to include them in your support network.

■ **BUILD A HEALTHCARE TEAM.** You don't have to do it alone. Doctors, nurses and nurse practitioners, diabetes educators, and behavioral specialists can help you solve the tough problems and feel more confident about caring for your diabetes.

CHAPTER 27

Traveling with Diabetes

Whether they're driving across the country or jet-setting off to an exotic locale, traveling, for many people, is one of the delights of their lives. They enjoy visiting friends and relatives in other parts of the country or traveling to foreign countries. They find the sights and sounds of new places, along with a break in normal routines, quite refreshing. You don't need to hesitate about taking a camping trip, visiting friends, or even taking an around-the-world cruise just because you have diabetes. With adequate planning, you can care for your diabetes while traveling just as well as you manage it at home.

Planning for Travel

The key to successful traveling is planning as far ahead as possible. Once you know your destination, how you are traveling there, and how long you'll be staying, you can make the following preparations.

- **A MEDICAL CHECKUP.** Visit your healthcare provider at least four weeks ahead of time to be sure that your general health is okay and that your diabetes is in good control. Ask your doctor to write a letter on letterhead stationery explaining in detail your condition and any complications that another physician would need to know to take proper care of you. The letter may also come in handy in case you are ever questioned about the medications, syringes, and other medical items you are carrying, particularly when going through airport security. You will want to ask your doctor about medications to combat motion sickness or diarrhea. Such problems can be very disruptive to your diabetes management. Figure 27-1 is a sample letter written by one of this book's authors.

Figure 27-1   Sample Travel Letter

To Whom It May Concern:

John Doe is treated for diabetes mellitus at the Joslin Clinic in Boston. It is medically necessary for him to carry insulin, syringes, and blood glucose testing equipment, including lancets and related supplies, at all times.

Sincerely,

Richard S. Beaser, M.D.

■ IMMUNIZATIONS. If you are traveling to areas of the world where immunizations are required, determine what's necessary for your destination as early as possible before your departure date. Some immunizations, such as the one for hepatitis, require multiple injections and may take some time. Vaccination requirements change constantly, so be sure to get the latest information. Also, check your medical records to determine which immunizations you've already had and when you had them. Certainly, influenza and pneumonia vaccinations may be recommended wherever you travel. If you don't have information about your immunization history, check with your healthcare provider's office. That way, your provider will also have plenty of time to deal with any effect the immunizations may have on your diabetes control. Many international airports and public health departments have phone-in lines to provide up-to-date information on necessary immunizations for various parts of the world.

- **EXTRA MEDICATIONS, SYRINGES, AND PRESCRIPTIONS.** Plan to take extra supplies of diabetes pills, insulin, syringes, and any other medications you may need. Take twice as much as you expect to use during your trip because the country you are visiting may not have the same medication and diabetic supplies. Also carry prescriptions for these medications, which you may need to fill if your supplies are misplaced. Ask your doctor to use the generic names of these drugs, because brand names may vary from country to country—for example, instead of Amaryl, your prescription should state the generic name, *glimepiride.*

    If the insulin you normally use isn't available in the area you plan to visit, your doctor can provide you with a prescription for an alternative form. Don't be alarmed if you encounter your form of insulin under a name you don't recognize. Also, be prepared to find it in concentrations of U-40 and U-80 rather than U-100. If the concentration of insulin is different from U-100, you should asked the pharmacist how to convert your current insulin plan in order to be assured that you are taking the correct amount. To measure these dosages properly, you'll need a U-40 or U-80 syringe. Such adjustments are necessary only if you lose your supplies or are planning to stay in another country for an extended period of time. For most trips, you will be able to carry all the supplies that you would regularly use at home.

- **INSULIN PUMP USE.** Insulin pumps can break, and supplies may not be readily available away from home. Pump users should consult with their healthcare team for "off pump" doses of injected insulin to use in case their pump malfunctions when traveling. You should also be sure to carry with you the needed insulin and syringes to take these doses.

- **TIME ZONES.** If you are traveling across time zones, consult with your healthcare providers before leaving. They can help schedule your medications, a topic discussed in greater detail later in this chapter.

When scheduling air travel, try to fly during daylight hours to minimize disruption to your schedule.

- **CONTACTING DOCTORS.** Your healthcare provider may be able to supply you with the name of a doctor who practices in the area you are planning to visit. Or consult with your local or the national office of the American Diabetes Association, which can put you in touch with people at affiliates along your travel route. They can also provide you with names of physicians in those areas.

   If traveling in foreign countries, ask the International Diabetes Federation for the names of diabetes associations, which will know diabetes specialists in the countries you are visiting. Once you arrive, American embassies and consulates will be at your service, and your hotels may also keep a roster of English-speaking doctors. In an emergency, you should go to the nearest hospital.

- **IDENTIFICATION.** Prepare a form of identification to carry in your purse or wallet that indicates you have diabetes. This card should also list your name, address, phone number, doctor's name and phone number, and the type and dose of insulin and other medications you use. Also wear a medical ID tag—a necklace or bracelet—that includes the name of your condition (diabetes) and an emergency phone number. This will help other people know how to assist you in an emergency.

- **BEFORE DEPARTURE.** Before departure, find out if your health insurance policy will cover you throughout your trip. Carry your health insurance identification card. If traveling to a foreign country, learn how to say, "I have diabetes," "Please give me orange juice or sugar," and "Please get me a doctor" in the appropriate language. You may also want to have these comments, written in the native language of the place you are going, on a card in your wallet.

- **AIRPLANE MEALS.** Call the airline to find out if a meal (or meals) will be served on your flight, what times the meal (or meals) are served, and what meal options you have. Today fewer airlines are providing meals, so you need to be prepared in case meals are not suitable or are served late or there are none! Be sure to carry a supply of snacks and glucose tablets or gel in case your blood glucose drops too low. Good snack choices include peanut butter crackers, granola bars, single-serving fruit cups, single-serving boxes of cereal, and small boxes of raisins.

- **PACKING A CARRY-ON BAG.** When the day comes for you to leave for your trip, include the following items in a small travel bag. Keep this bag with you at all times. Don't check the bag on public carriers such as planes, buses, or trains, as it might be misplaced.
    - **DIABETES PILLS.** If your diabetes is treated with pills, be sure you pack these in your carry-on bag.
    - **INSULIN.** Include all the insulin and any other injectable medications you will need for your entire trip. Watch out for temperature extremes. The insulin you are not using should be kept cool, but it should not be exposed to temperatures below 36°F (2°C). The bottle you have opened and are using is good for one month, so be sure to bring along enough for the full trip, plus backup. All unopened bottles are good until the manufacturer's expiration date. Don't put insulin in a bag that will be stored in the luggage compartment of an airplane, because high-altitude temperatures may cause it to freeze. Also, insulin should not be exposed to temperatures above 86°F (30°C) for any length of time. Avoid excess agitation, which can cause loss of potency, clumping, frosting, or precipitation. There are specific products you can buy to keep diabetes supplies cool and safe while traveling. A variety of travel packs can be purchased at your local pharmacy. If you use an insulin pump, bring extra batteries and supplies for the pump, but bring a bottle of insulin and syringes with you for emergencies. Also take your glucagon kit, and instruct a companion on how to use this medication in emergencies.
    - **SYRINGES.** Take all the syringes you will need during your trip. Use disposable syringes and be sure to dispose of them safely. Don't forget alcohol and cotton, to use in wiping off the top of the insulin bottles. Be sure to have a travel letter from your

physician authorizing you to carry these supplies, to facilitate your passage through heightened airport security.

■ **INSULIN PEN SUPPLIES.** If you use an insulin pen, be sure to bring enough prefilled pens or cartridges with you. And don't forget to bring enough pen needles, as well.

■ **MONITORING SUPPLIES.** Include all your supplies for checking your blood glucose. Take extra batteries or a second meter and glucose strips that can be read as a backup. If your travel will take you to higher altitudes, there's a possibility that your blood glucose meter may give an inaccurate reading—if this occurs, you should call the meter company's toll-free help line. If you have type 1 diabetes, be sure to pack ketone strips.

■ **SNACKS.** Prepare a snack pack containing carbohydrates to eat in case of low blood glucose. Travel often involves unexpected delays in your meal schedule, so always carry some carbohydrate foods, such as fruit or crackers. Cheese or peanut butter sandwiches are helpful if a meal has to be missed. If you use some of your food supplies, replenish them at your first opportunity.

■ **APPROPRIATE FOOTWEAR.** Traveling often involves considerable walking. If you plan to purchase new shoes and socks for your trip, do so several weeks ahead of time. This will give you enough time to "break them in." Purchase socks that will allow moisture to be wicked away from your skin to lessen the chance of developing blisters and fungal infections. Always pack an extra pair of comfortable shoes in your suitcase. Don't forget to take a mild antiseptic, moisture-restoring cream, antibiotic ointment, foot powders, and emery boards for proper nail care. Finally, don't take a "vacation" from inspecting your feet on a daily basis!

On the Way

■ **DO NOT SKIP MEALS OR SNACKS.** If traveling by car, be prepared to eat some form of carbohydrate when there are meal delays. Also, keep carbohydrate-containing foods in your car in case of a low blood glucose reaction. If this happens while you are driving, pull off the road, treat the low blood glucose (see Chapter 17), and wait at least 10 to 15 minutes before resuming driving. If you tend to have low blood glucose, you might want to eat a snack of one carbohydrate serving (15 grams of carbohydrate) every two hours.

■ **CHECK YOUR BLOOD GLUCOSE.** When traveling, check your blood glucose more often. When traveling long distances, be sure to check your blood glucose every four to six hours—even if you don't check that often at home. Stress and changes in activity, food intake, and sleep can affect blood glucose levels. Don't change your watch until you arrive at your destination; follow your usual schedule until then. Early in your trip, your readings probably won't be within target because of all the excitement and change in your usual routine. Once you've brought your blood glucose back to your target range, you can follow your usual routine with regard to checking your blood glucose.

■ **PLAN FOR PHYSICAL ACTIVITY.** Physical activity is important while traveling. If you are on an airplane or train for a long period, occasionally walk up and down the aisle to stimulate circulation. If on a car trip, plan to stop and stretch your legs every 1½ hours or so.

After you arrive, you may need to make some adjustments to your diabetes medications, and very possibly to your insulin dose, based on time-zone changes and anticipated variations from the usual pattern of food intake and activity. You will need more food (or less insulin) for walking, skiing, or a day at the beach than for sitting on a sight-seeing bus or going to movies and plays. If you take insulin, meet with your healthcare provider before your trip to discuss how you can adjust your insulin for extra activity and more or less food. If you take rapid-acting insulin before meals, consider learning carbohydrate counting, since the type, amount, and timing of food you eat in other countries may be very different from the way you eat at home. While people who use oral diabetes medications are less likely to need adjustments in their dosages, anticipation of considerable increases in physical activity might warrant a temporary change, and you might still check with your healthcare provider to be sure.

- **TELL YOUR COMPANIONS.** If you are traveling with relatives or friends, let them know about your diabetes. They can adapt their plans to meet your needs and can also be of assistance if you should need it.

- **ADJUST MEDICATION FOR TIME ZONES.** If you are crossing time zones, ask your healthcare provider if you should modify your insulin dose or injection schedule. A coast-to-coast trip within the United States means only a three-hour time difference, which usually requires minimal adjustment. But if you are crossing at least five time zones, with a time change of several hours, as a trip to Europe would entail, you may be advised to increase or decrease the amount of insulin in proportion to the time you will gain or lose. If you are not currently on a physiologic insulin regimen (see Chapter 15), discuss switching over to this kind of regimen with your healthcare team at least a month or so before you leave for your trip to allow enough time for adjustment—for example, a rapid-acting insulin at meals and insulin glargine as your basal insulin.

  If you take more than one injection, think of your travel day as being lengthened or shortened at the end. While your first dose will probably go unchanged, the later ones will be either increased or decreased. When traveling east, you lose several hours of the day. Taking a normal day's worth of insulin in this shortened day could cause hypoglycemia. So you typically need to take less insulin than you usually do.

  When traveling west, your normal insulin dose may not be enough for the lengthened day. Usually, you need to use more insulin than you normally would in a day. Work out the exact plans with your healthcare providers. The types and dose or doses of insulin you take and the timing and length of your flights all make a difference in your program.

  If you take diabetes pills, you may or may not be advised to omit a dose on a shortened eastbound travel day. This is more likely to be recommended for one of the medications that stimulate insulin secretion, such as a sulfonylurea, than for one of the medications that reduce insulin resistance, such as metformin or a thiazolidinedione.

However, you should certainly check with your healthcare provider on what to do if you are taking a long trip over multiple time zones. In general, having too long an interval between doses is safer than having too short an interval. If you are taking short-acting diabetes pills that are taken when meals are eaten, such as acarbose, repaglinide, or nateglinide, continue your usual dosing schedule. Talk to your doctor before your trip if you are taking nateglinide to determine whether you can take an extra pill if you eat an extra meal. By planning and working with your healthcare providers, you can manage your diabetes well no matter where you travel.

Sampling Local Foods

Become familiar with the carbohydrate, fat, and calorie content of different foods. If you're not sure of a dish's ingredients, be sure to ask. When experimenting with new foods, be sure to monitor your blood glucose, preferably before eating and two hours after the meal. You can feel free to take advantage of the native cuisine, but don't go overboard—you don't have to eat every snack and beverage offered. Just as you would at a restaurant close to home, ask how foods are prepared, and don't hesitate to make special requests, such as having your fish broiled with olive oil rather than butter. As always, go easy on the alcohol. Remember, alcohol without food can lead to hypoglycemia, so always eat something with alcohol.

Meet with your dietitian before you leave for your trip. Be sure you have a meal plan that will work with your travel schedule as well as the region to which you are traveling. Your dietitian can provide you with information on different kinds of foods to help you better plan your meals and more accurately count your carbohydrates. Use a carbohydrate counter book as a reference for food you may not normally eat at home.

Prevent Diarrhea and Motion Sickness

Diarrhea is an unpleasant problem for anyone. But for people with diabetes, it is especially dangerous because it can deplete the body of fluids and unabsorbed nutrients, upsetting the balance between your insulin dose and the glucose left in your system. To prevent "traveler's diarrhea" while on your trip, avoid eating peeled fruits, leafy vegetables, undercooked meats, and milk products like cheese and cream sauces, especially in Central and South America, Asia, and Africa. These foods may contain bacteria that cause intestinal upset. Also avoid tap water and ice cubes. Instead, drink bottled water and tea, which are usually safe because the water has been boiled. If you are traveling to a region where gastrointestinal upsets are an increased risk, check with your physician to see whether you should be taking medications with you, or perhaps even taking an antibiotic during the trip for protection.

If you do develop diarrhea and, in particular, vomiting that does not resolve quickly, you may need to follow sick-day rules and/or seek medical attention. Particularly if you treat your diabetes with insulin, prolonged vomiting will make diabetes management more difficult, or could signify diabetic ketoacidosis. Ailments like the ones you get at home might befall you on the road as well, such as bronchitis or an upper respiratory infection, a dental infection, or a urinary tract infection. Seeking medical assistance immediately is important, as infections can increase your glucose levels and potentially lead to serious consequences such as diabetic ketoacidosis. Be sure you know your sick-day routine (review it before leaving home) and follow it if you get sick. Motion sickness can also disrupt your normal eating schedule and fluid balance. Your healthcare providers can suggest medication to help you prevent this problem.

Prevent Sunburn

Avoid overexposure to the sun. Severe sunburn is stressful to the body and can raise your blood glucose levels, even to the point of the dangerous condition ketoacidosis. Be sure to use sunscreen, even on cloudy days. Also, be sure to wear a hat and sunglasses, and wear protective clothing if you'll be outside during peak sunshine hours.

By preparing in advance and taking the precautions suggested above, you'll be able to relax and have a wonderful trip!

CHAPTER 28

Good Diabetes Care:
What Is It? . . . How to Get It

Many people will be involved in caring for your diabetes—you and your healthcare team and members of your family or perhaps a special friend. You should know how to select the doctor who will oversee your care, as well as other professionals on your healthcare team and the services they can provide. You should also be aware of other resources that you and your family can use to find out more about diabetes.

Roles of Your Healthcare Team

Today's world of medicine is very specialized. In caring for your diabetes, it is likely that your medical needs will be met by a number of healthcare professionals in addition to your primary-care physician. If at all possible, you should find a medical setting in which your diabetes is cared for by a team of professionals, each an expert in a particular aspect of your total care. See Chapter 3, *Goals and Tools for Treatment*, for a description of who should be on your team and their roles.

Selecting Your Healthcare Team

Choosing a diabetes healthcare team may take some time but is well worth the effort. Such professionals are available at specialized centers, such as Joslin Diabetes Center in Boston and its Affiliated Centers in other parts of the country. First, ask a trusted doctor, nurse, or knowledgeable friend for recommendations and set up interviews with the potential choices. It is necessary to find a team of professionals with whom you feel comfortable and confident. Because the decision ultimately is yours, it is very important that you know something about diabetes care. As a knowledgeable health-care consumer, you will be better able to recognize the right team when you find one.

Below is a list of criteria that reflects desirable qualities to look for in a diabetes healthcare team. Use this list as a guide to help choose your team members.

- They are knowledgeable about diabetes and its care.
- They listen to your concerns and help you identify solutions to the problems.
- They return your phone calls within an appropriate amount of time.
- They consult you and consider your lifestyle, likes, dislikes, and abilities when developing your diabetes-care program.
- They work with you to help you maintain the best diabetes control possible.
- They help you learn as much as possible about diabetes and how to prevent complications.
- They routinely perform necessary tests and evaluations.
- They believe it is very important to keep your blood glucose, blood fats, and blood pressure under the best possible control.
- They participate in activities of the American Diabetes Association.

Questions to Ask Your Healthcare Team

Below are questions that should be asked of your primary care physician and of your diabetes team:

- What is my A1C level and what does it mean?
- How is my diabetes control?
- What are my blood glucose and A1C target levels?
- How should I be treating my diabetes?

What You Need to Do—and Know

People with diabetes must play a significant role in their care. Your diabetes team will consider your needs, concerns, and lifestyle when working with you to manage your diabetes. We began the book by emphasizing your key role on the diabetes team. And we end the book by reminding you again that it is your responsibility to carry out the treatment program—that is, to be involved with the "self-care" of your diabetes. On a daily basis you will be responsible for monitoring your blood glucose, selecting your food choices, participating in regular physical activities, and taking medications. You will interpret your blood glucose levels and make informed decisions daily about how to fine-tune your care. But along with responsibility for care, your have the right to be informed about your diabetes and your risks for developing complications. This right also includes knowing what options are available to care for your diabetes and any complications, along with your overall health.

There is a lot to know and remember when caring for your diabetes. Chapter 3, *Goals and Tools for Treatment,* also identifies clinical measures your healthcare providers should be addressing. The list below incorporates Joslin's Clinical Guidelines to help you ensure that your diabetes is being treated at an optimal level.

Appointments

Consultation with members of your healthcare team will vary with each individual, but should include at least the following number of visits:

> *Primary-care physician* — at least once a year for general care; more frequently if specific problems arise.

Diabetes specialist **may be called an endocrinologist or a diabetologist** — twice a year unless your physician recommends more frequent visits. The American Diabetes Association recommends that people using insulin see their diabetes specialist every 3 months.

Nurse educator — at least once a year you should receive educational training; you should receive it more frequently if you are newly diagnosed or changing your treatment program.

Dietitian — at least once a year to update and revise your food and eating program; you may need more help when you are newly diagnosed or changing your treatment program.

Exercise physiologist — at least once a year to review your fitness level and make any adjustments necessary for diabetes management.

Ophthalmologist (eye doctor) — once a year; more often if problems arise.

Mental health specialist — visits recommended: 1) when diagnosed with diabetes-related health problems, 2) when life with diabetes becomes disruptive to everyday life, 3) during any life crisis.

Guidelines for Office Visits

Following are guidelines for each visit with your diabetes specialist or your diabetes team:

Routine visits

— check your blood pressure
— review your blood glucose results; also test your A1C
— review and clarify your target blood glucose levels
— eye examination
— foot examination
— discuss other health problems you may be experiencing
— revise your diabetes treatment program, as necessary, including meal plan, physical activities, glucose-checking schedule, medications, and foot care

Annual visits

- all of the items under "Routine Visits" above
- complete physical examination
- review of self-care skills: how to use insulin or other diabetes medications, glucose-checking techniques, treatment of low blood glucose, sick-day care
- dilated eye exam by ophthalmologist
- tests to measure kidney function
- evaluation of risk factors for complications of diabetes: smoking, cholesterol levels, weight, and blood pressure

Tests by Professionals

You can use Table 28-1 to record your results from your office visit so that you can take charge of your diabetes. Ask your healthcare team to review your own personal goals and targets, as yours may differ from the suggested ones below.

Self-Care Skills

We've covered a lot of information in this book that will assist you in caring for your diabetes. Review the following list of knowledge and skills important to self-care and be sure that you have mastered each of them:

Self-monitoring of Blood Glucose

- use of glucose meter
- keeping a record of times that tests are performed, of results, and of other factors that affect diabetes management
- interpreting your blood glucose levels to make appropriate changes in your treatment program

TABLE 28-1	Goals and Results for Your Lab Tests and Exams					
Physical and lab results	Dates/results					
A1C (every 3–6 mos.) Goal: less than 7% or _____						
Review blood glucose records (every visit)						
Blood pressure (every visit) Goal less than 130/80 mmHg						
Weight (every visit) Goal: _____						
Foot exam (2–4 /yrs.)						
Total cholesterol (1/yr.) Goal: less than 200 mg/dl						
LDL cholesterol (1/yr.) Goal: less than 100 mg/dl or _____ mg/dl						
HDL cholesterol (1/yr.) Goal: greater than 40 mg/dl for men or greater than 50 mg/dl for women						
Triglycerides (1/yr.) Goal: less than 150 mg/dl.						
Microalbuminuria (1/yr.) Goal: less than 30 µg/mg creatinine)						
Dilated eye exam (1/yr.)						
Flu shot (1/yr.)						
Pneumonia vaccine						

Use of Medication

— knowledge of diabetes pills (type 2 diabetes)
— knowledge of types and actions of insulin (if using insulin)
— how to inject insulin or other prescribed injected medications
— site rotation for injection

— keeping a record of injections
— proper storage and refrigeration of insulin

Knowledge of High and Low Blood Glucose

— causes
— symptoms
— treatment
— prevention

Food and Meal Planning

— food and meal planning techniques
— special foods and occasions
— dining out
— portion control
— guidelines for low saturated and trans fat and low cholesterol
  eating
— weight goals

Physical Activity

— basic components of an activity program
— preventing low blood glucose
— adjustments for activity, including reducing insulin dose and
  carbohydrate snacks

Foot Care

— daily foot care
— emergency treatment
— preventing foot problems related to diabetes

Sick-day Management

— how to prevent life-threatening problems
— glucose-checking and medication schedule
— what to eat and drink

Testing for Ketones

— significance of ketones
— when and how to monitor
— how to interpret ketone tests

Ways to Learn More About Diabetes

- Classes and programs at diabetes centers
- Books, pamphlets, and magazines about diabetes by reputable organizations
- Internet sites from reputable organizations
- Support groups

Diabetes Resources

Joslin Diabetes Center and Its Affiliates

Joslin Diabetes Center is an international leader in diabetes treatment, research, and education. Established in 1898, and affiliated with Harvard Medical School, Joslin leads the field in both basic and clinical research, and is devoted to educating patients and professionals. Joslin is headquartered in Boston, Massachusetts, and has affiliates in prestigious hospitals and medical centers across the country and internationally.

Joslin Diabetes Center
One Joslin Place
Boston, Massachusetts 02215
Phone: (617) 732-2400

For more information about diabetes research, as well as innovations in clinical care and treatment, visit Joslin's website at www.joslin.org.

General Diabetes Information

American Diabetes Association, 1701 North Beauregard Street, Alexandria, Virginia 22311. Phone: (703) 549-1500, or toll free (800) 232-3472; www.diabetes.org

American Dietetic Association, 120 South Riverside Plaza, Suite 2000, Chicago, Illinois 60606. Phone: (800) 877-1600; www.eatright.org

Juvenile Diabetes Foundation 120 Wall Street, New York, New York 10005. (800) JDF-CURE; www.jdfcure.org

American Association of Diabetes Educators, 100 West Monroe Street, Suite 400, Chicago, Illinois 60603. Phone: (800) 338-3633; www.aadenet.org

International Diabetes Federation (IDF), Avenue Emile De Mot 19, 1000 Brussels, Belgium. Phone: 32-2-538 5511; www.idf.org

National Diabetes Information Clearinghouse, 1 Information Way, Bethesda, Maryland 20892. Phone: (301) 654-3327; www.niddk.nih.gov

Joslin Publications

This book is just one example of the variety of patient information and educational materials available from Joslin. Other titles that may be of interest include:

What You Need to Know About Diabetes—A Short Guide
Staying Healthy with Diabetes: Nutrition and Meal Planning
Staying Healthy with Diabetes: Physical Activity and Fitness
The Foot Book
Fighting Long-Term Complications

The Joslin Quick and Easy Cookbook
The Joslin Healthy Carbohydrate Cookbook
The Joslin Diabetes Great Chefs Cook Healthy Cookbook

To obtain a catalog, or for current prices and purchasing information, call (800) 344-4501; or order online at https://store.joslin.org.

APPENDIX

Food Choice Lists

Carbohydrate Foods

Carbohydrate Counting Guidelines: 1 carb choice = 15 grams carb
1 carb choice (15 grams) = 1 cup watermelon = 1 cup milk = ⅓ cup macaroni = _____
2 carb choices (30 grams) = 30 grapes = 1 English muffin = ⅔ cup rice = _____

Starch: Grains/Breads/Starchy Vegetables   *15 grams carb, 3 grams protein*

1 slice bread (1 oz.)	⅓ cup cooked rice	1 small or ½ medium potato
½ English muffin	⅓ cup cooked pasta	½ cup mashed potatoes
¼ large bagel (1 oz.)	½ cup cooked cereal	½ cup corn or peas
½ hamburger or hot dog roll	¾ cup dry cereal	½ cup lentils or beans
1 six-inch tortilla	¾ oz. pretzels	1 cup winter squash
2 pancakes, 4-inch diameter*	3 cups "light" popcorn*	4–6 crackers*

Fruit   *15 grams carb*

1 small–medium piece fresh fruit	½ cup canned fruit	1 cup berries
10–15 grapes	½ cup (4 oz.) juice	2 tbsp. raisins
1 small or ½ large banana	1 cup melon	¼ cup dried fruit

Milk   *15 grams carb, 8 grams protein*

1 cup low-fat or nonfat milk	⅔ cup light-style yogurt	1 cup reduced-fat milk*

---

* Starred items also have one additional fat serving (5 grams of fat).

Other Carbohydrates *15 grams carb*

½ cup frozen yogurt
¼ cup sherbet or sorbet
1 frozen fruit juice bar

2 small cookies*
2-inch-square brownie*
15 potato/tortilla chips*

1 cup broth-based soup
1 tbsp. jam, sugar, or syrup
⅓ cup hummus*

Vegetables *"Free" for 1–2 servings. 5 gm carb per serving; 15 gm carb for 3 servings.*

1 cup raw vegetables

½ cup cooked vegetables

½ cup vegetables

For Meal Planning

Meats and Meat Substitutes/Protein Foods

0 grams carb, 7 grams protein, 5 grams fat

1 oz., cooked lean meat,
    fish/or poultry

1 oz. low-fat cheese
2 tbsp. grated Parmesan cheese

¼ cup tuna or salmon,
    canned in water

¼ cup cottage cheese
2 medium sardines

2 tbsp. peanut butter*
    (counts as two fat
    servings)
4 oz. (½ cup) tofu
1 egg or ¼ cup egg whites

Fat Foods

0 grams carb, 5 grams fat

1 tsp. butter† or margarine
1 tbsp. reduced fat margarine
1 tsp. oil
1 tsp. mayonnaise

1 tbsp. salad dressing
2 tbsp. reduced fat
    dressing
10 peanuts
4 walnut halves

1½ tbsp. flax seed
2 tbsp. cream or
    half & half†
1 tbsp. cream cheese†
1 strip bacon†

Free Foods

A free food has no more than 5 grams carb and 20 calories per serving. Foods with a serving size should be limited to 3 servings per day.

1 tbsp. fat-free cream cheese
1 tbsp. liquid nondairy creamer
¼ cup salsa

1 tbsp. catsup
2 tsp. light/low-sugar jam
1 cup raw vegetables

Diet/sugar-free beverages
Sugar-free gelatin
Herbs, spices, seasonings

---

* Starred items also have one additional fat serving (5 grams of fat unless otherwise indicated).
† These items are sources of saturated fat.

Fast Foods/Combination Foods

Casserole/Hot dish (1 cup; example: chili with beans, lasagna)	2 carb choices, 2 meat/proteins
Cheese pizza (¼ of 12-inch pie)	2½ carb choices, 2 meat/proteins, 1 fat
French fries, thin (20–25)	2 carb choices, 2 fats
Burrito with beef (2)	4 carb choices, 2 meat/proteins, 2 fats
Chicken nuggets (6)	1 carb choice, 2 meat/proteins, 1 fat

DIABETES WORDS AND PHRASES

A1C — a blood test that measures average blood glucose over the past two to three months and is the best way to measure overall glucose control. It should be measured two to four times a year and the goal is less than 7 percent.

acanthosis nigricans — a thickening and darkening of the skin in patchy areas in the skin folds of the armpits, neck, or groin, ranging from tan to dark brown. This is usually a sign of insulin resistance.

ACE inhibitor (Angiotensin converting enzyme) — a type of medication used to lower blood pressure and help treat kidney problems related to diabetes.

antibodies — Antibodies are proteins that the body makes to protect itself from foreign substances such as bacteria and viruses.

ARB (angiotensin receptor blocker) — a type of oral medication used to lower blood pressure.

atherosclerosis — a process that involves thickening of the blood vessel walls thought to be related to inflammation of the vessel wall, which then leads to formation of plaques that cause partial blockages. If these plaques rupture, clots form on that rupture site, causing a more acute, total blockage. If the blood vessel is providing blood to the heart, the result would be a heart attack.

basal insulin — the insulin that controls blood glucose levels between meals and overnight. It controls glucose in the fasting state.

beta cells — cells that produce insulin. They are located within the islets of Langerhans in the pancreas.

biguanide — a class of diabetes medication (metformin) that reduces insulin resistance in the liver.

blood glucose (or just **glucose**) — a type of sugar that is created when the carbohydrate that one eats is broken down in the body. During digestion, glucose passes through the wall of the intestine into the bloodstream to the liver and eventually into the general circulation. From there glucose can then enter individual cells or tissues throughout the body to be used for fuel and provide energy.

blood pressure — the pressure against the walls of the blood vessels. High blood pressure is more common in persons with diabetes and increases the risk of stroke, heart attack, and kidney and eye diseases. It should be measured at every doctor visit, or at least once a year, with a goal of less than 130/80 mmHg.

body mass index (BMI) — a method of determining by the relationship between height and weight, whether or not a person is obese, overweight, underweight, or of normal weight.

bolus insulin — the insulin that is released when food is eaten. A bolus is a burst of insulin that is delivered by injection or by the insulin pump to "cover" a meal or snack or to correct for a high blood glucose level.

carbohydrate — the main source of fuel for the body. Carbohydrate includes starches and sugars, and is found in bread, pasta, fruits, vegetables, milk, and sweets. Carbs are broken down into a sugar called *glucose*.

carbohydrate counting — a meal-planning method commonly used by people with diabetes to plan their food and meal choices. Carbohydrate counting helps one achieve a balance between the amount of carbohydrate foods eaten and the available insulin.

cardiologist — a doctor who specializes in the heart and vascular system.

cardiovascular system — the heart and blood vessels. It is the means by which blood is pumped from the heart and circulated throughout the body. As it circulates, the blood carries nourishment and oxygen to all of the body's tissues. It also removes waste products.

Charcot foot — a condition in which the small bones of the foot become misaligned, leading to foot deformity. It is a problem that can evolve as a result of nerve damage.

cholesterol — a type of fat that is manufactured in the liver or intestines, but is also found in some of the foods we eat. (Only animal foods, such as eggs, milk, cheese, liver, meat, and poultry contain cholesterol.)

conventional insulin therapy — an insulin therapy in which the insulin regimen is decided first, and the person with diabetes has to eat and engage in physical activity according to the time actions of the injected insulins.

creatinine — a waste product derived from the activity of the muscles. Normally, kidneys can remove this substance from the blood. A buildup of creatinine in the blood signals that the kidneys are losing their ability to function normally.

dawn phenomenon — a rise in blood glucose levels that occurs in the early morning hours.

diabetes educator — a healthcare person who has the skill and knowledge to teach a person with diabetes how to manage the condition. Diabetes educators may be doctors, nurses, dietitians, mental health or fitness clinicians. Some also have the credential CDE (Certified Diabetes Educator).

diabetic ketoacidosis (also called **ketoacidosis** or **DKA**) — a condition that results from a lack of sufficient insulin in the body, leading to high blood glucose levels and ketone formation. It is an extremely serious and life-threatening condition that may lead to coma and death. The symptoms of ketoacidosis are nausea, stomach pain, vomiting, chest pain, rapid shallow breathing, and difficulty staying awake.

diabetic macular edema — a condition that can occur in either stage of diabetic retinopathy (nonproliferative retinopathy or a more serious stage called proliferative retinopathy) in which fluid collects in the central part of the retina, resulting in blurred vision. Macular edema can be treated with laser surgery when central vision is threatened.

endocrinologist — a doctor who specializes in diseases of the endocrine system such as diabetes.

fasting blood glucose test — a blood test in which a sample of blood is drawn after an overnight fast to measure the amount of glucose.

fructosamine test — a blood test that can detect overall changes in blood glucose control over a shorter timespan than the A1C test. Fructosamine levels indicate the level of blood glucose control over the past two or three weeks. Thus, when rapid changes are being made in a diabetes treatment plan, this test quickly reveals how the changes are working and whether other changes should be considered.

gastroparesis — a condition in which neuropathy affects the nerves controlling the digestive tract and causes difficulty processing or disposing of food. It can cause nausea, vomiting, bloating, or diarrhea.

gestational diabetes — diabetes that develops during pregnancy. During this time, some women will have only a minimal insulin deficiency and will be able to adequately control their blood glucose with a meal plan. Other women may have a more severe insulin deficiency and require insulin along with nutrition therapy to control their blood glucose. This type of diabetes usually lasts only through the pregnancy, but women who have it may be at greater risk of developing type 2 diabetes later on.

ghrelin — a hormone that relays messages between the digestive system and the brain. It works to stimulate appetite, slow metabolism, and decrease your body's ability to burn fat.

glucose — a simple form of sugar that is created when the body's digestive processes break down the food we eat. Glucose is the body's main source of energy.

glucose meter — a device that measures one's blood glucose levels.

glucose tolerance test — blood tests done every hour or at the two-hour point after drinking a sugar-filled liquid. This is one test used to diagnose diabetes. If at two hours your blood glucose rises to over 200 mg/dl, you have diabetes. This test is not as common as a fasting glucose test.

glycemic index (GI) — a system of ranking foods containing equal amounts of carbohydrate according to how much they raise blood glucose levels. For instance, the carbohydrate in a slice of 100% stone-ground whole wheat bread (a low glycemic index food) may have less impact on blood glucose than a slice of processed white bread (a high glycemic index food). The GI is an additional meal-planning tool to help one understand how carbohydrate foods can differ in their effects on blood glucose.

glycemic load (GL) — a system of ranking carbohydrate foods based on how much they raise blood glucose levels that combines the GI value and the carbohydrate content of an average serving of a food, of a meal, or of a day's worth of food.

glycogen — glucose that is stored in muscles and liver.

HDL (high-density lipoprotein—also called "good" cholesterol) — a type of blood cholesterol that sweeps excess cholesterol from the blood back to the liver where it is reprocessed or eliminated.

hormones — chemical messengers made in one part of the body to transfer "information" through the bloodstream to cells in another part of the body. Insulin is a hormone.

hyperglycemia — high blood glucose levels. Blood glucose is generally considered "high" when it is 160 mg/dl or above your individual blood glucose target.

hyperosmolar hyperglycemic state (HHS) — a serious condition characterized resulting from extremely high levels of blood glucose, causing excessive urination and severe dehydration, but without ketones. It is not very common.

hypertension — high blood pressure (when blood flows through the blood vessels with a greater than normal force) is defined as blood pressure equal to or greater than 140/90 mmHg and affects the majority of adults with diabetes. It increases one's risk of heart attack, stroke, and kidney problems.

hypoglycemia — a blood glucose below 80 mg/dl with or without symptoms or below 90 mg/dl with symptoms.

hypoglycemia unawareness — a condition in which one no longer recognizes the symptoms of low blood glucose.

impaired fasting glucose (IFG) — a fasting glucose level between 100 mg/dl and 125 mg/dl. Fasting blood test results between these levels mean that you have pre-diabetes.

impaired glucose tolerance (IGT) — a blood glucose level after a 2-hour glucose tolerance test between 140 and 199 mg/dl. This means you have pre-diabetes.

incretin — a hormone that helps stimulate the pancreas to make insulin.

incretin mimetics — a class of drugs that help stimulate the pancreas to produce more insulin. The first specific drug in this class to be approved is exenatide (Byetta).

infusion set — plastic tubing with a soft cannula at one end. The plastic tubing delivers insulin from a pump into the body through the cannula, which is inserted through the skin.

insulin — a hormone made in the pancreas that helps glucose pass into the cells where it is used to create energy for the body.

insulin pen — an insulin delivery method that looks like a writing pen.

insulin pump — an insulin delivery system; a small mechanical device, typically the size of a beeper or small cell phone that releases insulin into the tissues of the body by way of tubing and a needle.

insulin reaction (hypoglycemia) — low blood glucose resulting from either too much insulin, too much activity, or too little food.

insulin resistance — a condition that makes it harder for the cells to properly use insulin.

insulin sensitivity factor (also called the **correction factor** or **supplemental factor**) — the amount of blood glucose measured in mg/dl that is lowered by one unit of rapid-acting or regular insulin. The insulin sensitivity factor is used to calculate the amount of insulin you need to return blood glucose to within your target blood glucose range.

insulin-to-carbohydrate ratio — a method of determining how much rapid-acting insulin is needed to cover the carbohydrate eaten at a meal or snack. This is used as part of a more advanced level of carbohydrate counting.

intermediate-acting insulin — a type of insulin that begins to work to lower blood glucose within one to four hours and works hardest four to fifteen hours after injection. The intermediate-acting insulins are NPH and lente.

islet cell transplantation — transplanting islet beta cells that produce insulin from a donor pancreas into a person whose pancreas no longer produces insulin.

islets of Langerhans — cells found in the pancreas, the most important of which are *beta cells*—the tiny factories that make insulin.

ketones — acids produced due to lack of enough insulin to use the glucose in your bloodstream. Your body turns to its fat stores for energy. When this occurs, ketones are produced, which accumulate in the blood and spill into the urine. These ketones are made when fat is metabolized as a source of energy. The excessive formation of ketones in the blood is called *ketosis*, and the presence of ketones in the urine is called *ketonuria*. Allowed to go untreated, the combination of high blood glucose and ketones can lead to *ketoacidosis* (also called *DKA*).

ketonuria — the presence of ketones in the urine.

ketosis — the excessive formation of ketones in the blood.

lancet — a small needle used to get a drop of blood from your finger, arm, or other site. The blood is placed on a special strip, which is put into the meter. The meter "reads" the strip and gives a blood glucose reading.

lifestyle changes — changes made to one's eating habits and physical activity in order to control blood glucose.

long-acting peaking — a type of insulin that doesn't begin to work to lower blood glucose until four to six hours after injection. It works hardest from 8 to 30 hours after injection and continues to work for up to 24 to 36 hours. The long-acting peaking insulin is ultralente.

long-acting peakless — a type of basal insulin that begins to work to lower blood glucose within one to two hours after injection and works for 24 hours. The long-acting peakless insulin is glargine.

LDL (low-density lipoprotein) — a type of blood cholesterol that is considered "bad" because it can be deposited in the arteries, increasing the risk of heart attack or stroke.

medical nutrition therapy — a method of controlling blood glucose by working with a dietitian to assess one's food and nutrition needs and then developing and following an individualized meal plan.

Mediterranean-type diet — a type of eating plan that is low in saturated fat and cholesterol, high in fruits, vegetables, nuts, and grains and that also emphasizes controlling portion sizes to help in reducing overall calories.

metabolic syndrome — a cluster of conditions that increase the risk of developing vascular disease (heart disease, strokes, and peripheral vascular disease). The most recognizable components of this syndrome are abdominal obesity, high blood pressure (hypertension), high triglycerides (part of the lipid profile), low HDL (the "good" cholesterol), and glucose intolerance.

metabolism — the process by which the cells of the body change food so that it can be used for energy or so that it can be used to build or maintain cells and tissues.

microalbumin test — a urine test that measures the presence of small amounts of a protein called albumin.

microalbuminuria — the presence of small amounts of albumin, a protein, in the urine. Microalbuminuria is an early sign of kidney damage.

mixed dose — an injection that contains two or more types of insulin given in the same syringe at the same time.

necrobiosis lipoidica diabeticorum (NLD) — a skin condition believed to result from inflammation of the skin in which the skin thins out, becoming discolored and dimpled. This is the most specific skin problem among people with diabetes. It can be quite disfiguring.

nephrologist — a doctor who specializes in conditions of the kidney.

nephropathy — serious kidney disease that can occur in people who have had diabetes for a long time, particularly if their diabetes has been poorly controlled.

neurologist — a doctor who specializes in conditions of the nervous system.

neuropathy — damage to the nerves. It is a condition that can be very debilitating and painful. There are two main types of neuropathy, depending on which nerve cells are damaged. One type is called *sensory neuropathy*, which affects feelings in the legs or hands and is referred to as peripheral neuropathy. The other type is *autonomic neuropathy*, which affects nerves that control various organs, such as the stomach or urinary tract.

nocturnal hypoglycemia — low blood glucose that occurs in the middle of the night.

noncaloric or nonnutritive sweeteners — sweeteners that contribute few, if any, calories and have no effect on blood glucose levels.

nonproliferative retinopathy — the initial stage in diabetic retinopathy. High levels of blood glucose cause damage to the blood vessels in the retina. The blood vessels leak fluid, which can collect and cause the retina to swell.

nutritive or caloric sweeteners — sweeteners that contribute calories and can affect blood glucose levels.

ophthalmologist — a doctor specializing in conditions of the eyes.

oral glucose-lowering medications (also referred to as **oral antidiabetes medications**) — "diabetes pills," which are used in combination with a meal plan and physical activity as well as in combination with each other and sometimes with insulin to control blood glucose levels.

pancreas — a small gland located below and just behind the stomach that makes a specific kind of hormone called insulin.

physiologic insulin therapy (also called **intensive insulin therapy**) — an insulin program that attempts to provide insulin in the way that your body would if you didn't have diabetes. Insulin is adjusted to accommodate your food intake and your activity level, and as a result insulin doses change from one day to the next.

pre-diabetes — a condition in which either your fasting or two-hour post-meal blood glucose levels are higher than normal, but not high enough for a diagnosis of type 2 diabetes. Studies show that most people with pre-diabetes will develop type 2 diabetes within 10 years if they don't change their lifestyle. They also have a higher risk of developing cardiovascular disease.

proliferative retinopathy — a more serious stage of diabetic retinopathy in which there is a greater loss of vision or even total blindness. During this stage, abnormal blood vessels grow over the surface of the retina.

protein — one of the main nutrients from food along with carbohydrate and fat. The body uses protein to build and repair body tissue. Muscles, organs, bones, skin, and many of the hormones in the body are made from protein. As a secondary role, protein can also provide energy for the body if carbohydrate is not available. Food sources of protein include meat, poultry, fish, eggs, dairy products, and beans.

rapid-acting insulin — a type of insulin that begins to work to lower blood glucose within 10 to 30 minutes and works hardest 30 minutes to 3 hours after injection. There are three approved rapid-acting insulins — lispro, aspart, and glulisine.

rebound hyperglycemia (**high blood glucose** or the **Somogyi phenomenon**) — a condition in which, as a result of too low a level of glucose, the counterregulatory or stress hormones cause the liver to release too much glucose.

regular — the name for the common form of short-acting insulin.

relative insulin deficiency — a decline in insulin production that is usually a problem with or without insulin resistance early on in the course of diabetes.

retina — the thin, light-sensitive inner lining in the back of the eye.

retinopathy — damage to the *retina*, the thin, light-sensitive inner lining in the back of the eye. This damage occurs to small blood vessels in the retina that are easily harmed by high levels of glucose in the blood.

saturated fat — a type of food fat that is solid at room temperature. Saturated fats raise blood cholesterol levels by interfering with the entry of cholesterol into cells; this causes cholesterol to remain in the bloodstream longer and to become a part of the plaque that builds up in the blood vessels.

self-monitoring — managing one's diabetes by checking blood glucose, and being aware of how food intake, physical activity, and medication work together in order to keep blood glucose in good control.

SMBG (self-monitoring of blood glucose) — checking your blood glucose with a blood glucose meter.

short-acting insulin — a type of insulin that begins to work to lower blood glucose within 30 to 60 minutes and works hardest one hour to five hours after injection. The common form of short-acting insulin is called *regular*.

single dose — an injection that contains one type of insulin.

sugar alcohols or polyols — sweeteners that replace other sugars in foods causing slightly lower rises in blood glucose.

sulfonylureas — a class of oral diabetes medications that stimulate the pancreas to make more insulin.

thiazolidinediones — a class of oral diabetes medications that reduce insulin resistance.

trans fats — a type of fat formed from *hydrogenation*, a chemical process that changes a liquid oil into a solid fat. Trans fats are found in processed foods, such as snack foods, cookies, fast foods, and some stick or solid margarines. They can raise cholesterol levels and should be eaten in as small amounts as possible.

triglycerides — a type of fat stored in fat cells as body fat and burned for energy. High levels of triglycerides are linked with an increased risk of heart and blood vessel disease.

unsaturated fat (both *polyunsaturated* and *monounsaturated*) — fats that come primarily from vegetables and are liquid at room temperature. Polyunsaturated fats can help lower cholesterol levels. Monounsaturated fats also help lower blood cholesterol levels and may help to raise HDL cholesterol levels.

vitrectomy surgery — a process to remove the blood and scar tissue from within the eye that can frequently successfully restore vision.

INDEX

Page numbers in *italics* refer to tables and illustrations.